LIVING IN THE
POSTMASTECTOMY BODY

LIVING IN THE POSTMASTECTOMY BODY

LEARNING TO LIVE IN AND LOVE YOUR BODY AGAIN

BECKY ZUCKWEILER, MS RN CS

Hartley & Marks

PUBLISHERS

Published by

HARTLEY & MARKS PUBLISHERS INC.

P. O. Box 147   3661 West Broadway
Point Roberts, WA   Vancouver, BC
98281   V6R 2B8

Library of Congress Cataloging-in-Publication Data

Zuckweiler, Rebecca L.
      Living in the postmastectomy body : learning to live in and love
your body again / by Rebecca Zuckweiler.
            p.   cm.
      Includes index.
      ISBN 0-88179-152-0
            1. Mastectomy—Psychological aspects.   2. Mastectomy—Patients—
Rehabilitation.   3. Adjustment (Psychology)   4. Breast prosthesis—
Psychological aspects.   I. Title.
      RD667.5.Z83   1998
      618.1'9059'019—dc21   98-18466
                                                             CIP

Design and composition by The Typeworks
Illustrations by Sia Kaskaminidis
Set in SCALA and SCALA SANS

Printed in the U.S.A.

PERMISSIONS

Chapter 14, page 246. Paragraph from *Running in the Family* by Michael
Ondaatje, copyright 1982 by Michael Ondaatje. Reprinted with permission of
McLelland & Stewart Inc.

To my treasured friends, Dede and Ann,
who have fought their own battles with breast cancer,
and to my sister, Lisa.
In memory of the women in my family who were stricken with breast cancer
Marie Klietsch McQuade—Mother
Irene Hollihan Klietsch—Maternal Grandmother
Anna Shibutsky—Maternal Great Grandmother
Name Unknown—Maternal Great Great Grandmother
Helen Hollihan—Maternal Great Aunt

CONTENTS

ACKNOWLEDGMENTS

Shortly after I started writing this book, I wondered if I should be taking on this project. Then one evening at a Chinese restaurant, I opened a fortune cookie and the message read: "A book is in your future." Thanks, God, for your "sign."

I want to thank Drs. Alan Shons and Bruce Cunningham, my competent and compassionate plastic surgeons. I also want to thank Dr. Conrad Butwinick, the rheumatologist who offered me symptom relief and hope after my silicone implants ruptured.

Nancy Pascoe, my fitter, and Heidi's Mastectomy Shop in Edina, Minnesota, proved invaluable with helping me to make clothes work again and helping me to feel attractive following explant surgery. Nancy was also very informative about the postmastectomy industry.

Heather Wallace, my body therapist, assisted with restoring body movement. The exercises presented in this book draw from principles I learned from Heather.

I want to acknowledge the staff at Hartley & Marks Publishers, Inc. In particular, Victor Marks for believing in my vision, and Susan Juby, my editor, for her patience and writing talent. Considering my dyslexia and the emotional nature of the subject, Susan had no small task in completing this book with me.

I could not have completed this book without the help of my daughter, Carly, who was my constant computer-tutor and trouble-shooter. Thanks for never revealing that you thought Mom was a "dunce."

Last but not least, I want to acknowledge my husband and best friend, Jim, who provided me with tremendous support by wiping away my tears of frustration and by taking over many of the household duties while I wrote this book. I could never have come to accept my changed body without the unconditional love I have received from my cherished partner.

INTRODUCTION

I am one of those people who likes to get informed about difficulties I encounter in life. Learning about problems makes me feel empowered. A few years ago I was faced with a situation that I desperately needed to learn about. I had lived with silicone breast implants since undergoing a bilateral (double) mastectomy thirteen years before. Now, the implants had been removed and I did not have the faintest idea how to begin to reconstruct my life.

I went to the bookstore to find a book on postmastectomy care. To my surprise, one did not exist. I found an excellent selection of books on breast cancer, but I did not have breast cancer. I simply did not have breasts. I needed emotional support and validation for my tremendous feelings of loss. How was I going to get comfortable in this changed body? I also needed to find out what types of prostheses (breast forms) were available, as well as how to choose and alter clothing. What could I do about the persistent phantom pain in breasts I no longer had? I was faced with a whole set of questions for which I needed answers.

As I stumbled through the process of becoming accustomed to my new body, I discovered many very helpful people and supplies that assisted me. But I also concluded that much of what was available in breast forms and altered clothes did not work well for me. I became determined to find things that were a closer match with my lifestyle and how I wanted to look. My creativity helped me to solve practical problems and encouraged me to take action. My frustration led me to develop techniques to deal with some of the psychological issues that the loss of my breasts had brought about.

I believe that what is most needed for navigating the complex and often frightening journey after breast surgery is a practical book based on first-hand experience. Consequently, this is not a scholarly composite of research findings; rather it is a sharing of personal and professional knowledge designed to help women come to grips with, and eventually accept, their new bodies. It is also a guide to experiencing the joy that comes from taking charge of your own life and recovery.

This book is not about breast cancer, it is about losing a breast and the aftermath. However, I have included a brief chapter on breast cancer and treatment since most women have their mastectomies as a result of breast cancer. I strongly recommend that you supplement the information in this chapter with some of the other, more comprehensive resources available. There are new resources with the latest information coming out all the time.

I offer this book as a starting point for you to discover your own way to re-create your life after you have undergone a mastectomy. I hope that it makes your journey easier.

Because of my personal history and twenty-five years' experience as a psychiatric nurse, I place a great deal of emphasis on the psychological aspect of recovery. We are all unique but we have much in common as we come to terms with the loss of our intact bodies. All of us go through a grieving process of some kind, and we each have a history that greatly influences our particular needs and responses to life after a mastectomy.

One realization I came to as I tried to work through my grief was how much emotional pain I remained in because of the phantom pain I was experiencing. Every time I experienced phantom pain (sensations from the missing breast) it triggered a fresh, deep feeling of loss. Phantom pain has been viewed as an unfortunate neurological condition that follows the loss of a body part. I am delighted to tell you that I found a cure for my phantom pain and believe that you can also cure yours using the simple "image imprinting" technique I developed, which gives good results in a short time.

I am equally pleased to be able to offer you a new way to regain full use of your arm and shoulder. I found the postmastectomy exercises commonly recommended to be almost useless and replaced them with more effective ones. The exercises typically suggested for women recovering from a mastectomy, such as the wall climb, do not involve enough muscle groups and try to stretch the muscles where they are the most taut and painful, which I found ineffective. In Chapter 7, I explain how the mastectomy has affected your body and how to restore flexibility and strength.

By experimenting with clothes and different breast forms, I have learned to successfully alter many of my own clothes. Through trial and error, I have learned a lot about what works and what does not work. I encourage you to build on my ideas until you find a way to dress that allows you to feel comfortable and attractive.

I also learned a great deal about the process of becoming sexual again. Our breasts are a significant part of our sexuality. A mastectomy makes it necessary to speak openly about this very private and personal part of life. I found myself writing about this subject both from a professional and a very personal point of view. I have redefined what sexuality means to me as I have incorporated sex back into my life. Re-examining my attitudes and clarifying what is emotionally and physically satisfying has been an important part of reclaiming my sexuality.

The grief from losing a breast is often so intense many women worry that their reactions are not normal or are more than simply grief. I provide a thorough description of grief, depression, as well as sleep and anxiety disorders as they relate to having a mastectomy. This information will help you define what you are experiencing so you can seek the appropriate treatment.

Although this book focuses on women who use external prostheses, I also include a chapter on breast reconstruction. You should know your options and some of the benefits and possible negative consequences that go with each reconstruction choice. I do not intend this to be a comprehensive chapter and encourage you to look for other resources on the subject if you intend to explore it further.

Finally, I would not be where I am today without my sense of humor. After all our tears it is wonderful to be able to laugh again. I leave you with my final chapter of humorous stories that show it is possible to rediscover joy in living.

CHAPTER ONE

MY STORY

Most of you reading this book will have had your mastectomy as a result of breast cancer. My story is different in that my bilateral mastectomy was done as a preventive measure to avoid breast cancer. The choice to have an elective mastectomy may sound extreme, but with my family history it seemed a logical choice. There is currently not a consistent position in the medical community on the appropriateness of performing a double mastectomy on women with a strong genetic predisposition for breast cancer. I know that I have never regretted the decision. Fifteen years ago my sister made the same decision and she too has never regretted her choice. To understand why we decided to undergo double prophylactic mastectomies, you will have to understand the history of breast cancer in our family.

My maternal grandmother died when I was about ten years old. I hadn't known she was sick. The adults told us that Grandma died of lung cancer, and because she smoked it made sense. But I was confused because at her funeral I heard someone say that she died of breast cancer. Apparently, Grandma had had a mastectomy about ten years before she died of cancer. Hers was my first funeral.

About a year later, when I was in sixth grade, I happened to be in my mother's bedroom as she changed her clothes. She had a dressing over her nipple and was replacing the bandage. I remember telling her that she needed to go to the doctor right away. I do not remember the conversation that ensued, but somehow I knew she was not going to the doctor because she was afraid to find out that she had cancer and that she was going to die like her mother. I remember feeling as if I was the adult and she was the child. The helplessness and fear I felt for my mother were overwhelming and I felt trapped by her lack of action.

Finally, the following summer, Mom went into the hospital for a mastectomy. I was not told that Mom was going into the hospital. Dad returned to our summer cottage after dropping her off and told us that she was in the hospital to have a breast removed and would not be home for a while because she had to stay in town to receive radiation treatments.

One weekend, after she returned from her treatments, Mom called my sister and me into her bedroom and showed us her chest and prosthesis. It was a terrifying sight to me. She had undergone a radical mastectomy which was a far more disfiguring surgery than those performed today, so her chest was caved in, she had a long, thick, purple scar down her chest where her breast used to be, and a third of her armpit was gone. She had black Xs drawn on her chest and back which, she explained, showed the doctor where to direct radiation rays to kill the remaining cancer. There were burns on her skin from the radiation.

Her prosthesis was a plastic pouch which came with a little straw used to blow it up into a fake breast. Mom could blow the prosthesis up to a size that matched her other breast. It reminded me of an air mattress being inflated and deflated. She said she had to be careful when wearing it so it didn't accidentally pop from too much pressure. I remember Mom wearing the prosthesis in her swimsuit when going into the lake. This was in the early stages of her healing when she was trying to figure out how to make her clothes work again. With my preadolescent mind I concluded it was really cool that they had found a way to deal with not having a breast. I was glad she showed us her chest and her prosthesis; it made me feel included and less scared. Our family rarely talked about personal issues, and that afternoon was the last time we ever talked about her surgery or cancer. We never talked about my feelings or reactions to what was going on. I only knew that I felt incredibly sad for my mother as she tried to adjust to her changed body.

Returning to school that fall was hard. I was starting junior high with all new classes, teachers, and kids. I worried about how to tell my closest friend about my mom. I remember using the big name for it and then defining it. I said my mom had a mastectomy; she had her breast removed because she had breast cancer. Saying the word breast was terribly embarrassing. It was one thing to be proud of my own new breasts, but quite another to talk about something going wrong with a breast. Cancer was also a word that was way too big for my age and my friends. It was a scary word that to us at that age meant death, a concept none of us were ready to deal with yet.

After my mother's mastectomy I felt different from the other kids, too intense and very isolated—trapped inside my own head. I remember feeling incredibly betrayed by a cute, popular boy my age named Tommy, who lived a block away from me. One day as I was getting off the school bus he and a couple of other boys blasted me with snowballs and pushed me down in the snowbank. They ran away laughing, calling me a sissy for crying. I can recall thinking, "How could he do this to me? After all, his mom has cancer too, so he should know what I'm going through and be nicer to me." No one seemed to understand.

That Christmas vacation brought an enormous change to my life. The day after Christmas, Mom took the fully decorated tree and put it out on the curb saying, "We are never going to have Christmas again." A couple of days later my mother woke my sister and me at 7:00 a.m. and asked us if we wanted to leave Minnesota and move to California. We packed our things and were on a Greyhound bus by 11:00 a.m. that same morning. My dad was out of town selling insurance so my mother wrote him a note telling him we had moved to California and we hoped he would join us. My oldest brother was living in Iowa with my uncle, so my mom and her four youngest children headed off on the Greyhound for California.

My mother's emotional outburst with the Christmas tree and the impulsive move to California might seem crazy, and to a degree it reflected the poor coping skills of my family, but considering the context of her situation in the early 1960s, it makes sense. Cancer was a death sentence at that time. The methods of detection and treatment were quite primitive and had poor results in comparison to the many choices of readily available and very successful treatments and the significant survival rate that we have today. Back then, as now, many people did extreme things to find a last-resort cure. I remember hearing about people going to Mexico to get Laetrile in hopes it would cure their cancer. Recently, a woman told me she had to leave her small children in the early 1970s to go to Texas for nearly a year as her last hope to cure her terminal cancer. At that time, a facility in Texas was the only place that was using massive doses of chemotherapy which at that time was still at the experimental stage.

My mother was a decisive person and my father tended to resist change. She knew how much my dad loved her and she banked on that to convince him to follow her. She had gone from the absolute despair and defeat displayed in throwing out the decorated Christmas tree into a plan of action. She referred to California as the "Promised Land."

We first lived in Ventura, California for about three months until my dad sold the house in Minnesota and we moved to Santa Maria. Meanwhile, my mom's cancer was getting worse. Shortly after he joined us, I overheard my dad talking about a chiropractor who had been treating Mom for severe back pain without first taking x rays. When she went to another doctor who took x rays they discovered that the cancer had eaten away her spine. The chiropractor could have snapped her spine and totally paralyzed her. It terrified me to hear this story. I wondered if that could really happen to a person's back. It was also the first time I realized that Mom still had cancer. I thought her surgery had gotten rid of it.

Mom was in and out of the hospital after we moved to Santa Maria. I remember trying to give her a shampoo one day while she was in the hospital, using the dry shampoo that you sprinkle in and comb out. While I was rubbing the powder into her scalp, I came across some lumps and started to say something, then caught myself and stopped mid-sentence. I suddenly realized the lumps were cancer that had gone to her brain and I did not want to upset her. I felt numb and full of disbelief. A couple of days after I gave her the shampoo, on June 22, 1964, Mom died at the age of forty-two. I was thirteen years old.

We moved back to Minnesota, but rebuilding a future proved more difficult. In the eleventh grade a boy I was dating and I were passing notes in English class. I distinctly recall telling him in one of my notes that he should know up front that I would not be having any children when I got married because I was going to die at a young age from cancer and it wouldn't be fair to put my kids through that. I was completely serious when I wrote that note. I didn't believe that there was any hope of escaping cancer.

During my senior year of high school I began dating the boy who became my first husband. It was an instant attraction because we had cancer to bond us. His mother had a brain tumor so I felt right at home in his family. We married at nineteen after I had completed one year of a three-year nursing program. We moved in with my father-in-law so he could afford to pay for his wife's nursing home care. My mother-in-law went into a hospice program not long after we moved in and died soon after that. That first marriage lasted five years.

Shortly after my divorce I married Jim, with whom I had been good friends since high school. His first priority was family and he cared deeply about how I felt. My new husband was very affectionate. He could handle my feelings, encouraging me to be more open and helping me to build my self-esteem. Jim also encouraged me to believe in my abilities, so I went to the University of Minnesota and did a degree in social work. As an RN and social worker, I worked on the mental health floor of a hospital and later I moved to the chemical dependency unit at the same hospital. Two years later I entered a master's degree program in psychiatric nursing.

During this time I finally began to face my repressed grief over my mother's death. I wrote a letter to my mother and for the first time really cried over losing her. I was discovering that I did have feelings and it was much better to let them out. This helped me deal with my anger at God, whom I had been blaming for taking my mother away.

Meanwhile, when I was twenty-six years old, I had a tubal ligation. I had become panic-stricken at the possibility of having a child and abandoning it due to cancer. I convinced my doctor I wanted a tubal ligation because I was a career woman and did not want to have children. I had already had serious problems from five years of using the Dalkon shield and did not want to risk any more problems with birth control. With my family history of breast cancer, the birth control pill had never been an option for me. I knew that my husband wanted children but he never made an issue of it because I was his first priority.

Around this time my sister, who was an operating-room nurse, told me that some women with strong family histories of breast cancer were having preventive mastectomies. I made an appointment to talk to someone in the genetics department at the university, and I got a consultation with one of the finest surgeons in the nation. The surgeon gave me a breast exam, patted me on the head, told me I had nothing to worry about, and sent me on my way. Then I went to see the man in the genetics department. He was an older man in a tiny office filled to the brim with papers and books. He was very kind and took my concerns seriously. He listened to my story and sent me out to gather as much of my family history as I could. I wrote to an uncle, the only relative I knew from my mother's family who was still alive. He had a Ph.D. in sociology and a strong interest in genealogy so I hoped he could help.

He sent me a lengthy letter laying out the medical history of my mother's family and giving contacts for other relatives, whom I proceeded to call and write. I found out that my great-grandmother had breast cancer in her forties. Her sister also had some kind of cancer. My grandmother had breast cancer at the age of forty-four and died from lung cancer at sixty. Her sister had breast cancer and died at thirty-eight. My mother died of breast cancer at the age of forty-two. There was only one female that I knew of in this line of the family who escaped cancer, a sister to my great-grandmother, and she died of "old age" in her eighties. After I had compiled this information I took it back to the geneticist, who said that based on the information I showed him, I had at least a 60% chance of getting breast cancer before menopause. He referred me to an oncologist.

The oncologist asked me to write for my mother's and grandmother's medical records to try and determine what kind of breast cancer they had. After he received the records, he examined me, gave me a mammogram, and concluded that I had a greater than 60% risk because I had fibrocystic disease (lumpy breasts) along with the strong family history. (Today fibrocystic disease is considered a catch-all term for any variations in breast tissue density.) He recommended exploring the option of having a preventive bilateral mastectomy and referred me to the chief of plastic surgery. The plastic surgeon concurred with the geneticist and oncologist and agreed that preventive surgery was not an overreaction to my situation. He said he could remove all my breast tissue, skin, and nipples, and I could later have reconstructive surgery. The second option would be to remove the breast tissue and the nipples, leaving the skin, insert implants immediately, and construct new nipples later. The third option would be to remove the breast tissue, leave the skin and nipples, and insert implants immediately. He sent me away to think about it.

I spoke to my sister, who worked in the operating room with the surgeon. She assured me that he was an incredibly skilled surgeon who had performed this operation many times. Two years later my sister had the same surgeon perform her own preventive bilateral mastectomy.

By this time my panic level had risen and I felt like I was running scared. When I returned to see the surgeon I told him I should have the most extensive surgery possible. He said he would do that procedure if that was what I wanted, but he felt it was unnecessary. He recommended just removing the breast tissue and inserting implants. This would leave me with few breast cells, which would be close to the surface for easy, early detection. My husband wanted me to do whatever would put my mind at ease. He just wanted me alive and not constantly worried. I trusted my surgeon and decided to have the least extensive surgery.

The surgery took place one month after I completed graduate school. I felt I was taking control of my life and my future. One evening I came home to find Jim asleep. He had left me a note. It said, "I think we should buy a new TV and get a kid." I was totally shocked and delighted, and laughed until I cried. This was his way. We had never talked about having children after I'd had the tubal ligation but he knew I needed to hear that he was open to it and that he had faith in me to be a good parent. We immediately looked into adopting and started the paperwork. The proactive surgery made me feel as if I had a whole new lease on life by removing my omnipresent fear of breast cancer.

I went into the hospital on the evening of Tuesday, July 21, 1981, and had the surgery the following morning. I was discharged the following Saturday morning, which was then considered a short hospital stay. I was off work for about two weeks. I had expected to be away for three or four weeks, but because my job was not physically strenuous I was able to return sooner. Since I had the implants put in at the same time as the mastectomies, I did not have to figure out how to use prostheses. The physical recovery was quite simple, partly because I did not have a lymph node dissection since cancer was not suspected in my case. I will discuss the physical after-effects of removing lymph nodes later in Chapter 3.

For me it was the emotional recovery that was hard. I had already done significant grieving for several months, starting at the time of the genetic research and continuing right up to my surgery. By the time I actually went into surgery, I felt I was quite well prepared, except for my fear of being put to sleep. Yet I did a great deal more grieving after the surgery as I tried to accept my artificial breasts. It took time to accept them as part of me and find the pluses in the change. I liked having breasts the same size and I liked thinking they would not sag with age. But mostly I liked feeling I had a long, full future in front of me.

That September we completed the paperwork to adopt a Korean infant girl. By December our little girl had been identified and we just had to wait for the two countries to finish their paperwork so we could hold her in our arms. She arrived on February 10, 1982. I thought of the timing as very spiritual and truly orchestrated in heaven because our child was being brought into this world at the same time I was preparing to be an available mother. Her birthday is July 15, 1981, just one week before my surgery. Adopting our daughter has been the best decision we have ever made and it was made possible because of the confidence I gained from the preventive surgery.

The same year we became parents my husband decided to change careers. He did not want to be an absentee father who worked all the time, so he went back to school for a second master's degree in psychology. He claims that my surgery was the turning point that made him re-evaluate what is precious in life and helped him to see that the free worldwide travel passes and high salary he received from the airlines he had worked for were not enough to make up for the loss of time spent with his wife and child.

Jim and I resumed sexual relations shortly after my surgery, but it took at least another year for both of us to get used to and accept my new breasts. The first few months were difficult as we faced the difference between my natural, soft breasts with their full sexual responsiveness compared to the implants, which were stiff, not very pliable, and without sexual sensation. As time passed, most of the lingering pain from the surgery subsided and we settled into a new sexual routine with an attitude of acceptance.

I felt physically fine for a couple of years but complications gradually began to develop from my implants. One of my implants became hard and I was told that it had become encapsulated. The scar tissue around the saline- or gel-filled implants can shrink, which is referred to as a capsular contraction, and this results in a hard breast. I had done a lot of swimming almost immediately after my surgery, which my doctor had said would help keep the implants soft. He was very pleased that I had been able to do this and said my implants were in such good shape because I was physically active after surgery. He also thought that was why I had full range of motion in my arms. It had been very painful to swim right after surgery but I had forced myself anyway. The doctor told me there was nothing more I could have done to prevent the capsular contraction but, to prevent further hardening, I should squeeze and massage the implants many times a day. He suggested the capsule might even break if I massaged them enough.

Gradually my health worsened. I had many symptoms that seemed to suggest an overworked immune system. I was bothered with frequent colds, new allergies, headaches, and just didn't feel well. Eventually, I was unable to work full-time and felt miserable most of the time. My body hurt everywhere and I experienced terrible fatigue. I had charley horses (severe muscle spasms) that would start in the hip and run down my leg into my foot. My allergies grew worse and my body continued to have trouble fighting off infections that included yeast infections in my gastrointestinal and vaginal tract, mouth, and ears. As a result I itched everywhere.

Eventually, I discovered a newspaper article reporting that silicone implants were suspected to cause a lot of vague, unexplained health problems. For the first time I made a connection between my health problems and breast implants. I had seen numerous doctors about all my health problems but none of them suggested the implants may have been the origin of my failing health. In August 1993, I was helping my daughter practice basketball at the neighborhood park, and she did a body block on me that gave quite a blow to my chest. Shortly after that incident I noticed that one of my breasts had lost its shape, and over the next month I started to become very ill. l made an appointment with the surgeon, who immediately had an MRI (magnetic resonance imaging) scan done, which showed that both of my implants had ruptured. I was put on the surgery schedule to have the implants removed.

My surgeon did not recommend trying new implants because my body did not tolerate them well and he considered them a risk to my overall health. He suggested external prostheses or performing a reconstruction with my own tissue rather than implants. He explained the three possible tissue transfer procedures, latissimus dorsi muscle flap, transverse rectus abdominis muscle flap (TRAM), and free flap, which I cover in the chapter on breast reconstruction. But there was no way I would subject myself to any more surgery or risk using implants again because my poor body had already been through enough. My sister had had her implants replaced with new implants and I had no trouble understanding and accepting her decision. I had also heard of other women who had undergone tissue transfer procedures and were happy with the results, but I knew none of these choices was right for me. I felt comforted by my surgeon's willingness to recommend what was best for me. He directed me to some of the community resources for postmastectomy supplies, and referred me to a good rheumatologist who had seen a number of women suffering from implant-related health problems.

I had bilateral explant surgery with no reconstruction on March 17, 1994, through the outpatient department of my hospital. I was admitted at 5:00 A.M. and discharged the same day, late in the afternoon, with drainage tubes and suction bulbs, and two large bandages. My husband was given a quick demonstration on caring for my tubes and the incisional dressings. I returned the next week to have the tubes removed.

The explant surgery was just as traumatic to my body as the original bilateral mastectomy had been because the surgeon had to clean the spilled silicone from the chest area. Fortunately, the physical healing afterward went well. But unlike the last surgery, this time I had to cope with not having breasts at all, instead of having a different type of breast.

Even though my surgeon was able to use my original scars to remove the implants, I was still disfigured on both sides and that took some time to get used to. The first few months after my explant surgery were emotionally difficult and frustrating as I learned what products were available and how to use the ones that I had purchased. I experimented for the next eighteen months until I settled into a new, comfortable routine. As well, our sex life needed to be discussed and reshaped.

The period following the explant surgery was very hard. I was still plagued with fatigue, joint and muscle pain, short-term memory loss, and blurred vision. I developed a sleep disorder as part of the syndrome, and my grief and depression became extremely heavy and frightening. One thought kept going through my mind: "You can't fool Mother Nature." For a long time I'd felt that I had been clever enough to outsmart my genetic structure and rise above it. The timing of my failing health and surgery played a big part in my feelings of failure. I was forty-two when I had my explant surgery and my daughter was almost thirteen. My mother had died at forty-two years old when I was thirteen. For a short time before and after my surgery I felt so ill I truly wondered if I was going to die. I felt terrified and had no answers. My depression made this kind of thinking worse and my condition made my depression worse. I was trapped in a vicious cycle of despair.

The rheumatologist was the first person to give me hope. He started me on a low dose of an antidepressant that helped with the sleep disorder. He also put me on a very potent anti-inflammatory/analgesic medication for the muscle and joint pain. He encouraged me to use therapeutic massage, yoga, and stretching. He stressed the importance of taking short naps every day and pacing myself. His kindness, familiarity with my symptoms, and ability to help gave me hope and allowed me to move forward into believing in a future again.

Today I can honestly say that I have turned the corner and have returned to being a positive, determined person who has gone through a lot of trauma and come out stronger each step of the way. Writing this book to help others is the last phase of my healing process. When we come to the end of the grief cycle we naturally feel renewed energy and investment in life, and believe we have something to offer from the lessons we have learned. Even though I still battle with some chronic health problems, I have come to accept my body again. I am grateful that I have made it past forty-two, that I have not had to experience breast cancer, and that my daughter still has a mom. I now think Mother Nature and I are working together for the "good" of me.

A Husband's Reaction

Around the time of my thirtieth birthday, Becky and I came to a painful but necessary decision. Given her family history and the input we received from the oncologist, a preventive bilateral mastectomy seemed the only reasonable option. Not having the surgery would put her life at risk at a later date, and this meant that as far as I was concerned, there really was no decision-making process to go through. The surgery had to happen.

The primary feelings I experienced at this time were relief that we lived during a time in which preventive action could be taken, and fear that Becky could die during surgery. Any thoughts I had about what Becky would look like, and how the surgery would impact our sexual relationship were not even considerations then.

After the surgery was over and I knew that Becky was safe, I had a lot to keep me occupied. I spent time at the hospital, kept up our home, went to work, brought Becky home, and worried intensely about how she would be able to cope with this traumatic change to her body. As is the case with many people in a crisis, I focused on doing what needed to be done, rather than what was going on inside me.

As I look back on this difficult time, I remember being immensely grateful that action had been taken so my soulmate would not die from breast cancer well before her time. We are blessed to have a relationship anchored in love and in being each other's best friend, and knowing that we had taken steps to keep Becky alive longer was deeply satisfying.

Mixed with the relief and gratitude were feelings of anger, sadness, and loss. The anger was, and still is, rooted in the "Why do bad things happen to good people?" mystery. I can recall thinking, "We're a couple of decent folks who don't harm anybody. Why is this happening to us?" The grief was for the unwanted changes to Becky's body, the loss of sexual pleasure for both of us, and the fact that what used to be a simple process of expressing love was now encumbered with intrusive thoughts and feelings. I wished things could go back to being the way they were before the surgery.

The surgery produced scars under Becky's breasts, which were never repulsive or anything close to that, but they were a negative change. The skin around the scars was frequently irritated, red, and painful looking.

A second major change involved the replacement of her natural tissue with silicone implants. Breasts that were formerly soft, pliable, and stimulating to fondle and kiss were now stiff and decidedly less fun to incorporate into our lovemaking.

Another area of loss had to do with the sensations experienced by Becky. Touch which had previously been pleasurable for her was now painful, or at the very least uncomfortable. To make things even more complicated, sometimes a certain type of touch would be painful, while at other times it would be neutral. The end result was a decrease in erotic stimulation for Becky.

The sense of loss can manifest itself in many ways. Becky's breasts had been small, and not the same size. We used to kid around about "the big one" and "the little one." At the time of her surgery, she determined that she wanted her breasts to be of uniform size. This was a reasonable decision to make at the time; however, after the operation I found myself missing her natural body configuration. There was no longer any kidding between us about "the big one," and I missed that.

After more than a decade, we found out that the silicone implants had ruptured. There was no way to know for certain how much time had passed since the ruptures occurred, or what exactly the health implications were. The only things that seemed definite were that the implants needed to be removed, there would be the trauma of another surgery, and we would be forced to adjust to another major change in Becky's body.

I remember feeling angry about all of this, as it struck me as being very unfair. There was anger at the original physicians for not disclosing the risks of rupture and possible health consequences, and anger at the manufacturers for making money from a defective, and perhaps damaging, product. The "why us?" thoughts I had experienced at the time of the first surgery returned.

The choices open to us were all bad. Becky could be completely flat chested, tissue could be transplanted from her abdomen to create new breasts, or saline implants could be inserted. Only the first option appeared to be risk-free. This was another situation in which the decision really made itself. Becky needed to be able to go through life without wondering if she would someday be forced to endure yet another surgery to correct another problem with her breasts. Doing this twice seemed like more than enough.

Since the time of the first surgery, managed care had become much more established in Minnesota. As is the case with many things, managed care is a "good news/bad news" proposition. The bad news in this particular case was that Becky had surgery in the morning, recuperated after awaking by sitting in a chair for a couple of hours, and was discharged in the afternoon. I put on my "pretend nurse" hat, and helped get her home to bed.

One of the tasks that must be completed when someone has this surgery is the stripping of the drainage tubes which are inserted into the chest. It has to be done regularly and carefully, as the chest is very sore. It is not a fun activity for either person.

Since I was the one who stripped the tubes, I saw Becky's chest before she did. Although my main focus was on completing this job in a way that minimized her discomfort, I was struck by the absence of breasts. Everything felt incredibly permanent and very sad at that moment. An irrational thought zipped through my mind: "How do I keep Becky from seeing this?" Of course, that would not be possible. One more time we would have to count our blessings, adjust, and make the best of a difficult situation. We were both pretty tired of doing that.

The adjustment required in going from artificial to no breasts was, for me, more difficult than going from natural to artificial breasts. There was relief in knowing that we would never have to go through breast surgery again, but there was a profound sadness associated with the loss. For a man to attempt to disguise the sadness precipitated by this surgery in an effort to shield his wife or girlfriend is, I believe, both disrespectful and a waste of time. The woman is always smart enough to know better.

At the same time, it is essential that the man not "clam up" because he is afraid he will say the wrong thing. He should acknowledge the loss, while at the same time reassuring her that his love for her has not been affected, and that she remains feminine and desirable in his eyes.

Amidst all of the feelings of fear, relief, gratitude, anger, and sadness, I needed to make a decision of my own. I could choose to adopt a victim attitude and spend the rest of my life with Becky feeling cheated out of a normal sexual relationship, or I could decide to embrace the love and joy we share and "get on with it." I elected the second option.

The sexual part of a significant relationship, if it is to be about something more than brief physical pleasure, is one way in which two people express the richness of their emotional intimacy. Although natural breasts certainly add to the pleasure for both individuals, their presence or absence should never influence the depth of feeling which is the foundation of the relationship.

CHAPTER TWO

BREAST CANCER AND TREATMENT

Most women have mastectomies as a treatment for breast cancer. Of course, there are other reasons for having a mastectomy besides breast cancer or breast cancer prevention. Some women have suffered the loss of a breast as the result of an accident. Some women had implants for breast enlargement and did not tolerate them so are left with a partial loss of their breasts. But most women have mastectomies directly or indirectly as a result of breast cancer. My own bilateral mastectomy was done as a preventive measure to avoid the disease.

Breast cancer is a growing epidemic among women. Most of us know the frightening statistics: One in eight women will get breast cancer at some point in their lives. It is not my intention here to provide you with a comprehensive description of breast cancer and all of the available treatments, but because most of you will be coming to this book with at least some personal experience with breast cancer, I will provide a brief overview of the disease. Many excellent books are available which are devoted only to breast cancer and I strongly recommend that you take advantage of the information they have to offer.

Cancer

Cancer is a general word that describes over one hundred different diseases. These diseases all have as a common characteristic the abnormal and uncontrolled growth of cells. A tumor is caused by cells dividing out of control. Cell division is normal and necessary, but when cells mutate the normal control system breaks down. Depending on the type and stage of cancer, it may be contained in a tumor in a particular site, but as the cells continue to split the cancer cells will begin to move from their original site to other systems in the body. This movement from the original site is called metastasis. Cancer can spread through the bloodstream or through the lymph nodes and lymphatic system. Metastasis is the reason cancer can lead to death. When the cells multiply, creating colonies throughout the body, they become parasites, using up all the substances we need to keep us healthy and alive. Cancer cells consume all the nutrition, glucose, and oxygen needed to sustain a functioning body.

> Surgery is almost always required to treat breast cancer.

We are a long way from knowing all the risk factors for breast cancer and understanding exactly how they work. Lifestyles which are often reflected in different cultures, environmental conditions, and genetic structures are three very broad areas in which doctors are finding connections to the causes of cancer. Occupations that expose workers to hazardous chemicals; living in close proximity to a radiation plant or other toxic site; diets that include a lot of red meat, high fat content, and little fiber, are some of the conditions that seem to be related to the cause of breast cancer. It is believed that some families pass on a trait in the genes that produces mutant cells which lead to breast cancer. But the vast majority of breast cancer develops as various factors affect the genes' ability to produce normal breast cells. Having a first-degree relative (mother or sister) with a history of breast cancer increases a woman's risk by two to three times. When the family cancer occurred in both breasts or developed before menopause, the risk is six to eight, or up to 50%, greater.[1] If you have already had breast cancer, depending on its type, you have a 10–25% risk of developing it in the other breast.[2]

THE HEALTHY BREAST

Breast tissue covers quite a large area. It extends from the breast bone (the big bone that runs down between your breasts and anchors your ribs) into the armpits and up nearly to the collarbone. Breasts consist of fibrous, glandular, and fatty tissue that sits over the pectoris muscles (see Figure 2-1). Breast tissue is attached to the muscles by the suspensory lig-

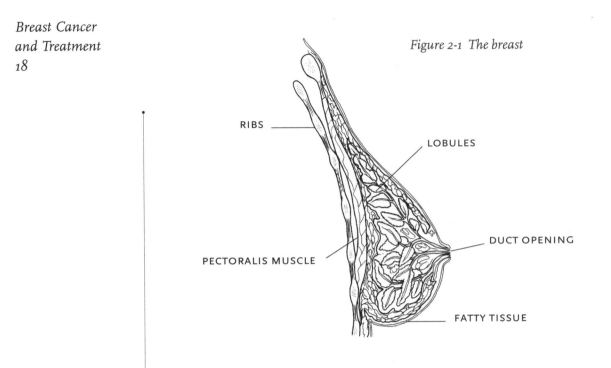

Figure 2-1 The breast

RIBS

LOBULES

PECTORALIS MUSCLE

DUCT OPENING

FATTY TISSUE

aments of Cooper, which are fibrous strands. The breast glands are padded with a layer of fat, and fat extends throughout the rest of the breast. The fatty tissue is what makes the breast soft and movable.

Besides the fatty tissue, the full part of the breast consists of glands, blood vessels, lymphatic channels, ducts, lobules, and sensory nerves. The lobules produce milk when the body is secreting enough of the right hormones and the ducts carry the milk to the nipples. The nerves run upward from the muscle layer and are highly sensitive in the area of the nipple and areola (the darker, wrinkled skin that surrounds the nipple). The nerves allow sensation or feeling in the breasts. Fluids come and go through the breast by way of the bloodstream and the lymph system. The lymph system consists of lymphatic vessels that carry fluid to the lymph nodes, which act as filters. The lymph system is a critical part of the immune system, which fights infection. When the body is fighting off a perceived invader, the lymph nodes will swell. The lymph nodes that are connected to the breast are located around the breast, near the breast bone and in the axilla (armpit).

Breasts come in all shapes and sizes. Some breasts are the same size but many women have one breast somewhat smaller than the other. Nipples can be erect or inverted. Some breasts are lumpier than others and some women's breasts swell more, or become more lumpy with the hormonal changes of the menstrual cycle. These variations are normal.

BREAST CANCER

There are approximately a dozen different types of breast cancer. The most common type (86%) is called ductal carcinoma. This type is located in the drainage ducts of the breast. The second most common type of breast cancer (12%) is called lobular carcinoma, and it is found in the milk glands (lobules). The other types of breast cancers originate in the surrounding tissues.

Breast cancers are classed as either noninvasive (precancer) or invasive. Noninvasive cancers can be considered "in situ" or in between cancerous and healthy cells. In the case of ductal carcinoma, these are called intraductal carcinoma, ductal carcinoma in situ, or noninvasive carcinoma. It is believed that breast cancer begins with a few abnormal cells and it takes between one and ten years for these cells to reproduce enough to make a detectable lump. When the cells begin to reproduce abnormally and move into the lining of the breast ducts, this is intraductal carcinoma. They spend some time in the ducts before beginning to spread to other locations. This is the best time to detect cancer because it is still contained, which makes it easier to reach and destroy.

Invasive cancer is so called because the cancer cells have spread from the duct or, more rarely, the lobule in the case of lobular carcinoma, into the surrounding tissue. After the cells have moved beyond the duct or lobule lining, they can be taken up into the lymph vessels and transported to the lymph nodes. The next level of invasion takes place when the cells are able to move into the bloodstream and are carried to other parts of the body, most commonly the bones, liver, or lungs.

Studies show that in many cases a lumpectomy with radiation and a modified mastectomy are equally effective treatments.

Stages of Breast Cancer

Breast cancer, like all types of cancer, is classified into four stages as a way of describing how far the cancer has spread. Treatment and prognosis are directly related to a particular stage of breast cancer; however, the stages are not absolute. You will need to find out what your physician means by asking for clarification of how your test results are being interpreted.

The four-stage system is called the TNM (tumor, nodes, and metastases) system and is based on the size of the tumor, the presence of cancer in the lymph nodes, and detection of cancer in metastasized locations.

- Stage 1: T-1 is a tiny tumor (less than 2 centimeters) with no lymph node involvement.
- Stage 2: T-2 is a small tumor with positive lymph nodes, a tumor between 2 and 5 centimeters with positive or negative lymph nodes, or a tumor larger than 5 centimeters with negative lymph nodes.
- Stage 3: T-3 is a large tumor with positive lymph nodes or a tumor with "grave signs".
- Stage 4: T-4 is a tumor that has obvious metastasis.

Treatment
SURGERY

Some form of surgery is almost always needed for the treatment of breast cancer. The only time surgery is not performed is when the cancer has spread throughout the body and is obviously untreatable. In that instance, putting someone through surgery would only be cruel. If there is even the slightest possibility of ridding the body of the cancer or greatly reducing it to prolong life, then surgery to remove the main source of cancer will be necessary.

There are four types of mastectomy, which vary in the amount of tissue removed. An axillary dissection, which is the removal of lymph nodes from the armpit, is done with all cancer-related mastectomies to determine if cancer has progressed into the lymph system. A section of tissue is removed, along with the lymph nodes that are present in that tissue.

The size and position of the tumor, as well as the surgeon's judgment and your personal preference, will determine which type of procedure is performed.

1. In a partial mastectomy, a wedge of the breast is removed. It is often referred to as a lumpectomy because the wedge is a small area where the lump, or tumor, is located. This procedure is used when the cancer is believed to be well contained in a very small area.

2. In a quadrantectomy, about a quarter of the breast is removed. It is a slightly more conservative approach than the lumpectomy because it takes more tissue from around the tumor site.

3. In a modified mastectomy, most of the breast tissue is removed. Along with removing lymph nodes to detect the presence of cancer, they can also be removed if it has already been established that the nodes contain cancerous cells.

4. In a radical mastectomy, as much as possible of the breast tissue is removed, including the pectoral muscles and all the axillary lymph nodes. This procedure was used exclusively for breast cancer many years ago. If your mother or grandmother had breast cancer, she probably had a radical mastectomy. This procedure is now the very rare exception. If the tumor has grown so that it has attached itself to the muscle then some or all of the muscle may need to be removed, but this seldom occurs.

RADIATION

Radiation is another localized method for killing cancer cells, in which radiation rays are lasered into a very defined area where cancer cells are believed to be present. Radiation kills both healthy and unhealthy cells and so it must be used carefully. This treatment is often used after surgery to clean up the surrounding area after the breast tissue has been removed. Radiation is commonly used with a lumpectomy because there is a lot of surrounding tissue. If cancer is present in the lymph nodes, radiation may also be used to kill it at that location. Radiation does not affect cancer cells that may be travelling through your lymph system or bloodstream.

Research shows that radiation does not affect the overall cure rate of breast cancer, but it can prevent local recurrence in the affected area.[3] Recurrence of cancer in the surgical area is very difficult to treat and can cause pain and bleeding, so radiation is an important part of the overall treatment regime. The radiation techniques and equipment used today are much more exact than in the past, resulting in fewer negative side effects and secondary problems.

A contralateral mastectomy is the removal of the remaining, non-cancerous breast. It is done for prevention or to achieve symmetry.

CHEMOTHERAPY

Chemotherapy is a systemic form of treatment that uses chemicals (medication/drugs) that travel through the body to kill cancer that has entered the lymph system and/or the bloodstream and other organs. There are a lot of horror stories about chemotherapy but, like many cancer treatments, it has improved over the years. Many people who have witnessed a loved one endure horrible side effects concluded that the chemotherapy was worse than the cancer, but the drugs used today are different and much more specific to cancer types and, therefore, much more effective. According to Dr. Susan Love, breast surgeon and author of *Dr. Susan Love's Breast Book,* chemotherapy reduces the risk of recurrence by about a third, meaning that the higher the chance of recurrence the greater difference chemotherapy will make to your survival.[4]

Chemotherapy can be accompanied by nausea and vomiting, fatigue, hair loss, and depressed bone marrow. The medical profession is now able to control the nausea and vomiting with medication more effectively. A friend of mine just went through a very potent course of chemotherapy during her stem-cell transplant procedure (see below) and only experienced about one day of severe nausea. She said she almost felt guilty because the other women in her cancer support group who had gone through this procedure had been very nauseated, but she had escaped the worst of the side effects because her doctors had just begun using a new combination of antinausea drugs. Much of the fatigue that accompanies chemotherapy is a result of the nausea and vomiting and an inability to retain enough nutrients.

Hair loss is another unfortunate side effect of chemotherapy, but even though it may be upsetting it should not deter women who are candidates for chemotherapy. The hair loss is not permanent and the hair often begins to grow back even before the treatment is finished. Many women are also surprised to see that their new hair growth has a natural curl. This curl is very common and it usually lasts for about a year. One woman thought perhaps it was nature's way of balancing the scales of life by giving her a ready-made permanent during a time when she most needed an easy-to-care-for hair style. Wearing a wig while she did not have hair also gave her the opportunity to discover a new hair style that she has since replicated with her newly grown hair.

Bone marrow transplant and stem-cell transplant are complex forms of chemotherapy. Allogenic bone marrow transplant is the term used when someone else donates some of their bone marrow, the part of the bone that produces all blood cells, to a cancer patient who has undergone very high doses of chemotherapy, which kills bone marrow as well as cancer cells. Autologous bone marrow or stem-cell transplant, or transplant, means that the patient's own stem-cells, a specialized part of the bone marrow, are used for the transplant. Allogenic transplant is used to treat lymphoma, leukemia, and multiple myeloma. At this time only autologous transplant is used to treat breast cancer. Prior to chemotherapy, the patient is hospitalized, bone marrow taken from the bone or stem-cells are harvested for later use. After the chemotherapy is completed, the stored stem-cells are transfused back into the body to restore its immune system defenses. In some places this procedure is considered experimental, while in other areas it is commonly used for women with more advanced forms or recurrent breast cancer. I have two friends and one client who have undergone the stem-cell transplant procedure within the last year.

HORMONE THERAPY

Hormone therapy is a treatment given when breast cancer has been shown to be fed by the presence of estrogen. An estrogen receptor assay is a test to determine whether the tumor is nourished by estrogen. If the test is positive, tamoxifen (Nolvadex) may be used to block estrogen.

Making the Choice

Many women are given the choice between a lumpectomy with radiation or a modified mastectomy. This can be an extremely difficult decision to make. What we really want is to have the doctor tell us there is one procedure that is guaranteed to get rid of the cancer. But unfortunately, medicine is not that exact, and scientific progress now allows women different treatment options. Research shows that lumpectomies with radiation are just as effective as a modified mastectomy.[5] Some women respond to their choice by feeling empowered. They tend to be the same ones who gather as much information as they can, as a way of coping. Other women feel overwhelmed and confused by their choices. They need to make life simple again by limiting the amount of input they receive and recruiting the help of others to make the decision. Both reactions are common and neither one is better than the other.

Because the two procedures give the same result, your decision will come down to which approach is going to give you the most peace of mind. Carol had a lumpectomy with radiation in both breasts. She found the first lump when she was a university student so she had access to a medical library, which she used to study breast cancer and the treatment options. She concluded the lumpectomy was a safe method that would best fit her life as a single woman in her forties. A second cancerous lump occurred about five years later, which was unrelated to the first incidence, and Carol underwent a second lumpectomy. She came to me for psychotherapy at the time of her second occurrence because she was depressed. Although she had a lot of feelings to process about her cancer and lumpectomies, she did not question her choice of procedure. She felt good about taking an active role in her medical care. Some time later a questionable mammogram gave her another scare. A needle biopsy was performed, which showed no evidence of cancer, so she did not have to have another surgical procedure. At this time Carol questioned whether she should have had a bilateral mastectomy when she had the first lumpectomy. She wondered whether she would have been spared all the worry and extra procedures. However, this was a momentary reaction, and overall Carol says she has been and is comfortable with her choices.

Carisa, who came to see me for depression following a modified mastectomy, confessed she was obsessing that she had made a mistake by not having a lumpectomy. She said she would never admit this to anyone else, but she worried that she had made a bad decision. Her doubt re-

sulted from the extreme discomfort she was experiencing from numbness and pain. Her phantom pain cleared in a few days, but she was left
with numbness that interfered with her daily living. As we talked, she re-
membered that she had chosen the modified mastectomy because she
believed it was her best chance for getting rid of the cancer and it would
help her not to worry as much about a recurrence. She had not wanted to
go through radiation, and by choosing a modified mastectomy and hormone therapy she was able to finish her cancer treatment and get back to
normal living sooner than if she had radiation. Because she would have
had a node dissection regardless of the type of mastectomy she chose,
her numbness would probably not have been any less with the lumpectomy.[6] Research shows that there is no difference in the amount of pain
or numbness a woman has with a modified mastectomy versus a
lumpectomy. As Carisa moved through the grief process she was able to
focus on the positive aspects of her decision and realize that her mastectomy had been the right choice for her.

> "I would have
> preferred to have
> both off. It was
> having just one and
> being lopsided that
> was hard."

Contralateral and Bilateral Preventive Mastectomies

Contralateral mastectomy is the removal of the remaining non-
cancerous breast. Many women struggle with the decision of whether to
have the other breast removed, to prevent further incidence of breast
cancer and for cosmetic reasons, for those who are troubled by asymme-
try. Your risk of getting breast cancer in your remaining breast is increased once you have had breast cancer, but how much is determined by
your previous risk factors, as well as the type of breast cancer you had. If
you had lobular breast cancer, your chance of getting a new occurrence
in your other breast goes up by 25%. I encourage you to talk with your oncologist or surgeon about your type of cancer and what it means in terms
of your risk of recurrence.

There are conflicting view on the effectiveness of preventive mastectomies. Some surgeons offer this option and present it as the cure-all for
avoiding recurrences of breast cancer. Many surgeons offer preventive
contralateral or bilateral mastectomies, but explain there is no guarantee
that they will prevent breast cancer. And, some surgeons, such as Dr. Susan Love, strongly discourage preventive mastectomies because they be-

lieve the surgery has not been shown to prevent breast cancer. There are no currently definitive studies to provide us with a clear-cut answer about whether or not preventive mastectomies are effective for preventing breast cancer, or to what degree they do reduce the risk. We are now working from the assumption that our risk level will be reduced by the same percentage as the amount of breast tissue we reduce. This may not be true. But on the other hand mastectomies are the treatment for breast cancer.

Dr. Love suggests that there may be a difference between removing already existing cancerous tissue and removing tissue before cancer has developed. Mutations that can develop into breast cancer may be contained in any existing breast cells. Breast cells exist in more than the bulge of tissue that we consider a breast. There are breast cells in the surrounding muscle and connective tissue that includes the armpit, some of the back as far up as the collarbone and down as far as the bottom of the rib cage.

My surgeon told me before my preventive bilateral surgery that I would have some remaining breast cells and would still have to do monthly checks for lumps. He put my implants under my chest muscles so I could easily feel the muscle to detect a lump. After my surgery, my gynecologist ordered a mammogram and instructed the mammogram reader to look for the presence of remaining breast cells. The mammogram showed very few remaining breast cells and they were in the bit of fatty tissue I have in the upper-outer chest area next to my armpits. When I examine myself I am especially careful to check these areas. I received this medical care in the early 1980s, and I have since read a lot about the progress that has been made in preventing and treating breast cancer. I now know that the mammogram I had back then could not have shown all of my breast cells.

A preventive mastectomy may be the best way for some women to feel safe from the recurrence or onset of breast cancer. Living in constant fear of breast cancer can affect a woman's quality of life as well as her overall health. A recent study done at Ohio State University found that the breast cancer patients with the most anxiety about their medical condition had the lowest levels of white blood cells, those that normally attack cancer and combat infection.7 Women with the highest level of stress had 20% to 30% fewer immune system cells of the kind used to kill cancer cells. Gamma interferon, a natural protein that enhances immunity, and T_4 cells, a key lymphocyte in the body's defense against infection, were shown to work less effectively in women with the greatest level of stress and worry about their health. Cancer phobia may be successfully treated through psychotherapy, but some women may not be able to be rid of their fear until they can do something active that makes them feel they have changed their risk level. The important thing is that you listen to yourself and take whatever measures you think will help you to reach the greatest comfort level.

I do not regret having a bilateral preventive mastectomy. It gave me peace of mind and allowed me to open up to having a full life, including raising a child. I regret getting silicone implants, but not having the mastectomies. Even though I know I still have a risk of getting breast cancer, the surgery was my way of dealing with the mental obsession about getting breast cancer. Fear no longer runs my life and I have defied the odds—I haven't developed breast cancer even though my chances of getting it were very high.

Be aware that surgeons will each have their own belief. You are in a vulnerable position and so may be easily influenced by their attitude. If your surgeon sways your decision to have or not have a preventive mastectomy and you feel comfortable with that, then that is fine. But if you have to struggle to accept your surgeon's recommendation I strongly encourage you to research the question through further reading and by consulting other surgeons.

My friend Allison who is in her early fifties is struggling with the question of whether or not she should have a bilateral preventive mastectomy. She has extremely dense breast tissue that is difficult to read accurately on a mammogram, and she has numerous painful cysts. Both her mother and sister have had breast cancer. She lives six hours away from a breast clinic and has to drive this distance twice a year for breast exams. Each appointment takes several hours because the mammogram

The four types of mastectomy are: partial mastectomy or lumpectomy, quadrantectomy, modified mastectomy, and radical mastectomy. All vary by how much tissue is removed from the breast area.

has to be repeated many times before the technicians feel they have gotten an accurate film. She sits in the waiting room in a patient gown in a state of extremely high anxiety. Each time the doctors question whether to make her into a pincushion by doing biopsies to provide a more accurate picture of what is going on. Allison comes away with little reassurance. She feels that she could cope fine after preventive surgery and would gain a great deal of relief from stopping the nerve-wracking process of trying to detect breast cancer in its early stages, but does not know how well her husband would adjust. Allison knows he would love her just as much but she has observed him to be very squeamish over medical conditions and worries that he would react to her postmastectomy chest with anxiety and discomfort. The breast cancer detection methods she is currently using greatly affect her quality of her life and are putting her at risk of poor health from all the worry. Her doctor has presented surgery as an option and she is getting a second opinion. Allison is also preparing to make her decision by talking to women who have had mastectomies, educating herself through seminars and literature, and discussing her thoughts and fears with her medical team.

A contralateral mastectomy is often performed as a means of reaching an esthetic goal or a lifestyle that is most comfortable for the postmastectomy woman. Contralateral mastectomies are often done to achieve symmetry, and make breast replacement less complicated. The decision to have the remaining breast removed is most always done some time after the first mastectomy in reaction to the problems that come from trying to reach a balanced look. Women who have preventive surgery done on their remaining breast are tired of having to worry about normal weight fluctuations and the affect they have on keeping a balanced look, and feel burdened by the cost and bother of having to come up with accessories that will keep both breasts looking even. Having both breasts reconstructed makes it easier to match them, and having both breasts gone allows more choices in clothing and prostheses. It is possible to go without prostheses, wear different sizes, and use different types of prostheses depending on your activities.

One serious downside to having a contralateral mastectomy is the loss of all of your erotic breast sensation. The women I have talked to said the biggest concern they had about removing the other breast was whether they would be cheating their sexual partner by not having at least one breast left for lovemaking. They also knew they would be cheating themselves out of erotic pleasure, but this tended to be a secondary concern in comparison to their partner's loss.

CHAPTER THREE

SURGERY

The Surgical Team

Preparing for a mastectomy is no different from preparing for any other type of major surgery. The process starts in the doctor's office as you begin to establish a relationship with your surgeon and the medical staff. You were probably under the care of your family doctor or gynecologist when you first discovered a lump and were then referred to the surgeon. It is important for you to try to make a connection with the surgeon. You are putting your life in this person's hands. Most of us come to the situation with a certain amount of trust in the doctor who referred us. It may be helpful to remember the trust you have in your primary care physician and realize that your doctor must have referred you to this particular surgeon for a good reason.

While becoming comfortable with the person who will perform your surgery, ask yourself what you need your surgeon to do for you. Obviously, you want a skilled surgeon, and you probably also want information about the operation and about your treatment and condition.

You are likely to receive a teaching pamphlet from the surgeon's office or the hospital. This will answer many of your questions and help you to formulate other questions. At this stressful time it is likely that your anxiety level will be high, which can make your memory function poorly. Therefore, it is a good idea to write down your questions. It is also helpful to have someone come with you during the office visit to assist you with remembering and interpreting what the doctor has said. The person you choose to accompany you should be someone who can comprehend the information without having his or her anxiety interfere with the ability to retain the answers to your questions.

Some questions that you will probably want to ask are:

1. How will my choice of mastectomy affect the treatment I will need to have to get rid of any remaining cancer after the surgery?
2. How will my choice of mastectomy affect my risk level of recurrence?
3. What will I look like after the surgery?
4. How long will I be in the hospital?
5. When can I return to work?
6. When and how will I get my pathology report?

Another resource for getting your questions answered is the nursing staff. The surgeon usually has a nurse in the office who will be available to you during your office visit and by phone. There will also be nursing staff around during your hospital admitting time. They have been through the operation with many women and will be able to answer most of your questions, and if they don't know they are in a good position to be able to get an answer for you.

Most people do not realize that it is not the surgeon who usually makes the difference as to whether or not you come out of surgery alive, it is the anesthesiologist. If you are having open heart surgery, the surgeon plays a huge part in bringing you through it, but in the case of a mastectomy the greatest risk is with being put to sleep and then returning you to a conscious state. It is extremely rare for an anesthesiologist to make a mistake. How many people do you know who have had surgery? How many are not here today because the anesthesiologist did a bad job? I personally know of no one and I have been in the medical profession for twenty-five years.

My biggest worry in undergoing surgery was being put to sleep, for fear I would not wake up. I dealt with this irrational fear by remembering the facts. I have gone under general anesthetic five times in my life, dating back to age two, and I am still here to tell about it. In fact, one of the best parts of my surgery experiences has been the nurse anesthetists and anesthesiologists who have cared for me. They always seemed to show

The nursing staff in your surgeon's office or in the hospital are an invaluable resource for answering your questions.

Even with the tightest of managed health care plans there is room for more than one choice of surgeon.

up right when I needed someone the most, and were always incredibly sensitive to my fear and could anticipate what I needed to hear. They knew I was terrified that I would not wake up and they were not uncomfortable addressing the subject honestly and openly. Each time the anesthesiologist asked me how I was doing and if I had any questions, and took the time to explain what I would see in the operating room and what I would experience during the procedure.

After you have considered the whole team that will be getting you through your surgery, you need to ask yourself whether the surgeon is acceptable to you. Does the surgeon appear competent and respectful? How were your questions answered? It is important not to delay surgery because some forms of cancer progress quickly, and it is hard on you psychologically to have to wait. But this does not mean you cannot afford to take the time to go to a second surgeon if you do not feel comfortable with the first one. Even with the tightest of managed care medical plans, there is room to have more than one option for a surgeon. Do whatever is necessary to allow you to go into the operating room with confidence in the medical team. I do, however, want to caution you against getting too much advice, resulting in too many choices. Right before a mastectomy, decision-making can be extremely difficult, so spare yourself unnecessary anguish by keeping your choices to a manageable number.

PREPARING FOR SURGERY

There are a few things you can do to prepare for surgery. First of all, you should prepare your home so it is the way you want it when you return. You will be in no shape to do housework for some time after the surgery, so make sure your immediate space is clean and comfortable. You may find the cleaning "busy work" takes your mind off things and helps to work off nervous energy, or you may feel overwhelmed and tired, in which case you might consider asking for help. Friends often feel helpless to know how they can support us through this time and appreciate the opportunity to help. It is very appropriate to ask your children, spouse, or a good friend for help in getting your house in order before your surgery.

I would like to suggest some things to leave home and some to bring with you to the hospital. All of your jewelry will be removed before surgery. A wedding band can be taped to your finger but hospitals prefer you don't bring valuables with you. If you bring glasses or special jewelry that will have to be removed, I recommend that you give them to a friend or spouse to hold for you. You will need your medical card and ID, but the rest of your purse should stay home where it will be safe.

After surgery you will need clothes that can be buttoned up the front. You can use the hospital gown, but you may also want your own pajamas. Don't bring any clothing that is snug or has to be pulled over your head. A man's pajama top works great. You will want the clothes you wear home to be easy to slip on and big enough to disguise your lost breast. The bandage you will be wearing immediately after surgery is quite thick, which will help. Remember that you will not be wearing a bra home.

As you will probably only be in the hospital overnight, you will not need a lot of toiletries, but your own toothbrush and toothpaste, hairbrush, and comb will make you more comfortable. And last but not least, make sure you bring a few things from home that help you feel loved and secure. A family picture, a special pillow, headphones with relaxing music, or a stuffed animal are all examples of things you may want to bring.

Leave your valuables at home before your surgery. If you must bring some items with you, such as glasses or a wedding ring, leave them with a friend or spouse to hold for you when you go in for the operation.

THE LIVING WILL

Do not be alarmed when you are confronted with the living will. Most hospitals want to respect your wishes about how you want to live and how you want to die, and that is the purpose of the living will. It is merely a statement that declares what kind of medical care you wish to receive or refuse if you should reach a state where you are deemed unable to breathe and circulate your blood on your own and it is expected that you will never return to a condition where you would be able to do so without the help of a respirator. It is standard practice for hospitals to ask you to sign a living will indicating the type of care you would want under such conditions, and is done for all patients, even for such simple procedures as a tubal ligation or tonsillectomy.

There are two ways to approach the living will. One is to simply wait until you go to the hospital and sign their standard living will. The other

Don't forget to bring
some momento from
home that will make
you feel safe and
loved, such as a
family photo or
stuffed animal.

is to prepare your own. I chose the latter method. I purchased a blank living will form from a stationery store. The form came with an instructional booklet that explained the purpose of the living will and how to complete it. My husband and I wrote my living will together, which allowed us to feel more prepared and in control. I brought a copy of the living will with me to the hospital and it was placed in my medical record.

Just having to sign a living will often makes you aware that death is possible and brings you face to face with your mortality. When I prepared my living will I had two reactions. One was a very intellectual, rational reaction in which I was able to reason with myself that of course I was not going to die. The second reaction was purely emotional. I could not help but consider what it would mean to be dead and the effect on my husband and my daughter. This triggered some grief about losing my mother to breast cancer at the same age as my daughter would be when I had my surgery. It also made me think about the type of care I would want in the event that something went wrong. I would not want my family bankrupted to keep me hanging on for a while, only to die later. It became a time to reaffirm my spiritual beliefs and put my life in perspective. I am glad I faced those feelings, hard as they were to go through, because I was much more prepared to go into surgery. The living will helped bring my fear of dying into the open, and it allowed my husband and me to talk about our fears openly. By the time I went into surgery I felt strong and confident that I would make it through just fine.

MENTAL PREPARATION

It is important to build a positive attitude to take with you into surgery. Pleasant, positive thoughts have been shown to influence the outcome of surgery. Try role playing a positive attitude. First, close your eyes and go through the whole surgical experience, seeing your medical team doing a great job every step of the way. See yourself calm and confident, and see your medical team, compassionate and competent. Hear the team saying things that indicate the operation is going well, such as, "She's doing fine. The bleeding is surprisingly minimal for this type of surgery. It looks like we got it all. Wouldn't it be great if all surgeries could go this well." Then see yourself waking up, relieved that the surgery is over.

After you have visualized a successful surgery, set aside that image and create a new image of yourself surrounded by people who love you and who comfort and protect you. You might think of a partner or a friend, or both, or you may see yourself in the arms of a guardian angel or in God's arms, or floating on a cloud. You may see yourself in your mother's arms or in the arms of the Virgin Mary. The particular image is not important. What matters is that the image comforts and calms you. As you practice, you will find that there are some images that seem easier to create and more comforting. These are the ones you should use. If you find yourself having to work to create a particular positive image, that means you should try a different one. Use this imaging the night before surgery, while you are waiting to go into the operating room, and just before you are anesthetized for your surgery.

The anesthesiologist plays an essential role in your surgery.

Putting positive thoughts into your mind through these types of mental imagery exercises can affect the level of tension in your muscles, breathing patterns, and action of your heart. Calm thoughts will relax your muscles, slow and deepen your breathing, and keep your heart from racing. For example, you will be less sore from lying on a hard operating table for a couple of hours if you start out with relaxed muscles. However, even if you cannot calm yourself using mental imagery, the medical team will manage the functioning of your body to keep it safe and produce a good outcome. Too often people learn about mental imagery and feel if they cannot make themselves relax they have only themselves to blame. Remember that mental imagery is an aid to make you feel more comfortable; you should not feel a sense of failure if it doesn't work for you.

The Operation

You will be told to not eat or drink anything for several hours before surgery. This could be for as long as twelve hours if you are told to not consume anything after midnight and your surgery is not scheduled until noon the next day. There is a very good reason for this. If you have anything in your stomach while you are under general anesthetic, the food or liquid could come back up and, because you are unconscious, could get into your lungs, which would be life threatening. If you have forgot-

"In my experience the anesthesiology staff always seem to show up at the time I most needed someone. They were always incredibly sensitive to my fears and took the time to explain the procedure I would be undergoing."

ten and eaten something, it is very important to tell someone when you are checking into the hospital so they can determine whether it is safe to proceed or if your surgery will need to be delayed or postponed to another day.

Often you will be checking into the hospital the morning of your surgery. You will complete your registration, if you have not already done so over the phone, and then you will have to wait for quite a while before anything more happens. During the wait you will likely want someone to talk to. Many people are too anxious to be able to focus on a book at this time and find the distraction of conversation a relief.

Either during your wait at this time or the night before you go into the hospital, you will be instructed to scrub your chest and armpit area until it feels like the skin is going to fall off. This used to be done by a nurse at the hospital, but now the patient usually does it at home. The scrubbing cleans the skin so bacteria cannot get into the open area once the incision is made.

When it is time for you to be taken to the operating room, you will be given a hospital gown, then be rolled on a gurney to a new waiting area. My husband always accompanied me to the pre-op waiting area and stayed with me until I was taken into the operating room. It can be very comforting to keep someone with you for support right until you go into surgery.

When you are waiting outside the operating room, the operating room team, which consists of a registered nurse, an anesthesiologist (MD), a registered nurse trained in anesthesiology (CRNA), and your surgeon will probably visit with you. These visits help to pass the anxious waiting time. Your blood pressure, pulse, and temperature will be taken to see what your baseline is for comparison while you are going through the operation. An intravenous drip (IV) will be started in your arm or on the top of your hand. The IV is used to keep enough fluids in your body to maintain a stable blood pressure and to administer medications, which will be added to the IV throughout the operation. The insertion of the IV doesn't hurt much because the needles used are tiny and the operating team is very skilled at starting them.

This is the time to use the protective, positive images that you practiced before you came to the hospital. If you are very anxious during this pre-op waiting time you may be given some anti-anxiety medication. You will have a choice about this. Some people like help to relax, and some, including myself, do not like feeling any loss of control and find that anti-anxiety medication actually creates a feeling of panic. I like to be fully alert and in control until it is time to go to sleep. Make sure your needs are met and tell the staff your preference. Your support person may be able to assist you with asserting your needs if you are having trouble doing so for yourself at such a vulnerable time. But make sure your support person doesn't take over rather than help you to be heard.

Finally, you will be wheeled into the operating room, which will be very cold. The room is cold to keep it sterile and prevent infection, since bacteria can only thrive in a warm environment. You will be moved to a hard operating table. The nurses will cover you with heated blankets until you are anesthetized. Fear also makes you feel cold, which can add to the discomfort, so don't hesitate to ask for more blankets if you are still cold. Once your surgeon comes into the room the anesthesiologist will tell you to start to count down from one hundred or from ten and to think of something pleasant. After you have counted a couple of numbers you will suddenly be asleep. It feels just like falling asleep for a good night's rest. It is a good idea to ask someone to hold your hand as you go under. Most people are glad to help and it can be a real comfort.

> The operating room is kept very cold to keep it sterile and prevent infection. Ask for extra blankets if you need them.

After Surgery

When you wake up in the recovery room you will be surprised that the operation is over because it feels as if you just went to sleep. Anesthetic has been greatly improved over the years. Not only is it much safer, but it is also easier and more comfortable to wake up from than it used to be. The drugs do not last as long in your body, so you do not experience a long, heavily sedated period after surgery. Once you completely wake up after the surgery you will be fairly alert and coherent. You will feel very tired but not drugged.

You will spend about an hour in the post-operative recovery room. Once you are awake and alert and your vital signs are stable, you will be taken to another room, which is where you will probably stay until it is

"I found imagery and meditation helpful. I would imagine I had little Pac-mans running through my body eating up cancer cells."

time to be discharged. In 1981, when I had both breasts removed and implants put in, I was operated on Wednesday morning and went home on Saturday morning. This was considered a fast discharge at the time. In 1994, when I had my implants removed, I had my surgery in the early morning and went home about 5:00 P.M. the same day.

Doctors consider it unsafe to send women home on the same day after having a mastectomy, but in the U.S. insurance companies with managed care practices have insisted on this. Since 1997, however, in the state of Minnesota, it has been determined that women should be kept in the hospital for at least one night after having a mastectomy, and I expect other states to follow suit if they have not already done so.

I definitely feel that after my second surgery I should have stayed overnight. My husband told the surgeon that I was concerned about going home too soon. The surgeon told him that if I really felt I should stay, he would deal with the insurance company to have them pay for the overnight stay. I did not want to be a bother. After all, I thought, if all the other women could go home the same day I should be able to, too. Before I knew it, I was on my way home. I felt weak and vulnerable and we lived out in the suburbs far away from the hospital. I silently worried I would start to hemorrhage and be too far away to reach the same hospital. I worried that I would end up at a different hospital, treated by doctors I didn't know or trust, and who did not know exactly what had been done during my surgery. I also knew that any unusual bleeding would happen soon after the surgery, so staying overnight in the hospital would be enough to help me feel safer. If I had to do it over again, I would have stayed in the hospital.

Despite my fears, the chances of complications from a mastectomy are extremely low. My anxiety came from a previous surgery nearly twenty years before, when I'd had a tubal ligation and one of the cut blood vessels had not been cauterized properly. I experienced a fair amount of bleeding and had to go back to the doctor's office the next day. Staying in the hospital overnight after my explant surgery would have spared me unnecessary emotional strain.

Some people wake up after anesthetic feeling very sad and tearful.

The medication can cause this through its interaction with the nervous system. These emotions are just a temporary reaction that will go away as the medication clears your system. But sometimes the medication opens you up to your grief about the losses associated with your surgery. You will be too drugged immediately following your surgery to make much sense out of your emotions. They will become part of your long process of emotional healing.

DRESSINGS AND AFTERCARE

One thing you will have to deal with immediately at home is changing your dressings and draining the drainage tubes. You will have a big bandage, or dressing, over your incisions. Regardless of the type of mastectomy you have had, if cancer is suspected you will need to have lymph nodes removed from your armpit. If you have a lumpectomy you will have two incisions, one in the breast area and the other in the armpit. If you have a more complete mastectomy your surgeon may remove the nodes by reaching into the armpit from inside your chest, so a second incision is not necessary. Some surgeons prefer to make a second incision. This varies based on the surgeon's preferred technique, skill level, and your particular needs. The nurses will tell you how often to change the dressings, and show you how to do it, and will very likely send you home with the necessary supplies for changing the bandages.

You will probably have drainage tubes in your incisions. Some surgeons put a drainage tube in both incisions, and some only put one in the mastectomy site. The drainage tubes drain off fluids that build up in the surgical area which, if left undrained, can interfere with healing and lead to infection. Draining also relieves the uncomfortable pressure that results from a build-up of fluid. The fluid will be a mixture of clear and bloody liquid. It looks like watered-down blood. As it dries somewhat in the tube, it may turn a dark blood color.

The drainage tube will have a bulb attached to the bottom that collects the fluid. This tube will need to be stripped, or "milked," to help the fluid drain and the bulb will have to be emptied. To strip the tube, hold the top of it tightly with one hand and use the other hand to milk the tube by

The hospital staff will show you or your companion how to drain the tubes left in your incisions.

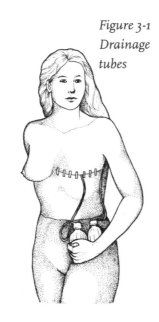

Figure 3-1
Drainage
tubes

pinching it between your thumb and index finger as you pull down the entire length of the tube until you reach the bulb (see Figure 3-1). You can do this in sections by holding tight and pinching the tube as you move to a lower portion. After you have finished stripping it a couple of times, open the bulb and drain it. Your doctor will probably want you to measure the amount of drainage, so the hospital will send you home with a container for measuring the fluid. After you have measured the drainage, it can be disposed of in the toilet.

Before you close the bulb, you should deflate it to create a suction that will draw fluid down the tube. The nurses will teach you how to do this, but right after surgery is generally not the best time to try to absorb information, so it is helpful to have a spouse or friend with you when the nurse is explaining the dressing changes and care of the drainage tubes.

If you find blood around your incision site, your tube may have gotten clogged with a blood clot at the top where you cannot see it. Milking will help to clear the tube so the fluid will go out the tube instead of seeping out of your incision.

Don't worry about pulling the tube out when you are stripping it or moving around. The tube is usually anchored with a stitch. If you accidentally pull out the stitch, the tube extends several inches into your incision, so even if it comes out a bit there will still be enough left in to do its job. The tube will probably be removed during your first return visit to your surgeon, generally about a week after your surgery.

The tubes are extremely annoying. They are always in the way and you have to be careful when you move. They are particularly burdensome when you have to go to the bathroom or are trying to wash up. The best way to deal with them is to pin them to your shirt or the waist of your pants with a big safety pin. Be careful to not pin them too high because they need to be lower than your incision so gravity can help with proper drainage.

Having the tubes removed is no treat, but neither is it horrible. Just take a deep breath while the doctor quickly pulls them out. I don't know what caused me more pain, the tubes being pulled out or the pain from my husband holding my hand, supposedly for comfort. He squeezed it so hard I thought it would break. I am sure the procedure was more painful for him than for me. He looked green when it was all over. I was doing fine, but he needed a bit more time to recover.

You probably won't have any stitches, or sutures that need to be removed because the incisions are usually closed with dissolvable sutures and a special type of tape. If there are a few stitches that are not dissolvable, you should feel only slight discomfort when they are removed.

> The chances of complications following a mastectomy are very low.

COMPLICATIONS

Numbness

You may notice numbness in the surgical area after your mastectomy. This can occur in a very small localized area, or extend into surrounding tissues. There is a major sensory nerve in the armpit and nerves in the chest area that can be cut or injured during surgery. This usually happens when lymph nodes are removed, but can also happen without the removal of lymph nodes. It is usually described as a numb sensation, but that is not how my friends, clients, or I describe it. Numbness implies that all sensation is gone, but what I experienced after surgery was a mixture of numbness and an unpleasant feeling that was very uncomfortable, distracting, and annoying, but not exactly painful. I experienced quite a bit of this unpleasant sensation after my double mastectomy and, even though my surgery was preventive with no lymph nodes removed, I still had the sensory problem. Some of the numb sensation went away over time but some of it has stayed. After I had my implants removed, even more of the area was affected. Some of that numbness has remained, and been added to the permanent feeling loss from the first surgery. The numbness seems to come and go with changes in weather and is influenced by how much the area is rubbed by clothing. I have noticed that fatigue makes it worse. The numb/unpleasant sensation comes and goes across my chest, into my armpits, down the inner parts of my arms to my elbows, and into my upper back. In Chapter 6, I will discuss treatment for this discomfort.

Lymphedema

Another possible complication after a mastectomy is lymphedema, which can result from having lymph nodes removed. Lymph nodes carry fluids through your tissues. When there are fewer nodes available and built-up scar tissue in the armpit, fluid can get trapped in the arm. Because there is less available lymph system action in the armpit and arm, it is important to watch for this fluid build-up and go to your doctor immediately if you suspect a problem may be developing. I explain lymphedema and its treatment further in Chapter 6.

Basilic Vein Discomfort

The final side effect you may experience after surgery is tightening and pain running down your arm. This pain comes from your basilic vein, a long vein that runs from your armpit down into your hand. The basilic vein can be shortened by surgery and cause a pulling sensation. One of my friends had such tightening that she feared the vein would snap. Your veins are very elastic, however, and they will not snap. Eventually the vein will stretch out again. In Chapter 6, I describe techniques to help ease discomfort and stretch the basilic vein.

CHAPTER FOUR

COPING WITH GRIEF AND OTHER EMOTIONS

Before we can move on with our lives after a mastectomy we need to take time to acknowledge our grief over the loss of our breast. Grief after a mastectomy is not an indication of superficiality or vanity. Grief is a natural, human response and a natural process which allows us to feel, and eventually recover from, loss.

Stages of Grief After Losing a Breast

Grief is an unfolding process that consists of five basic stages. We start the grieving process as soon as we learn that a mastectomy is a possibility and continue grieving long after the surgery is over. Grief for an impending loss is referred to as *anticipatory grief*.

When we first experience loss we go into the *denial* stage, during which we may feel shock, disbelief, and numbness. The denial stage is nature's way of cushioning us from the bluntness of reality. Denial allows us to gradually absorb the painful truth. Many women who have grieved the loss of a breast describe their response in the denial stage as hearing the information the doctor is telling them as though the physician is talking about someone else. They find themselves thinking that cancer and mastectomies happen to other people, not them. This response can give you time to intellectually attend to the details, such as making appointments with the surgeon and oncologist, before emotion floods in.

As our initial shock wears off we move into the *protest* stage, a phase of intense emotion, including anger, sadness, and confusion. As the facts start to sink in, our thoughts set off an emotional reaction. Our fear

Grief consists of five
basic stages: denial,
protest,
disorientation,
detachment, and
resolution.

of surgery and of cancer is probably foremost in our minds. Before we are even sure we have cancer, we often start to think about dying and leaving our loved ones behind. We feel sad for ourselves, our kids, and partner. We often feel betrayed and angry at our body. My clients consistently ask me what they did to deserve breast cancer. This is the time during which we tend to blame ourselves or others as we try to make sense of the loss. Anger at God, our doctors, or the relatives who passed on the bad genes is very common during the protest stage. Besides feeling the need to direct our anger at someone, it is also common to engage in unrealistic mental bargaining, such as promising to go to church every Sunday if our breast is spared. This bargaining is a combination of denial and our need to feel that we have some control over the situation. During this time, it is also common to experience physical symptoms from stress, such as diarrhea, constipation, neck and shoulder pain, restless sleep, and fatigue. Your stomach may ache or you may find yourself with a splitting headache that makes it hard to think. Your body may seem to be screaming out a message of emotional pain

The third stage of grief is the *disorientation* stage. This stage is often accompanied by restlessness, confusion, and depression, as we have to change our routines and adjust to the changes the mastectomy has brought. We may also continue to experience the physical symptoms of stress during this stage. Disorientation is very natural after your chest has healed enough to begin to wear more normal clothes and you are feeling strong enough to go out in public. You can't just go to your closet and pick out an outfit like before. Throwing on a bra and a T-shirt is not an option at this point. Now, selecting an outfit means finding a top that your tender chest and restricted arm can tolerate, plus finding a way to fill in the missing breast. You have lost a breast, the freedom to wear a variety of clothes, the movement in your arm, trust in your body, some of your sexuality, restful sleep, and physical comfort, to name a few of your many losses. And even though most of these losses are temporary or become easier with time, making the adjustment to them is likely to cause you to feel confused and disoriented.

Following the disorientation stage we move into the *detachment* stage. During this stage we tend to isolate and withdraw ourselves, and possibly feel resigned and apathetic. It is as though we have to go off quietly by ourselves and sit with our loss. Too much contact with other people at this time often feels like an intrusion and a lot of work. We often feel we need to be left alone in our misery to fully absorb our loss and get used to the fact that a mastectomy has forever changed our life.

The last stage of grief is *resolution* and it is during this stage that we enter a renewed state of reorganization and acceptance. We are not happy about the loss or our breast, but we see that we can live without it. The resolution stage often brings us insights into ourselves and our lives that build character and produce wisdom. During the resolution stage our mood lifts and we find we are able to experience joy again. This is also a time when we become grateful for what we have and want to give back. Volunteerism, such as in breast cancer support organizations, frequently accompanies this last stage of grief. If you give yourself the room to go through the emotions, you will move forward into the resolution stage of grief where you begin to feel acceptance. You will want to take back control of your life by becoming pro-active again. Priorities become redefined and life goals are re-established. Your overall reaction may actually be a blend of loss and gain. Initially it may have felt like a horrible loss but, as you move through the process, you discover some advantages that come along with your body changes (see Chapter 8).

There is also something called *automatic behavior* that often accompanies the grief process. This is what is happening when we don't get our routine behaviors quite right and we start to feel like we are going crazy. As we process our loss we become distracted from life's little details, and this natural preoccupation results in poor concentration while attending to daily tasks. As a result of automatic behavior you may find yourself putting the cereal into the refrigerator and the milk into the cupboard, squeezing a tube of skin cream instead of toothpaste onto your toothbrush, or seeing that the traffic light has turned red but not really registering it, and driving right through. Your short-term memory will also be affected because good concentration is required for the memory to work well. Do not panic over these lapses. They are temporary. However, it is

If you find yourself putting the cereal in the fridge and the milk in the cupboard then you are probably experiencing automatic behavior. Pay special attention when driving a car or doing any task that requires concentration as you are likely to make mistakes.

helpful to remember that automatic behavior can occur during the grief process, so you can safeguard yourself. When you set out to drive, remind yourself that you are prone to poor concentration and constantly remind yourself to tune into the "here and now." During this time you should stay away from dangerous machinery until you feel your focus and concentration return.

Each of you will go through the grief process in your own way. The stages of grief are meant to give a general description of the grief process, but in reality they are not as clean-cut as I have described. You will move back and forth through the various stages and can experience more than one stage at a time.

The significance you attach to your loss will determine how long your grieving process will last and how intensely you will feel it. Grief from losing a small purchase you just made may last only minutes, whereas a significant loss such as the death of a close friend, a divorce, or a house burning down may take years. Significant losses are often brought to mind by special events and seasons associated with the loss and these triggers can create new emotional pain. Most women take about two years before they report feeling fairly resolved about the loss of a breast. Your most intense grieving will probably happen close to the time of your surgery but you will likely continue to experience some grief from your mastectomy for the rest of your life. You may feel that you have just nicely accepted your loss just when something seems to set it off again. It may be three years later, when you are faced with having to find an evening dress for an elegant wedding, that you suddenly feel the tears bubbling up again. You may want to scream and stamp your feet at the unfairness of only being able to consider a quarter of the dresses because of the changes to your body. Twenty years after your surgery your best friend or daughter may be diagnosed with breast cancer and you may find yourself reliving some of your own pain as you walk through the process with her.

Defining Our Loss

Each one of us will have a unique set of losses associated with the loss of a breast based on our personal histories and our relationship to our breasts. The size of the breast does not determine how much we miss it. For example, very large breasts can be a big part of one's identity, and hence a huge loss. On the other hand, a woman with very large breasts might welcome the opportunity to get rid of a lifetime burden by having a double mastectomy and using smaller prostheses, or to get a welcomed breast reduction in the remaining breast. In the same way, a woman with smaller breasts has also defined herself accordingly and she may miss her little breast. Or, the mastectomy may offer a woman who has always wanted larger breasts the option of "up-sizing."

How big a part of your identity were your breasts? How did they fit into your image of yourself?

WHAT OUR BREASTS HAVE MEANT TO US

The way we define our loss and grieve after our mastectomy is influenced by the meaning we have given to our breasts as a result of our experience of developing a woman's body. Breasts are a significant part of our identities as women. Our worth as a person, of course, is not defined by our breasts but they are certainly included in our self-definition.

As we passed through the developmental stages of physical maturity we experienced many different phases. When we were small we anticipated growing up to look like Mommy, which meant having breasts. When our breasts began to bud we often became shy and wanted to hide them. Many of us walked with a hunched posture to keep others from seeing those little bumps pushing through our T-shirts. As our breasts continued to grow, our attitudes began to shift from shyness to pride. A mixture of anxiety and delight often accompanied the purchase of that first bra. We all have a story about what it was like to come into our breasts. I recall feeling grown up and proud because I was one of the first girls to develop enough to require a bra, yet not so early that I stood out in a negative way.

After puberty we discovered exciting new sensations in our breasts. Moving into the late junior and senior high school years, our breasts became a significant part of our new womanly definition, but may also have been a source of discomfort and fear as we considered the role our breasts played in our sexuality.

As we continued to mature and develop deeper, intimate relation-

What was it like to mature into your breasts? Was it a positive or negative experience?

ships, many of us came to know our breasts as much more than an erotic source of pleasure. We learned that a precious part of a deeper relationship that occurs as we relate to each other's body. In the privacy of our intimate relationships, some of us were given pet names for our sexual parts, including the breasts. Many of us established comfortable and stimulating sexual routines of which our breasts were a significant part. And some of us experienced the special bonding that comes from breast-feeding a child.

The way our families handled our development will probably influence the way we feel and respond to our grief after a mastectomy. Many women had mothers who were comfortable with their bodies and quite at ease when it came to talking with their daughters about their breasts. Other women relied on friends to help them get a bra because they found it difficult to communicate with their mothers about their development. Women have shared stories with me about mothers who bought them a bra and left it on their beds without a word.

The reaction of an older sister or brother, and of our fathers, also played a part in our acceptance of our breasts. An older sister who guided us, or a brother who protected us from sexual harassment, and a father who could let us know our body changes were attractive but off limits for him, all made it easier to grow into a woman's body. Hurtful, embarrassing teasing, or sexual abuse in the family can have a strong negative effect on a young woman's acceptance of her femaleness.

Growing up in an environment that was accepting and supportive of our development would have given us positive attitudes and coping skills to help us through the grief process after a mastectomy. If we were raised in an environment that taught us to not talk about our bodies and to feel shameful about having breasts, we are going to have a more difficult time processing the grief. Healing grief requires that we think, feel, and talk about what we are experiencing. Some women have to break through old beliefs that it is not acceptable to talk about their breasts before they can process their grief. Some of the grieving for women who have not had open, supportive families will include feelings about how painful it was to grow up in a non-nurturing environment. They may feel sad over never having been shown how to love and accept their bodies, in addition to the grief about losing part of their bodies.

Growing up with a mother and/or grandmother who had breast cancer will also influence how a woman feels and relates to her breasts and how she grieves after a mastectomy. The pride I had in my breasts came before I had started to understand that I too could die from the breast cancer that was so prevalent in my family. The way our families handled breast cancer provided us with role modelling on how we should deal with it. If our families never talked about what was going on when there was cancer in the family we may react the same way, or we may do just the opposite because we remember how hard it was to never be able to talk about it. Going through our own mastectomy may also trigger unfinished grief about our mother's or grandmother's mastectomy years ago.

I encourage you to take a journey through the past of your physical development to recall the positive and negative aspects of growing breasts. This walk down "memory lane" will be helpful as you process your grief by providing insights into how you feel and think about your breasts and how you arrived at these reactions.

Blocks to Grieving

There are a number of reasons people encounter difficulty in moving through the grieving process. Having a limited support system, holding certain beliefs or attitudes, and lacking adequate emotional development can all play a part in blocking grief.

LACK OF SUPPORT

Some people do not have adequate support for their feelings and do not want to have to go through their pain alone, so they avoid facing their emotions. If you do not have many people in your life or enough people who will sincerely take the time to listen to you share your story and what it means to you, then you may find yourself "shutting down" and withdrawing.

Conversely, sometimes our loved ones watch us too closely because

"Right after my surgery I only wanted close friends and family around. I didn't want to be left alone. They did a good job of keeping my spirits up."

they are worried we will not be able to cope with the pain and grief from our mastectomies. This can make them hover over us at a time when we need a little space. We may need to withdraw a bit to wrestle with our apathy and despair. Telling our partners we are okay, we just need some time to ourselves, can help them to not close in or try to "fix" our feelings.

If you find yourself without an adequate support system, I strongly recommend that you seek out a support group or an individual counselor. Your doctor, clinic, or the local Cancer Society office should be able to help you find appropriate professional support (see Chapter 13 for further discussion and resources on support groups and individual counseling). The women in a support group are going to understand what you are going through and you will feel less alone with your trauma. Many women go to a group because their pain is so extensive they do not want to wear out their family and friends. A lot of women have loving, close partners, but they realize that their partners are going through their own set of losses associated with the mastectomy and can only be so strong. Your home life needs to normalize before the stress will settle down, and taking some of your pain to a group can balance your relationships. Also, friends and partners, as much as they want to understand, cannot fully appreciate what you are going through because they have not gone through it themselves.

I want to caution you, though, when you are looking for a support group that the group is only as good as its members. If the group consists of women who are fairly well matched with your circumstances, you will probably find it to be very helpful. However, if it is not a good match it will be a waste of your time and only reinforce your feeling that you are truly alone in your pain. One woman I spoke with found her first group a disastrous experience. She was a young, Jewish, professional woman with small children who ended up in a small group of kind, older women who could not relate to her concerns as a young working mother and wife. To make the situation worse, one of the group members tried to convert her to Christianity by telling her that there were "Jews for Jesus." She quickly saw this group was not going to benefit her and she tried a new one. The next group was made up of young professional women who met at a time of day that least affected their family time. She has built a warm, comfortable, supportive network with her second group and has remained in it for several years.

HINDERING ATTITUDES

There are many attitudes that we bring to the grief process that can get in the way of resolving the loss of our breasts. Many people are told to count their blessings, which invalidates our feelings of loss. It is helpful to keep our grief separate from our gratitude. I believe being grateful is an important part of having a positive attitude about life. I am truly grateful I am not dying from cancer. It is very easy to look around and see how we are, in many ways, more fortunate than others. However, we need to round out the picture. Lots of other women are more fortunate than we are because they have not had to have a mastectomy. We have suffered a loss and we are entitled to a normal human emotional reaction. We feel angry, scared, confused, and incredibly sad.

I cannot stress enough that we need to accept our reactions as valid no matter what they are. It's our body, our loss, our change, our gain, depending on who we are and what attitudes and history we bring to the situation. Finding compassion for ourselves and room for our feelings is how we can move forward. I find that when I try to make myself feel grateful when I am faced with a disappointment, it makes me feel worse. I still have the feelings about my disappointment that are being ignored, plus I think I am a bad person for not feeling sincere gratitude. When I give myself room to be honest about my feelings I naturally seem to end up feeling grateful for what I do have. Grief and gratitude can be experienced at the same time; the important thing is to not prescribe one or the other for yourself. I felt incredible grief over the loss of my breasts and health, but I also felt appreciative for the good care I was receiving from my doctors and the love I was shown by my friends and family.

EMOTIONAL REPRESSION

If you were raised in a family that was uncomfortable and confused about what to do with their emotions, and have not had an opportunity in

"I had a certain amount of time on my own when my husband was at work and my children were at school and I needed it. I couldn't have coped with having people around all the time. I was so tired."

your adult life to learn about your own emotions, you will be faced with recovering from your mastectomy with limited skills to assist you with your grieving.

Some people believe they will be "emotionally well" when they no longer feel anything "negative." They have the mistaken belief that reaching the state of health means never feeling scared, angry, or sad. The truth about mental and emotional health is that it entails being comfortable with your emotions. To become emotionally well we have to learn to suspend judgment about our feelings as either good or bad, and accept them as simple human responses associated with living in this world in a body.

Once you learn to not fear your emotions, you become free to experience life. Because I went through many losses as a child and was raised in a family that could not teach me how to cope with my emotions, I started my adulthood with strong denial and emotional repression. Subconsciously I believed that releasing my emotions would result in a complete loss of control and disintegration that I would never recover from. Once I realized I had this fear-based belief, I was able to work through it, allowing myself to admit that I came from a dysfunctional family and to feel the emotions that went along with growing up with a lot of emotional pain. As a result of opening up my emotional side, I found that my body felt less tense and I was taking more risks in life. Doing this emotional processing allowed me one of my greatest joys in life, becoming a parent. Working through our grief as we come to accept our changed bodies puts us in a better position to be available to our daughters and granddaughters as they come into their womanly bodies.

Operating as an Integrated Whole Person

I understand humankind to be spiritual "beings" in physical bodies. We experience human, earthly life through our mind, emotions, and body. When we are using all of our entities we feel integrated and complete.

The order in which we respond to life is as follows: an event happens, we formulate a thought about the event, an emotional response produces an energy form in the body, and the body reacts by releasing the emotional energy. We have the capacity to feel four basic emotions: anger, sadness, joy, and fear (mad, sad, glad, and scared). We have lots of words to describe our feelings, but they can all be traced back to these four basic emotions. Irritation, annoyance, frustration, or rage are all forms of anger. Each emotion runs on a continuum from mild to intense. For example, a little bit of sadness may be called disappointment, whereas intense sadness might be expressed as devastation, and a little bit of joy might be called feeling pleased, whereas a lot of joy could be called elation.

An illustration of what it might look like when we are operating in a full, integrated way goes something like this: A close friend has just died (an event happens); you think, "Susan is gone from me forever. I'm going to miss her so much. What am I going to do without her?" (thoughts are formulated); deep, sad energy develops in the front, visceral side of your body (emotional energy is generated); and lastly, the sad energy rises through the body into the face, causing sobbing and tears (body release). Until a certain amount of time has passed and your routines that included your friend have been eliminated or altered, thoughts will continue to be formulated which generate emotional energy that your body will need to release.

Not seeing your friend and not routinely connecting with her through phone calls reduces the amount you will think about her. Gradually you will think about her less often and eventually you may go for a long time without feeling grief, but grief can be triggered again by memories and thoughts indefinitely.

RELEASING AND INTEGRATING EMOTIONS

Emotions might be seen as energy forms that flow along our internal electrical system, which is regulated by our breathing patterns. Emotions are a normal, physiological reaction to thoughts. According to the theory of bioenergetics analysis and other somatic forms of psychotherapy in which psychological issues are understood and treated through the body, each of the four basic emotions is expressed along its own physiological pathway. Following is a description of these emotions and their

"I was very controlled. I didn't let other people see I was sad. I left my crying sessions to my bedroom at night."

pathways of expression, and how you might safely go about releasing each feeling.

If your grieving process is blocked because of a lack of emotional development, it is important that you become knowledgeable about the basics of how emotions operate in the body. This information will allow you to reason with yourself about fear-based attitudes that may be holding you back from expressing your emotions. Integrating your emotions into your whole self so they work in conjunction with your mind and body will help you feel more connected to yourself and less restricted.

Mad

Anger typically moves up the back of the body along the spine, over the top of the head, and out through the eyes and mouth. It travels down the arms and goes through the hands. The tendency anger has to move along the back side of the body is reflected in such expressions as "a pain in the neck" or "pain in the butt." You have probably had the experience of becoming so angry with another person that you instinctively tightened your fist in response to anger moving through your arm and hand. If you closely monitor your body before you make an angry statement you are likely to sense a surge of energy coming through your eyes and a tightening of your jaw.

All emotions follow a pattern of buildup and natural discharge within the body. Saying that you are angry, blowing out air while making a groaning sound, and smacking your fist into the palm of your other hand are examples of anger releasing from the body.

As with all other feelings, anger is felt in various degrees. On one end of the continuum is mild anger, which might be described as irritation or annoyance. At the opposite end of the continuum is rage, a form of anger that might be characterized as blinding, or out of control.

Once you experience a thought in response to a situation that you feel angry about, you will have angry body energy that needs to be released. Altering your thoughts in order to perceive the situation differently may help you to not produce any additional anger, but you will still be left with the original anger-energy. If the amount of accumulated energy is relatively small, simply saying you are angry may be enough to let it go. If you have a lot of anger, you may feel a need for a more complete release.

Because anger is an emotion that women have been socialized to repress, many women find anger distasteful or frightening. Many women have an intuitive fear that allowing themselves to be angry will lead to loss of control. Women often keep a tight lid on their anger, which creates tension headaches and frequently painful knots in their upper back muscles. Women need to learn that they have a right to be heard and anger is a part of having a voice and asserting ourselves. Anger can energize us and give us the inner strength to tackle a problem instead of adopting a passive, victim mentality, particularly as we go through the process of recovery from a mastectomy. It was my anger and frustration with postmastectomy supplies that energized me to find new ways to alter my clothes after my mastectomy.

Releasing anger in a healthy, productive way involves expressing it in a safe, useful manner. It is not okay to splatter other people with your anger. Verbally abusing others, screaming, or breaking things are not necessary to release anger, nor are they appropriate or acceptable. Anger is not the same as violence. Remember that anger is simply an emotion. Violence is an unhealthy, destructive method of releasing anger.

If you are only somewhat angry, techniques such as saying how you are feeling, tightening and squeezing a fist while perhaps making a short grunting sound or sighing, and pounding your fist down once on a soft surface or into your other palm are all potentially effective ways of giving your angry energy an outlet. It is important that the physical release be performed while thinking of the reason you are angry in order to integrate the experience of knowing you are angry, understanding why you are angry, and then releasing the anger. This ensures the coordination of mind, body, and feeling.

For more intense feelings of anger try hitting a racquetball or tennis ball against a backboard. Standing up while angry makes some people feel more at risk of losing control, so another option is to lie on your bed with your eyes open (so the energy has an outlet for discharge) and allow your fully extended arms to alternate going up and down onto the mattress in a forceful fashion. Pounding your fists on the bed is only an op-

Your mastectomy can present you with the opportunity to change old ideas about grief and how you handle your emotions. It is essential to acknowledge your loss and to grieve.

Emotions can be
seen as energy forms
that flow along
certain pathways.
That explains why
anger gives us a
"pain in the neck."

tion when you are dealing with your anger before surgery or after you have healed from your mastectomy. Remember that you will not be able to do this with your affected arm after surgery due to the possibility of developing lymphedema. Another anger-releasing technique is to bring your legs up and down onto the mattress. In other words, have a safe, well-contained temper tantrum. When your arm and chest can tolerate it, you can also do this exercise while lying on your stomach, but be certain to place a pillow under your abdomen in order to give your lower back necessary support.

A variation on this approach involves using an old tennis racquet to hit a pile of pillows stacked on the floor or on a mattress while you kneel on the floor. Let your head and neck move to be at the same level as your arms; if you keep your head up while your arms come down it will create a bend in your neck where the energy can get stuck instead of being released along an open pathway. Kneel on a soft surface with your legs apart to give you a solid base of support. Keep your eyes open at all times when releasing anger or you will get a splitting headache. If you should forget to open your eyes and develop a headache as a result, simply open your eyes and hit a few more times. This should be sufficient to release the energy. Let words and sounds come out as you are hitting.

In addition to the anger-release methods described above, you might also find stomping your feet and making noise very satisfying. Small children frequently release their frustration by stomping. This is because a child's body is a smaller container than adults so the anger tends to flow up the body as with adults, but it also runs down their legs. If some of your anger is coming from thoughts about how your early childhood years repressed and stunted your emotional growth, releasing the anger as a child does may feel very fitting.

If you have children, you can teach them how to release anger in a healthy way. If you have exposed them to safe, nonviolent anger release, it will make it easier for everyone when you find you have to release your anger. With an open attitude about anger within your family, you can say to your children, "Mommy is really mad right now so I'm going into my room to get rid of it. If you hear some noise you don't need to be worried or scared." Then, as soon as you have moved beyond your anger, it is a good idea to reconnect with your children so they can see for themselves that everything is really okay.

Infants, toddlers, and small children are often terrified by the sounds of released rage, so I advise against releasing this intense form of anger where they can see or hear it. Screaming into a pillow will muffle the sound in a way that avoids distressing vulnerable children while still allowing you to discharge your feelings.

Sad

Sadness is a tender emotion that comes up the front of the body, through the throat, into the face, and up to the eyes. It is released through crying. It is normal to feel the need to cry a lot before and long after your mastectomy. The deep sorrow we feel as a result of the many losses we suffer from a mastectomy is usually released as sad energy through our tears.

The flow of sad energy is most frequently blocked by restricting the breathing so the diaphragm muscle (the essential muscle for breathing) constricts, thereby holding the sadness in the gut, or by constricting the throat muscles. You will recognize this latter technique for blocking sadness from the feeling you have experienced as a thick lump in the throat from holding back tears. Blocking the release of sadness can lead to very tight throat muscles and a chronic, painful ache in the throat.

An effective way to correct blocks to sadness is by taking a *slow,* deep breath through the nose and down into the abdomen, filling the chest to expand the diaphragm, then exhaling through the mouth. This will help throat constriction, but you may also need to open your mouth, tilt your head back and suck in air to open up your throat.

Peeling onions will help to open up tear ducts if they have become clogged from lack of use. Sad songs or television programs can also be used to trigger sadness. You might find yourself attracted to sad, intense books, movies, songs, poems, or newspaper articles, as a way of assisting you to connect to the sadness associated with your own loss.

Some people are more comfortable expressing sadness than anger, and find that they start to cry as soon as they try to release anger. This may well be helpless despair coming up as they try to assert their anger. It is very important if this happens to push ahead and continue with the

All emotion has to be released somehow, usually through an action or a noise, such as a sigh or a yell or stomping our feet or crying.

"I have a lot of anger. It's kind of strange. I found out when we went to Hawaii on vacation that I was jealous of the women who had two breasts. Even now, the summer time really affects me."

anger work even if you are crying and want to stop. If you move forward, your anger will strengthen you and pull you out of the despair. On the other hand, sadness is frequently hidden behind anger, so it is not unusual for a person to break into sobs after releasing anger. If you have sadness hidden behind your anger, then releasing that anger can help you connect with a deep sense of grief. After you have cleared out the angry energy and reached your sadness, allow yourself to curl up and sob like a baby while holding onto someone, or something soft and nurturing such as a soft blanket, pillow, or stuffed animal as you continue to release your pain. Bringing in a nurturing protector through the use of imagery described in the mental preparation for surgery in Chapter 3 can feel very supportive and healing at this time.

Glad

As with sadness, joy is experienced primarily on the front side of the body, running up and down the full length of the torso. Joy can be experienced as sexual energy in the genital region or it can be experienced higher in the body, as in that funny feeling you get in your stomach from swinging on a swing or going over and down a hill while riding in a fast-moving car. Dancing, singing, smiling, and jumping are all outlets for the feeling of joy ("jumping for joy"). Sometimes the energy of joy is also released through tears, as happens sometimes when a person feels overwhelmed with happiness.

Accepting kind gestures and gifts from those who support us through the painful process of our mastectomies is likely to create feelings of joy. Being told by the doctor that the cancer has not spread to the next level will result in a feeling of relief, which is a form of joy. Accomplishing each step of our healing process is likely to be experienced as joy that your body is going to want to release.

People tend to block or hold in joy if, like many children, they were constantly instructed to "settle down" when they were merely happy and moving to release the joy. Kids love to jump, sing, and dance out their joy. Unfortunately, an emotionally constricted family will not tolerate too much of any emotion, whether it be happiness, sadness, anger, or fear.

Another powerful reason for holding in joy is the fear that expressing joy will precipitate an unleashing of emotional pain as well. Sometimes emotional constriction stems from a belief that the individual does not deserve to feel good, but it can also result from an attempt to avoid pain if a person lacks adequate skills for dealing with their emotions.

Joy is held in by shallow breathing and by holding the breath. Regular deep breathing will allow joyful energy to move through the body. This process can be frightening and intimidating if a woman is not comfortable with her sexual feelings because the energy can drop down into the pelvic area.

One way of getting used to the sensation of joy is to go to the neighborhood playground and do some slow swinging. Swing slowly and work on paying attention to your body. Gradually build up your "tolerance" for joy by adding a little more height.

You can also open up your breathing by singing while driving in the car. You do not have to have a good voice in order to feel the joy from singing. The movement of breath will create the sense of joy. I have a terrible voice but singing the high notes along with Barbra Streisand really makes me feel alive and joyful as it opens up my breathing. Dancing will do the same. As your constriction begins to loosen, the feeling of joy will flow more and more naturally.

Scared

Fear is typically felt in the pit of the stomach. It can move along the front side of the body or it can travel along the spine.

When I ask my clients what happens in their bodies when they are scared, the most common response is that they feel "tight." Stiffening the body is an attempt to avoid feeling fear, which is released through trembling or shaking. Think about a child giving her first book report in front of the class. She might experience shaking, trembling legs and hands that are incapable of holding the paper still. This child is likely to feel shame in response to her fear if other students notice the trembling and call attention to it by laughing. As a result, she will learn to keep her breath shallow and to tighten her muscles to prevent the trembling. Fear is a very common emotion that will surface many times for women going through the experience of losing a breast. There will be moments of

> Anger and sadness often go hand-in-hand. If you uncover one, the other is usually not far behind. If you don't let anger, sadness, and fear out, joy will also be blocked.

"I really don't know if
I have ever really felt
happy or carefree
since my surgery.
Every time I change
or look in the mirror I
am reminded of what
I have lost."

very intense fear, such as when you are waiting on the surgical table wondering if you will come out of the surgery alive, to less intense times when you are worried about how you will look when you go back to work. I remember making the surgical table vibrate with my intense trembling as my body shook out my fear of dying.

Fear will actually pass more quickly if you allow the energy to be released through the trembling, as long as you are in a safe situation. If you are still in a frightening situation, you will continue to experience thoughts that tell you you are not safe, thereby generating new fear to be released. Once your thoughts are consistent with being safe, the terror or fear will pass much more quickly if you take some slow, deep breaths and permit your body an opportunity to shake out the fear by not tightening your muscles. While lying on the surgical table, I remember trying to take slow deep breaths to open my muscles and as I did my body released the fear through the trembling. I was able to observe how the trembling lessened as I told myself I was not going to die and I would be okay. I released the fear that had already been generated but prevented additional fear by putting comfortable, positive thoughts in my mind.

You can reach the point where you are capable of opening and closing your emotions almost at will. You need not deny your feelings nor allow them to run your life. When you have developed the skill of handling your emotions and have learned deep breathing, you will understand that, although your thoughts create emotional energy that your body needs to release, you can decide when and how you are going to do the releasing.

For clients who have trouble processing their feelings, I often recommend setting aside a certain amount of time each week to focus on the emotional self. This exercise allows for deepening feelings while also creating freedom from constant emotional intrusion into daily living. If you are at work and sad, angry, or scared thoughts keep intruding into your concentration and interfering with the task at hand, say to yourself, "I have set aside Tuesday from 7:00 to 8:00 P.M. for this. I'll think about it then." If you are faithful to yourself and follow through on your commitment to address the disturbing issues, you will be amazed at how your psyche will let up on you. If you fail to follow through, distracting thoughts and feelings will continue to creep into your mind as your psyche's way of forcing you to deal with your emotions. Your body wants to be healthy and it works jointly with your mind to keep you on the path to good health.

Making a date to address your feelings can also be very helpful with sleep problems. When you are trying to sleep but your mind is spinning, ask yourself if you can do anything about the problem at that time. If not, identify a time when you can give the problem some attention. Once you have done so your mind is more likely to quiet down so you can get some rest. Your support group, individual therapy time, and/or regular journaling can be ways of devoting time to your emotional needs.

The price we pay for holding in our pain is shutting out our joy. Opening up your breathing will give you access to your entire emotional self. Avoiding your emotions will limit your ability to express yourself, which prevents closeness in personal relationships and puts you at risk for having your feelings come out in ways you didn't intend. We may find ourselves taking our anger out on the doctor or our partner by being sarcastic, or hiding our fear, or sadness by being evasive. Learning to express my emotions allowed me to do past and present grieving, which led to an openness about these losses. Because my family repressed the grief of my mother's breast cancer and death, we were never able to talk about her or the experience we had gone through. We had to bury all our memories so we could keep from having to release our feelings. Once my sister and I each finally grieved over our mother's death we no longer had to avoid talking about our past, including our memories of our mother. I now think of my emotions like waves I have had to learn how to ride as they come and go. The more we learn to accept, experience, and release our emotions without judgment, the more we will feel whole and complete and find the inner strength and optimism to move on.

CHAPTER FIVE

PHANTOM BREAST PAIN
AND TREATMENT

Phantom Pain

It is very common to experience phantom breast pain after losing a breast. To help you understand this phenomenon I will start with a brief description of the discovery of phantom pain and what we have learned about it over the years. Phantom pain is best known as a condition following a limb amputation. The phenomenon of feeling the presence of a missing limb occurs in two different forms, phantom sensation and phantom pain.

PHANTOM SENSATION

In 1551, Ambroise Paré first described the phenomenon of phantom limb sensation.[8] After the American Civil War (1871), Silas Weir Mitchell wrote a classic essay about his work on phantom sensation. His observations resulted from his work with ninety amputees of the almost 15,000 individuals who were estimated to have lost limbs during the war. He found out that phantom sensation was remarkably constant, and was almost universally experienced following a major amputation.[9]

The term "phantom sensation" is usually reserved for those individuals who have an awareness of the missing portion of their limb, in which the only subjective sensation is mild tingling. It is described as rarely unpleasant; in fact, the majority of amputees describe their phantom sensation as painless. The experience of this phenomenon is commonly described in terms of numbness, pressure, position, temperature, or needles and pins. The type of sensation and intensity level vary by individual patient. Since phantom sensation is considered to be painless, treatment is deemed unnecessary.

PHANTOM PAIN

Phantom pain is different from phantom sensation in the type of feeling it produces. The three most commonly described symptoms of phantom pain are:

1. Cramping or squeezing sensations that occur with a change of posture.
2. Burning pain.
3. Sharp, shooting pain.

Phantom limb pain has four other major characteristics:

1. The pain lasts long after the healing of the injured tissue and may last for years.
2. Stimulating certain points in the surrounding healthy tissue can trigger pain in the absent limb.
3. Phantom limb pain is more likely to occur in patients who suffered pain in the limb for some time before the amputation occurred.
4. Phantom pain may be abolished by producing physiological changes in the stump.

The cause of phantom pain remains controversial. Explanations have tended to focus on irritation to nerve endings in the remaining tissue, the part of the brain that allows us to experience sensations, and psychological factors. Many people who work in the field of managing phantom pain operate on the assumption that all three factors play a part in phantom pain. Recently a team of researchers in Toronto, Ontario, discovered that the hiding place of phantom pain is the cells that represent the missing part in the brain.[10] These cells remember their old job and if they are stimulated in certain ways they will continue to indicate that the absent part is feeling pain.

There are a number of ways to produce a physiological change in the stump. Short-term treatment for phantom pain sometimes consists of using drugs that increase the blood flow to the stump to alleviate chronic stump pain, or a sympathectomy, which increases blood flow to the re-

Phantom pain occurs in between 17%–61% of mastectomy patients.

maining portion of the limb to decrease the burning sensation. Less invasive forms of treatment that cause physiological changes include gentle manipulation of the stump with massage or a vibrator, stump wrapping, baths, and application of hot packs or ultrasound. Certain "trigger points" on or near the stump may be injected with local anesthetics, but the relief is only temporary so treatment has to be repeated often. Transcutaneous electrical nerve stimulation (TENS) has also been somewhat successful in treating phantom pain. A TENS is a tiny machine that sends low-level stimulation to the nerves in order to interfere with the pain messages going to the brain. Wearing an artificial limb can also decrease phantom pain.

It was originally believed that nerve pathways were permanently formed during infancy, but recent research has shown this is not true. Nerve pathways do change as other aspects of the body change. Researchers are finding that when a limb is lost, the sensory cortex in the brain gets rewired, and sensations from the intact body parts seem to be coming from the missing limb.[11] This rewiring often results in pain. Researchers are working diligently to determine how the rewiring occurs. Currently Vilayanur Ramachandran, a neurologist at Scripps Research Institute and at the University of California at San Diego, has been able to offer relief to amputees by using a mirror box that allows patients to "see" their phantom.[12] Amputees slip their intact limb into the box and mirrors make it appear as if the missing limb has slipped into the box as well. This results in phantom pain relief, but only while the limb is in the box.

Phantom Breast Pain

Phantom pain was never considered to be a problem after the loss of a breast because such pain was only associated with the loss of a limb. The few studies that exist on phantom pain after a mastectomy have primarily come from the observations made by oncology nurses working with women receiving care for breast cancer. The studies I reviewed indicated that phantom breast pain occurs in between 17% and 61% of mastectomy patients.[13] The study showing 61% drew from the largest number of subjects and is probably the most reliable. Each of the studies indicated that phantom breast pain was far more common than expected, and explained that the lack of recognition of the problem was due to women's hesitancy to report the pain and health providers neglecting to ask about it specifically because they did not expect it to exist. Most women experiencing phantom breast pain are also being treated for breast cancer, so the focus of concern tends to center around the illness. In that context many women feel that their phantom pain is petty and some women fear being labeled crazy for experiencing pain in their missing breast.

Phantom breast pain is a combination of pain and itchiness in the missing breast that is caused by nerves and a mental image that tells our minds the breast is still present. Phantom breast pain is different from the incisional pain which can be present, off and on, for many years after surgery. Aching, stabbing pain, itching, burning, tingling, numbness, or throbbing in the incisional or surgical area comes directly from the remaining tissue, so these sensations match reality. Phantom pain, on the other hand, is physically uncomfortable, but also emotionally unnerving, because it occurs in a part of us that no longer exists. Just as with phantom limb pain, phantom breast pain is a combination of phantom pain and phantom sensation, which can be felt separately or simultaneously.

One of the times women may experience phantom sensation after a mastectomy is when they roll over to lie on their side. For many women it is an instinctive reaction to move their breast so it is not pinched between their arm and their side. Once the breast is gone, it is no longer necessary to move it when turning, but our brains do not know that. When we roll over we instinctively reach to pull the missing breast out of the way until we remember, "Oh, that's right, I don't have a breast any more," causing us to retract our hand. One woman who is very small-breasted said she could not relate to having to move her breast as she rolled over, but noticed that the change in position would set off the phantom sensation of having two breasts instead of one.

We are most likely to experience phantom sensation at times when

"In some ways I like the phantom sensation. It is better than having no feeling at all, like in the places where I am numb."

routine is part of our activity. We humans are creatures of habit and become very routine in our activities, especially when it comes to caring for our bodies. For example, each one of us can probably describe the step-by-step process of how we shower. Maybe you shampoo your hair first, then shave your legs, and lastly wash your body, and you probably wash your body parts in a particular order. Getting dressed can also be another very sequential, orderly behavior pattern. The more an activity becomes a routine pattern, the more the brain comes to anticipate it. The brain remembers the usual time to wash the breast, clothe it, or have it touched during sex. Our brains still have a mental picture of our breast as it used to be and so messages are sent by the nervous system that create sensations as if the breast were still there.

PHANTOM BREAST SENSATION AND GRIEF

I disagree with the old premise that phantom sensation in postmastectomy patients does not need to be treated because it is not painful. Phantom sensation needs to be treated because it has a psychological impact on our ability to complete the grief process. Phantom sensation is emotionally distressing because it gives us constant stimuli that reminds us of our loss. For instance, if you are grieving the loss of your dog, and both the dog and the daily routine of caring for him are gone, the reminders are gone.

With the loss of a body part, the mental mechanics are different. You have a picture in your mind of what your body looks like that incorporates your experiences with your movements, followed by nerve impulses and sensations. Because your old body image is still present in your brain, it sets off a wave of grief every time you do something as simple as rolling over. As you roll over and try to move the breast you experience phantom sensation (event) and your mind says, "Oh, that's right. I no longer have a breast" (thought), creating sadness or anger (emotional energy) that leads to tears, a lump in the throat, or verbal expression, neck pain and headache (body's attempt to release emotional energy). This cycle, in which routine behaviors set off waves of grief because of an unchanged internal body picture, can go on for a lifetime if the brain pattern is not changed.

So what can we do to avoid dealing with phantom breast pain for the rest of our lives? My own recovery process has resulted in discoveries about how to treat phantom pain after a mastectomy.

After a lot of crying and feeling devastated after being told by my surgeon that I could expect to live with phantom pain for the rest of my life, I found myself responding with anger and a determination to conquer the problem. I set out to change the distressing way my body and mind were working.

I brought some unique experiences to the problem of phantom pain and sensation. First of all, as a psychiatric nurse working as a therapist, I had explored body image issues with sexual abuse victims and women with eating disorders for many years. I found certain attitudes and mental imagery exercises very helpful in assisting women to learn to live more comfortably in their bodies. Second, I knew what it felt like to have my own breasts, what it felt like to have implants, and what it felt like to have no breasts, and could compare the differences between each state.

As I retraced my experiences with my body changes, I remember feeling a lot of grief over the loss of my real breasts and hatred for my fake breasts. They felt stiff and unnatural, but they did feel like part of me, and gradually I began to accept my new self and came to like my new breasts. For the first time, I did not have to dress to accommodate different-sized breasts. I also filled bras and swimsuits much better because I was now a standard size.

Thirteen years later, when I had my ruptured implants removed and began using external prostheses, I found myself going through the same intense grief as when I originally had my mastectomies. The implants were now part of my self-definition and body image. My sense of loss was accentuated by the phantom pain that began when my implants were removed.

When I began to look for a way to get rid of the phantom pain, I was struck by the fact that I'd never had phantom pain with my implants. When I spoke to other women who had implants at the same time as their mastectomy, they also reported experiencing no phantom breast pain. I searched my mind to see what ideas and images I was holding

"When I feel cold I still feel it in both breasts."

Phantom breast pain
can set up a cycle of
physical and
emotional feelings of
loss and distress.

that might offer some clues to the differences in sensation, and found a picture of my body intact with breasts. My conscious thoughts said I did not have breasts, but my brain continued to hold onto a picture of a body with breasts. As I continued to explore my mental image of myself, I realized that I thought of myself as occupying a certain amount of space and that space included breasts, whether real tissue or implants. With the implants gone, my body no longer matched the image in my mind. That is why my brain was still sending messages of sensation for breasts that were not there. Dr. Love suggests in *Dr. Susan Love's Breast Book* that the brain needs to be reprogrammed before the phantom pain will go away.

Once I had identified the inconsistency between my actual body and my old body image, I was well on my way to resolving the problem. I intuitively knew that these two parts had to match. I decided to focus on creating a new body image. I visualized the energy that circulated throughout my body. I visualized my body as it was without breasts, and saw my energy retracting back into my existing tissue. I did this throughout the day as often as I could remember, particularly when I had phantom pain or sensations.

I was delighted to discover that the visualization worked. After two weeks of working with my mental body image, the phantom pain and sensations were 95% gone. I was able to match my self-image with my actual body. I still had incisional pain and discomfort but I no longer had any phantom pain. The incisional pain was much easier to cope with because I could make sense of it, and it did not make me feel crazy or send me back to thoughts of loss and grief.

The old methods of treating phantom pain do not reprogram the brain to correct the inconsistency in body image. Probably the reason that wearing an artificial limb decreases phantom limb pain is that a limb is put back into the space where the real limb is missing. The mirror box used by Dr. Vilayanur Ramachandran likely works because a limb is being put back in place to match with the original body image that is still in the mind. But it only works as long as the limb is in the box.

In order to have a permanent remedy, we need to reprogram the brain to fit our body by giving it a correct body image. Trying to give the mind back a missing part is coming at it from the wrong angle. It does not last because you have to keep tricking the mind into thinking it still has the missing body part. Constantly wearing an artificial limb or putting your arm or leg in a box is not practical. Using the previous researchers' reasoning of replacing the missing body part would suggest we could only expect to get rid of phantom breast pain by replacing the missing breast with an implant or reconstruction. Reprogramming the mind to match your new body makes all that unnecessary.

IMAGE IMPRINTING

I call this treatment approach I have developed the *image imprinting technique*. It is not enough to have a general thought or general awareness that you have lost your breast. The change in your body needs to be imprinted into the part of your brain that holds your body image. We can reprogram our body image by changing the pictures we hold in our minds. My own experience offers an example of how treatment for phantom breast pain works. However, it will work differently for each of you.

If you are at a point in your healing where you are ready to begin working to get rid of phantom pain, try the following mental exercise. There is no one right time to begin. It is best to wait until after you have gotten through the most intense physical pain from your mastectomy and have had some time to get used to the idea that you no longer have your breast. For me, it came about eight months after my surgery, when I had emotionally accepted my loss and was tired of thinking about it every time the phantom pain set off a grief reaction. For you, the right time may come two months after surgery or two years after surgery. Be respectful of your personal time frame.

Creating a New Body Image
Sit quietly by yourself when you can devote fifteen to thirty minutes of uninterrupted time to reprogramming your brain's body image. Close your eyes or stare at a fixed point in the room and ask yourself what image of your body you have in your mind. Look carefully at the image that comes to you.

As you begin to work with your mental images you need to under-

The key to treating
phantom pain is the
picture of your body
that you hold in your
mind.

stand how mental imagery works. Each person has her own unique way of imaging. Your images will show you how you relate to the world. Most people have one or two dominant senses: vision, touch, smell, taste, or hearing. There is no right or wrong way to image the world.

To learn which sense or senses dominates your perception, pay attention to the words you use as well as the way your image appears. Since I am strongest visually (sight) and kinesthetically (touch), I will often say such things as: "Yes, I can see your point" or "Yes, I feel strongly about that." I am not likely to say, "Yes, I hear what you are saying."

Before trying to get an image of your body, you may want to experiment a little and image something simple and neutral, such as an apple or a flower. In your mental picture, do you actually see a picture of a flower or do you just sense its presence? Notice the color, texture, smell, and weight of it. If you have had limited or no experience with mental imaging, practice imaging simple objects at first to make your body imaging more effective. Try to take a light-hearted attitude and be playful when you are working with imaging. The more you work at developing your imagination, the easier it will be to create images.

Now let's go back to exploring the body image you hold in your brain. As you focus on the question, "What do I imagine my body looks like?", you will start to hear thoughts about your body and see and/or sense what your body looks like to you. Your thoughts may match what you mentally see or they may contradict each other. You may have the thought that you have a chest with a missing breast, but you may visualize a chest with two breasts.

Don't try to change anything about your body image or thoughts yet. At this point you should just try to get a good sense of the concepts and images you have about your body. I found that my mind consciously was aware that I no longer had breasts, but my mental picture was of a body with breasts, and I discovered that I believed I occupy my physical space with energy. These three insights showed me what I had to work with and where the inconsistencies between my mental and actual self-image existed.

Once you have defined how your brain is piecing your self-perceptions together, you can begin to decide what needs to be changed to make your thoughts, body image, and actual body shape match.

Start with an accurate statement about the state of your chest, such as, "I now have a chest with only one breast." Next, create an image in your mind that reflects the truth about your body. Last, try to feel yourself inside your body image. In other words, try to feel real and alive in your body as you visualize it in your mind. Maybe your image consists of energy or maybe you experience yourself as hot and cold; your living self feels warm but where your body ends, becomes cold.

While doing the image imprinting make sure your thoughts are non-judgmental statements that merely describe your existing tissue. Try to make your self-description clinical, as if a doctor were describing it. It won't be helpful to use such thoughts as, "I have an ugly, deformed chest." We all battle with low self-esteem and negative thoughts as we get used to our changed bodies. Don't ignore these thoughts and feelings: acknowledge them, cry, and get mad until you can shift to a more positive attitude. Trying to pretend you don't have negative thoughts will only make things worse, because they tend to retreat to our subconscious and are then expressed indirectly. Repressing negative thoughts will result in unresolved grief and a lack of acceptance of your loss. This psychological block is likely to show up in restrictive behavior, such as being unwilling to venture out in public, wearing only loose-fitting clothes, sexually shutting down, and avoiding looking in the mirror.

It is not necessary to have all your negative thoughts resolved before working on an accurate body image. The more your negative thoughts are reframed into positive thoughts, the more you will feel an overall acceptance of your loss. However, negative thoughts about your body will probably come and go throughout the rest of your life because they are part of your grief process and grief is a lifelong process. To work on image imprinting, you need to be able to set your negative thoughts aside temporarily and use neutral, factual statements about your body. A neutral statement is not the same as a positive statement. A neutral statement is: The breast tissue is gone. A positive statement is: I like my body, it serves me well.

Image imprinting enables you to reprogram your brain to stop phantom pain.

Think of pulling
phantom sensations
back into your actual
tissues.

Once you have re-imaged your body, the next step is to incorporate the new, updated mental picture into your life. Whenever you start to experience phantom sensation or pain, go into your mind to reinforce your new body image. When you get the sensation that the breast is still there, just say to yourself that the breast is no longer there and image your body as it now exists. Then gently imagine pulling the phantom sensation back into your remaining body where it belongs. See the itch or stabbing sensation coming from the tissue as it exists, not from the area that used to be a breast.

It should not take long to develop an accurate body image and to pull the sensation back to where it should be. If it is taking a long time to do the imaging, you are probably trying too hard. Initially, it may take a couple of fifteen- to thirty- minute sessions before you have a clear picture of how your new body looks and how you experience sensation. It will also take a couple more sessions to get the new picture set in your mind. If you see an accurate picture most of the time, but sometimes the old picture appears, go back to the first part of the process, in which you created the new image. Do not take this as an indication that you are image imprinting incorrectly.

Once you have a new image to work with, reinforcing it mentally should only take between fifteen seconds and a few minutes. If you try to remind your brain of the change every time you feel phantom pain or sensation, imaging will become easier, and you will be free of phantom breast pain faster. You may get to the point where it takes only a couple of seconds to flash the new image into your mind after you experience a false sensation.

Our experience of phantom breast pain and how quickly we move beyond it is influenced by a lot of different factors. If you try to get over phantom pain when you are still in the early stages of grief and recovery, you may find it takes a long time. If you have reached a place where you consistently feel accepting of your body, the mental imagery work will probably go faster. On the other hand, some women discover that using mental imagery very early in the recovery process is helpful for gaining overall acceptance. They combine the healing of acceptance with building a new picture in the brain.

The degree of body awareness and body image varies tremendously from woman to woman. Some women are very in tune with their bodies. They know what their body is feeling, they look at it often and freely, and over the years develop a very accurate picture in their mind of how their bodies look. But many women have very little body awareness. They operate primarily from their heads in an intellectual way and pay very little attention to what is going on with their body. These women usually require a very loud signal from the body that something is wrong before they will notice pain or abnormalities. Women who are not very in touch with their bodies generally have a more difficult time revising their mental image. They will be able to create a new picture of the body because that is an intellectual process, but pulling the sensations back to the actual tissue will be much harder, because that requires the awareness of body sensations.

The amount that we use our body is not actually a good indicator of our amount of body awareness. One athlete can have a lot of body awareness and be constantly "reading" her body, while another athlete may almost totally ignore what her body is saying and focus only on performance. Most women are somewhere in between the two extremes.

Body awareness differences can play a part in how much phantom breast pain you might have and how much work is needed to get rid of it. It will help to adopt an attitude of curiosity about how you are put together and how you can reshape your self-image to fit the body in which you are living.

Ginger, a friend of mine, used the image imprinting technique and got fairly good results but was left with some phantom breast pain. As I reviewed how Ginger was doing the image imprinting I could see how much her personality was influencing the results. We have a standing joke between us about how Ginger likes to avoid emotionally uncomfortable things by "putting her head in the sand." Ginger is a very successful, intellectual, perfectionistic businesswoman who has a track record of avoiding going to the dentist because it was painful and scary when she was a kid. When she had her mastectomy I kept asking her if she had looked at her chest and the answer was, "not yet." She had planned to do that at her next doctor visit but somehow it had not happened then either.

"The surgery made me more aware of my body. I am more aware that I have to be in charge. I can't leave it up to anyone else or expect a doctor to take care of me."

She eventually worked up the courage to look at herself so she could check it off her list of things she needed to do to recover.

Ginger could do her scheduled time to practice her body imaging but she did not reinforce it at the spontaneous times when she felt phantom pain. She was so used to ignoring her body that focusing on her phantom pain enough to treat it was too difficult for her. Since most of her phantom pain was gone, the remaining amount was not a serious concern. Ginger had her mastectomy over two years ago and when I recently asked her about phantom pain she said she only experiences it for a few seconds on a very infrequent basis.

Working with a client who was referred to me for depression six weeks after her mastectomy showed me how the timing of treating phantom pain could vary greatly. When I asked Carisa if she was bothered by phantom pain she said she had experienced it for only a couple of days and it was gone. When I asked her how she had changed her body image she explained that she had developed a clear picture in her mind of her altered body. As a way to prepare herself for the loss, Carisa had asked the surgeon for pictures of what she would look like after her mastectomy and made herself look at them over and over again. She tried to imagine herself looking like them. She'd had no idea that this was going to prevent phantom pain; she was doing it as part of her psychological acceptance. Carisa was a very practical, matter-of-fact woman who identified problems and faced them head on.

CHAPTER SIX

TREATING SURGICAL COMPLICATIONS AND FIBROMYALGIA

Treatment for Surgical Complications

As I mentioned in Chapter 3, numbness, lymphedema, and a tight basilic vein are three surgical complications commonly seen after a mastectomy. The following are simple and effective treatments for each problem.

NUMBNESS

Numbness can occur in a very small localized area or it can extend into the tissue surrounding the surgical site. The major sensory nerve in the armpit and nerves in the chest area can be cut or injured during surgery. This usually happens when the lymph nodes are removed but it can also happen without the removal of lymph nodes. The sensation that results when these nerves are affected is usually described as numbness, but neither I nor any of the women I know who have undergone mastectomies describe it that way. Numbness implies that all sensation is gone, but what is most often experienced is a mixture of numbness and pain. It is best described as an uncomfortable, distracting, and annoying feeling. Many of us call it the "icky" sensation. I had quite a bit of this unpleasant sensation after my double mastectomy even though I had no lymph nodes removed. Some of the feeling went away over time, but some remained. After I had my implants removed, I experienced even more of this sensation. The numbness and pain seems to come and go with changes in weather, and is affected by how much the area is rubbed by

75

"The numbness is
really frustrating. I
can tell I have an itch,
but scratching
doesn't help."

clothing. I also have noticed that fatigue makes it worse. I experience it across my chest, into my armpits, down the inner parts of my arms as far as my elbows, and into my upper back.

It has been my experience that medical professionals do not appreciate the extent to which numbness affects us after a mastectomy. This is probably because they have not experienced the sensation themselves, they think there is nothing they can do about it, and they see no reason to mention it before surgery since the mastectomy has to happen regardless of the side effects.

For one of my clients, Carisa, this sensation was the worst part of the mastectomy and she wondered if she had made the right decision to have the mastectomy instead of a lumpectomy, as she thought the lumpectomy might have resulted in less numbness. It was terribly bothersome while she did her job as a nurse. She tried many types of bras with different pressure points and in varying fabrics. But it wasn't until she began wearing a stockinette on her upper arm, which prevented her bra and sleeve from rubbing against her arm, that she really felt comfortable. I was able to reassure her that some of the numbness would quiet down in time. I spoke with her about fifteen months after her mastectomy and she was glad to report that the numbness had lessened and she was no longer so troubled by the annoying sensation.

Another thing I have found particularly helpful in treating the numbness is rubbing the affected area. I initially had a strong aversion to having the skin on the numb area touched because touch made me acutely aware of the sensation. However, I kept hearing an inner voice suggest that I should stimulate the area by rubbing it.

I used a bath sponge that was soft on one side and rough on the other. While in the shower, I started out with the soft side of the sponge and then switched to the rough side. On the sponge I used body shampoo which cleansed the area and prevented any harmful friction. I discovered that when I stretched to make the affected area taut before rubbing it, the rubbing was a very tolerable sensation and it felt healing. I started doing this a few times a week and now I do it whenever the numbness or severe itching becomes a problem.

Rubbing to counteract numbness works for two reasons. The first is that the stimulation increases circulation to the tissue and the second is that rubbing stimulates the nerves. Rubbing works on the same principle as the nerve stimulator machines (TENS or transcutaneous electrical nerve stimulation) that I mentioned in Chapter 5, which inhibits pain messages by sending electrical impulses along the nerves, thereby competing with the pain messages. We also know that stimulation to damaged nerves can help them regenerate.

Be careful not to begin stimulating the numb area until it is completely healed. If you are listening to your body, common sense will guide you. Initially you will have acute pain from the tissue damage, and as that heals you will notice the numbness. When rubbing you also need to be careful not to set off lymphedema (see next section). It is not necessary or desirable to rub deeply into the muscles of the numb area because the nerves you are trying to stimulate are close to the surface. Instead you should try a brisk light rubbing.

In addition, I find that I sometimes develop an itch in my surgical area that is not eased with the type of scratching I use elsewhere on my body. The itch seems to have something to do with nerve damage, as it is generally in the area of my incision where my bra rests. I find that rubbing also helps with this itch. Occasionally the skin in this area becomes inflamed and warm to the touch, as well as itchy. I have discovered that if I wrap my index finger with a wash cloth and dampen it with cold water, then vigorously rub the area, the inflammation and itch go away. It takes about five to ten minutes after rubbing it before the sensation is no longer noticeable.

LYMPHEDEMA

Lymphedema is another common complication after a mastectomy. As I researched lymphedema and how to treat it, I was referred to Dr. Sandra Rosenberg, medical director of the Physical Medicine and Rehabilitation Department at United Hospital in St. Paul, Minnesota. Her interest in the area came from her personal and professional background. Dr. Rosenberg had breast cancer and underwent a bilateral mastectomy with

"Before my surgery I could feel every part of my body. Now that has changed and there is nothing I can do about it."

Rubbing can help
ease numbness by
stimulating the
tissues. Be careful
about rubbing the
surgical side in order
to avoid lyphedema.

lymph node dissection followed by six months of chemotherapy. Six months after the mastectomy, her right arm began to swell until it was a third bigger than her left arm. Frustrated with the existing treatments, she created her own.

Dr. Rosenberg was able to draw from her history as a ballet dancer and her medical specialty of physical medicine and rehabilitation to go beyond the European massage method, which was the usual treatment for lymphedema and is often referred to as Complex Decongestive Physical Therapy (CDPT). Dr. Rosenberg knew how important it was for her to be with her husband and children following her surgery, and with a clinic to run as well, found the European treatment required too much time. She has developed an approach that allows the patient to be as independent as possible. It allows women more control of their swelling with less need for medical personnel, which I discuss later in this chapter.

Lymphedema is the swelling of a body part caused by an abnormal accumulation of lymph fluid due to a malfunction of the lymphatic system. The lymphatic system is much like the blood circulatory system in that it has many vessels throughout the body. An extensive webbing of tiny vessels, called superficial lymphatics, lies very close to the surface of the skin. They maintain a healthy environment for the cells, clearing such things as toxins, bacteria, viruses, and particles that enter the body through absorption and breakdown of the skin. The lymph fluid travels through the lymph vessels to the lymph nodes, where it is detoxified and later added to the blood circulation. The lymph fluid is moved through the vessels by the spontaneous contraction of the muscles surrounding the vessels. There are bundles of lymph nodes in at least a dozen different locations throughout the body. The nodes that surround the breasts, line the collarbone, and reside in the armpit are those most affected by breast cancer.

Swelling occurs when there is more fluid present than the lymph system can handle. When lymph nodes are removed from the armpit to determine whether the cancer has spread to the lymph system or been destroyed by radiation treatment, this compromises the lymph system's ability to handle the buildup of lymph fluid. According to Saskia R. J.

Thiadens, a registered nurse and founder of the National Lymphedema Network in San Francisco, if lymphedema is untreated it can cause skin breakdown, infections, and loss of limb.[14] During a recent lecture, Dr. Susan Love explained that if lymphedema is not treated in the early stage and soon after its onset, the built-up fluid will cause the skin to lose elasticity, which is an essential part of facilitating the movement of the fluid back to the heart. With her great sense of humor, she related the arm with lymphedema to a pair of pantyhose at the end of the day, in that they both lose their shape and the tautness that is supposed to hold everything in. But unlike pantyhose, you cannot simply wash your arm to restore the shape because the elasticity is permanently lost.

As Dr. Rosenberg lectured across the country to her colleagues she repeatedly heard doctors say that lymphedema does not hurt. Her response has been to laugh and say, "You have obviously never experienced lymphedema." The type of pain that goes with lymphedema is usually an ache. Women know how much breasts can hurt when they swell from PMS or pregnancy. Swelling causes discomfort by pushing on the nerves in the swollen area.

Dr. Rosenberg believes that anyone who has had lymph nodes removed from the armpit will have lymphedema at some point, but not all women will be bothered by it or even notice it because a little more than half a cup of liquid must accumulate before lymphedema will be recognizable. The number of nodes you were born with, the number of nodes that are removed with the tissue sample, and how you heal, as well as whether or not radiation treatment was used, will significantly influence how great a problem lymphedema will be. Lymphedema can occur any time after a lymph node dissection. It can be a problem immediately following your surgery, not show up for many years after, or surface off and on in varying degrees over the rest of your life. A number of things can be done to prevent or minimize the development of lymphedema.

The key to preventing lymphedema, or keeping it under control, is practicing good skin care. You want to protect your affected extremity from injuries such as infection, muscle strain, sunburn, overheating, and constriction.

Lymphedema often follows a lymph node dissection which is part of surgery for breast cancer. It is the swelling of a body part caused when there is more fluid present than the lymph nodes can handle. It can be very serious if left untreated.

Always carry your purse on your non-affected side. It should never be heavier than five pounds.

The following instructions provide a detailed description of preventive care:

1. *Daily skin check*

This should become part of your daily hygiene routine. If you suspect an infection, you should contact your doctor immediately.

- Examine your arm for cuts, burns, or insect bites because these can be a potential source of infection. Make sure you check all skin folds and between your fingers.
- Treat any open area by cleansing it with antibacterial soap and water, applying an antibiotic ointment, and covering it with a BandAid.
- Watch for redness, warmth, tenderness, and red streaks because these could be signs of infection.
- Inspect hands carefully for hangnails, cracked or torn cuticles and ingrown nails.

2. *Avoid infection.*

- Keep your arm meticulously clean, especially between fingers. Keep all of the creases on your arm and between fingers dry because bacteria and fungal infections grow in moist areas.
- Keep your cuticles moist and push them back without cutting them. If you go to a manicurist, make sure she knows you have lymphedema and the instruments are sterilized.
- Wear gloves when doing the dishes or loading the dishwasher (bacteria begins to grow within ten seconds), handling sharp objects, and cleaning the house and especially while cleaning the bathroom, diapering, and gardening. Dr. Rosenberg was told that postmastectomy patients should never garden for fear of causing lymphedema. She told me that she would sooner cut off her arm than go without her roses and so she continues to garden but uses precautions such as protective gloves and long sleeves, and she washes very well when she is finished.
- Never allow injections (except under emergency circumstances) or blood tests to be done on your affected side. Be assertive!
- Use an electric razor under your arms. This is especially necessary because this area is frequently numb, and hence prone to cuts.

- Use a thimble or finger guard when hand sewing.
- Use a low pH lotion such as Eucerin or Curel regularly to keep the skin from drying out. Avoid lotions with perfumes because they can cause irritation.

3. *Avoid muscle strain.*

- Use your arm as normally as possible.
- Avoid heavy lifting, greater than 12 to 15 pounds.
- Exercise moderately. Start out slowly with a new exercise program. Monitor your arm carefully and watch for swelling. It is normal to experience slight soreness or discomfort when beginning an exercise program, but this should not be long-lasting. It is best to avoid contact sports or sports that put you at risk of sustaining skin or muscle damage that can lead to swelling. For instance, Dr. Rosenberg no longer plays competitive volleyball, and when she is biking and her arm starts to ache from too much exertion, she tries to reposition her arm so it is not hanging down and ends the activity as soon as possible. Then as soon as she gets home she puts on her compression bandage and elevates her arm. She emphasizes that the key to preventing serious symptoms is to listen to your body. When her arm starts to ache she knows it means to back off from the activity she is doing for a while.

4. *Avoid sunburn and burns.*

- Use a high SPF sunscreen (15 or higher) whenever you're in the sun. Make sure to cover your face, chest, and back as well as your arms and legs (Eucerin has a lotion with SPF 25 that works well under makeup.)
- Use extra-long oven mitts to protect hands and forearms from cooking burns.
- Be extra careful with curling irons.

5. *Avoid overheating.*

- Exercise moderately, take rests, and cool down afterward.
- Hot tubs, saunas, and steam baths are likely to increase swelling, so the temperature should not exceed 95° to 96° F.
- Showers and baths should not be so hot that it causes a reddening of the skin.

The key to preventing and controlling lyphedema is practicing good skin care.

"Sometimes when I play tennis in the sun my arm gets huge welts on it. I worry a lot about it getting big so I have a massage once a week."

6. *Avoid constriction.*

- Carry your purse on the shoulder of your nonaffected side or across your body. Your purse should not weigh more than five pounds. A fanny pack is safest.
- Underclothing should not bind at the chest, underarms, groin, or waist. A bra should not be so tight that it causes an indentation.
- Clothes should also be loose at the wrists, ankles, and waist. (A tight girdle is not a good idea.)
- Do not allow your blood pressure to be taken on your affected side.

7. *Take special precautions when flying.*

- Wear compression bandages or garments.
- Walk around frequently.

Along with patient education in lymphedema and good skin care, Dr. Rosenberg starts patients out with a basic exercise program that mimics the patterns of lymphatic massage. The exercises look a lot like ballet dancing. These exercises are then done at home for six to eight weeks. At the end of this time, patients return for an evaluation and if further treatment is needed, lymphatic massage, medical compression bandages, skin care, and exercises are done in the clinic for two weeks.

Dr. Rosenberg does not typically recommend the use of lymphatic fluid pumps to drain the excess fluid. Some research has suggested that the pump can force too much fluid at one time into the lymphatic system. The overload can damage the vessels and cause poorer lymph drainage of the surrounding area, which can lead to infection and further swelling. A more gentle and effective method is to do exercises that stretch and stimulate the torso to create better drainage throughout the body so it can help compensate for loss of nodes in the affected area. The final stage of Dr. Rosenberg's program is to fit the patient with a compression garment and give further instructions on home exercises. Dr. Rosenberg will be publishing the details to treating lymphedema in the near future.[15]

BASILIC VEIN DISCOMFORT

Some women are bothered and frightened by tightness in the vein that runs down the arm on the surgical side. After surgery it often hurts, feels hot and too tight.

This vein is called the basilic vein. It is the largest of the superficial veins in your arm. The basilic vein receives blood from small veins of the hand, the forearm, and the arm. It starts at the base of the underside of your hand and runs up the inside of your arm, through the armpit, and into the shoulder.

The basilic vein is often uncomfortable after surgery because it is shortened during the mastectomy and the removal of lymph nodes from your armpit. Shortening makes the vein tight and can cause inflammation. It also makes the vein come closer to the surface of your skin and therefore become more noticeable.

What you need to know is that even though it may feel like it, your basilic vein is not going to snap. Yes, the vein is tighter than it was before, but it will not snap because veins are extremely elastic. Eventually your basilic vein will stretch out so it feels normal again.

There are a few simple things you can do to make yourself more comfortable and to stretch out the vein. Applying ice to the armpit and along the path of the vein can relieve inflammation. Make sure you do not place ice directly on your skin. Since you have lost some sensation in the area where the lymph nodes were removed, you will be more prone to frost burn, so place a thin cloth between your skin and the ice. The same principle applies to stretching the basilic vein as any other tight area; use the area that is less tight to give stretch to the tightest part. The tightest point in the basilic vein is in the armpit area, because that is where it will have been pulled up during surgery, and the armpit is where inflammation will be the worst.

You can stretch the basilic vein by "milking it," from the hand up to the armpit. Place the tips of the fingers on your opposite hand over where the vein starts close to your wrist. Then, applying light pressure, slide your fingertips up your arm along the vein until you reach your armpit. It should feel as if you are stripping or milking the vein. You are stretching it out by bringing the extra tissue from the looser, lower part of your arm up to the tight area in your armpit. Applying ice right after you stretch the vein will reduce the inflammation and hence the pain. You can do this several times a day, but you need to listen to your body for signals that you are overdoing it. Your arm should not hurt after stretching the vein. If it does, you have applied too much pressure.

"At first the tightness in my vein reminded me of when you try and thread a drawstring through a waistband; only there wasn't enough string."

Fibromyalgia is a
chronic pain and
fatigue condition that
is frequently seen in
women who have
experienced adverse
reactions to breast
implants.

Analgesics can be helpful until the basilic vein stretches out and settles down. Immediately following surgery you should not take analgesics such as aspirin (Bufferin) or Ibuprofen (Advil) because they have an anticoagulant agent in them which can interfere with blood clotting. You should use whatever painkiller your doctor has prescribed or use acetaminophen (Tylenol) as an over-the-counter medication until you have your first return visit to your doctor and you are given the go-ahead to use other types of analgesics. However, by the time you notice and are bothered by your basilic vein, it will probably be well past the point where it is not safe to take an analgesic with an anticoagulant. The most helpful type of analgesic for pain in the basilic vein is either aspirin or Ibuprofen because they kill pain and reduce inflammation.

Coping with Fatigue and Chronic Pain after Ruptured Silicone Implants

If you have been involved in breast implant litigation you know that there are a number of conditions that are suspected to be associated with silicone implants. I am not going to enter into the debate about the links between certain health problems and silicone implants (see Chapter 12 for further information on breast implants). Many women report incredible fatigue and chronic pain along with many other symptoms and conditions, after getting breast implants regardless of what has been proven. Many of you who have chronic pain and fatigue that you attribute to breast implants probably fall into either the "atypical connective tissue disease" or "atypical rheumatic syndrome" category. These categories may make us feel validated for our experience, but they do little for us when we seek treatment. What many of us are figuring out is that we have a condition called fibromyalgia as well as other symptoms.

WHAT IS FIBROMYALGIA?

Fibromyalgia syndrome is a common form of generalized muscular pain and fatigue that has been associated with an adverse reaction to breast implants, among other factors. "Fibromyalgia" means pain in the muscles and the fibrous connective tissues, which consist of the ligaments and tendons. Fibromyalgia is a form of "soft-tissue" or muscular rheumatism rather than arthritis of a joint. Rheumatism refers to pain and stiffness associated with arthritis and related disorders of the joints, muscles, and bones. Fibromyalgia primarily affects muscles and their attachment to bones. It feels like a joint disease but is not a true form of arthritis and does not cause deformities of the joints. There is some inflammation with this condition but not nearly as much as with arthritis. Fibromyalgia is a chronic illness and is very similar to chronic fatigue syndrome but with CFS fatigue is more pronounced than pain.

There are a number of excellent books available on fibromyalgia (see resources listed at the back of the book). You can also contact the Arthritis Foundation for further information at 1-800-283-7800.

SIGNS AND SYMPTOMS OF FIBROMYALGIA

Pain is the most prominent symptom of fibromyalgia. The pain is felt all over but usually starts in one part of the body and spreads to the rest of the body over time. The pain is described as burning, radiating, gnawing, sore, stiff, and aching. It varies according to time of day, activity level, weather, sleep patterns, and stress, and there is some degree of pain always present. Fibromyalgia can feel a lot like having the aches and chills of a persistent flu. For some people the pain is quite severe.

About 90% of people suffering from fibromyalgia describe moderate to severe fatigue with lack of energy, decreased exercise endurance, or the kind of exhaustion felt with the flu or with lack of sleep. Most people with fibromyalgia have an abnormal sleep pattern, and especially interruptions to their deep sleep. (See Chapter 13 for more information on sleep disorders.)

Many people with fibromyalgia feel "blue" or "down," although only 25% are truly depressed. (See Chapter 13 for more information on depression.) Generally, depression and anxiety seem to follow the onset of fibromyalgia symptoms and may be the result of fibromyalgia rather than its cause. People with fibromyalgia frequently report having difficulty concentrating or performing simple mental tasks. They may also feel numbness and tingling in their hands, arms, feet, legs, or sometimes in their face. Muscular headaches and migraine headaches are also common with fibromyalgia, as well as blurred vision, abdominal

Figure 6-1 Location of tender points

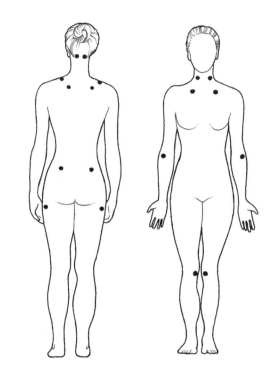

pain, bloating, and alternating constipation and diarrhea. This may resemble "irritable bowel syndrome" or "spastic colon." The skin and circulation of those suffering from fibromyalgia are often sensitive to temperature and moisture changes, resulting in temporary changes in skin color.

DIAGNOSING FIBROMYALGIA

Fibromyalgia is diagnosed by the presence of widespread pain, in combination with tenderness at specific locations as shown in Figure 6-1. Although a general physical examination is usually normal, and individuals may look well, a careful examination of their muscles demonstrates very tender areas at specific locations. The presence and pattern of these characteristic "tender points" is what separates fibromyalgia from other conditions.

A rheumatologist is a physician specifically trained in treating inflammation and pain in muscles and joints, but there are other types of physicians who are also knowledgeable in diagnosing this condition. You will know if you have been properly examined for fibromyalgia if the doctor applies pressure on the spots indicated in Figure 6-1.

TREATING FIBROMYALGIA

Like many chronic illnesses, fibromyalgia treatment must be individualized to fit the patient. Some people have mild symptoms and need very little treatment once they understand what fibromyalgia is and what worsens their condition. Most people with fibromyalgia benefit from a comprehensive program.

Medications Medications that diminish pain and improve sleep can be crucial to getting relief from fibromyalgia. I know many people with fibromyalgia and we are mystified when we hear that studies have shown that inflammation does not play a big role in fibromyalgia, because we all have gotten such relief from taking an analgesic/anti-inflammatory medication. There are some prescription analgesic/anti-inflammatory medications that can be taken once a day, such as Oruvail and Relafen, which are ideal because one of the keys to coping with chronic pain is learning to ignore your pain. Needing to remind yourself to take medication every four hours or waiting until your pain is bad enough to remind you, keeps the pain in focus and can result in despair and a depressed mood.

I don't recommend that you try to treat your own pain with over-the-counter medication because excessive use of these drugs can cause medical complications. You should have a physician who knows how to treat fibromyalgia working with you to find the most effective and safest treatment for your symptoms. Narcotic pain relievers, tranquilizers, and cortisone derivatives have been shown to be ineffective and should be avoided because of their potential side effects.

The most important fibromyalgia symptom to treat is the accompanying sleep disorder. Medications that promote deeper sleep and relax muscles help many people with fibromyalgia. Flexeril, a muscle relaxant, is sometimes prescribed. The drugs most used for fibromyalgia-based

Those who suffer from fibromyalgia are often misdiagnosed and the disorder itself is still under controversy in the medical community as to whether it exists.

"Stretching has been
my salvation from
fibromyalgia."

sleep problems are Elavil, Sinequan, Prozac, Trazodone, and Paxil, all of which are antidepressants. Although these medications are also used to treat depression, they are generally used for people suffering from fibromyalgia in low doses at bedtime to treat the sleep deprivation. It is believed that the lack of deep sleep that occurs with fibromyalgia does not allow adequate muscle relaxation, resulting in muscle pain and the other symptoms listed above.

Exercise and Physical Therapy Two main treatments for fibromyalgia are increasing cardiovascular (aerobic) fitness and stretching affected tight, sore muscles. It is a matter of faith for fibromyalgia patients to believe that exercise is what is needed because for most of us it seems like an impossible task to exercise when our muscles hurt so much, and we are so tired. Low or non-impact aerobic exercises, such as brisk walking, biking, swimming, or water aerobics, are generally the best way to start such a program. It is important to exercise on a regular basis, such as every other day, to gradually reach a better level of fitness. Gently stretch your muscles and move your joints through a range of motion daily and particularly before and after aerobic exercise.

Stretching has been my salvation. Like many people with fibromyalgia, I have had severe leg cramps that start in the hips and run all the way down to my feet, ending in charley horses. I learned that stretching my hips is my best way to relieve the cramps in my feet. After several years of slowly stretching out my tight muscles I seldom have severe cramps any longer. I have learned to recognize and avoid activities that can set off the muscle spasms. I have also learned to tell if my body is starting to get tight and I work on loosening that area before it gets out of hand. Physical therapy can be very helpful to get you started on a safe stretching program. Just learning correct posture from a physical therapist can be helpful because poor posture pulls on your muscles, which can cause your muscles to spasm.

Heat, ice, massage, whirlpool, ultrasound, and electrical stimulation may help with pain control. Many people with fibromyalgia get relief from a whirlpool. I have found that a few minutes in a whirlpool feels good, but if I stay in the warm water too long I will have severe leg cramps and aches a few hours later. If my body is hurting a lot I have discovered that resting on the couch with a blanket wrapped around my legs helps the most. I sleep with an electric blanket most of the year and always warm my bed before I get in because cold sheets can cause muscle spasms. If I become chilled during the night I curl up too tightly, which does not allow my muscles to relax and so I end up with more pain and not feeling rested.

Massage usually needs to be done differently for someone with fibromyalgia than for someone without the syndrome. You may be able to tolerate a very deep massage but a few hours later can develop muscle spasms that may last for days. You are most likely to notice problems in your upper back and neck and with headaches if you have a massage done too deeply. Only get a massage from someone who has experience working with fibromyalgia patients and make sure the massage therapist starts out very gently. Once you find someone who helps, stay with that person because he or she will come to know your body and remember what does and does not work. It may initially feel like you didn't get much of a massage but if it was done well, over the next few hours and into the next few days, you will notice your muscles letting go and relaxing.

Yoga can also be helpful for fibromyalgia. Start with a beginners class and let the instructor know your limitations. Because fibromyalgia is likely to be with you for the rest of your life, building a structured exercise program you can do alone or with a group, such as yoga, will assist you in preventing your fibromyalgia from getting the upper hand.

Fatigue and Stress Management The fatigue that comes with fibromyalgia can be extremely debilitating and depressing. Once we have been reassured that our pain does not indicate that our bodies are undergoing continuous structural damage, we can learn to do a lot of things in spite of the pain. But the fatigue is different. I know that the more fatigued I become, the more I hurt, and the less clearly I think. I may have energy for several days and then for no apparent reason I will bump up against several days of exhaustion. It feels like there is lead in my muscles, it is an effort to move, my head becomes heavy, and I can't keep my eyes open. I usually see clients between eight in the morning and one o'clock in the afternoon and only work four days a week, yet many days I

If you have fibromyalgia you have to be aware of your limits and not overdo things, even if you are feeling well.

have to fight to stay awake for the fifteen-minute drive home. I have found that a short nap can help me to feel rejuvenated enough to get through the rest of my day (see Chapter 13 for more on napping), but if I have to go out in the evening, I really struggle with fatigue the next day.

Learning to pace yourself is imperative when you have fibromyalgia. We have to learn to make priorities and set limits to accommodate our chronic illness. We no longer have a body that will allow us to volunteer for every good cause or interesting project. We need to learn to incorporate periods of rest into our schedules so our bodies don't collapse. It has taken me a while to become realistic about how much I can accomplish in a day. While I have been writing this book I have had to learn to ask for help. My husband and daughter have been extremely accommodating by taking on more family responsibilities and by lowering their expectations of me as their way of supporting me. Make sure to put your health first in your schedule.

Learning to live with fibromyalgia has entailed additional grief over my lost breasts. As I have put together a new life that accommodates my limitations, I have grieved the loss of my health and my breasts. I still have days when I have a good hard cry over my pain and the results of living with fatigue, and I expect I will have those moments of sadness and anger for the rest of my life, but I do not let negativity control my life.

Many people with fibromyalgia have used biofeedback, meditation, and relaxation tapes to learn how to relax their muscles and their minds. There are also many support groups, local newsletters, and specialized treatment programs available for people with fibromyalgia. There are a number of professionals who might help with your fibromyalgia, including physical or occupational therapists, medical social workers, rheumatology nurses, mental health professionals, rehabilitation counsellors, and sleep specialists. A type of physical therapy you may want to seek that is especially helpful for fibromyalgia, is called the "myofascial" approach. I recommend you ask your surgeon or doctor for the name of a rheumatologist who treats women with muscle pain and fatigue.

CHAPTER SEVEN

RESTORING BODY MOVEMENT

When we first come out of surgery it is instinctive to want to keep our bodies absolutely still to avoid further pain. But as time passes we discover that we need and want to move because the lack of motion makes us stiff and sore and prevents us from doing essential everyday activities, such as feeding ourselves, changing our clothes, and brushing our hair. As we slowly return to normal activities we begin with gross body movements, then focus on moving the affected arm.

Your mastectomy and lymph node dissection will have caused significant tissue damage resulting in inflammation and swelling in the affected area. Inflammation is usually experienced as a hot burning sensation. The swelling comes from lymph fluid that rushes to the injury to fight infection when the body begins its healing process. Swollen tissue can cause pain from the buildup of pressure in the swollen area that pushes on nerves. Your nerves will have been overstimulated and damaged during the operation, which also leads to pain. The swelling and inflammation are temporary conditions that your body will resolve fairly quickly on its own. The pain that comes from nerve involvement is addressed in Chapter 5, as well as at the end of this chapter.

Once your surgical area has healed, much of your pain will come from tissue or nerves that are pulled too tight to allow full range of motion. If it hurts when you move your arm, it is because there is not enough give or stretch left in the tissue of your armpit and shoulder to allow the same flexibility you had before the surgery. The tight areas will

Fascia is connective tissue that surrounds our bodies and all of our organs and glands. It contracts after surgery and is part of the reason we feel stiff and sore after an operation.

have to be stretched or chronic pain will result, along with limited use of your arm.

Another reason that you will feel stiff and sore after surgery is that your fascia will have contracted. The fascia can be thought of as the "bag that holds the body together." If you think about taking the skin off a raw chicken breast, there lies a thin, almost transparent, white membrane between the skin and the meat. Humans also have fascia under our skins and it surrounds our whole bodies. All of our muscles and all of the fibers that make up each muscle are covered with fascia. Our organs and glands are encapsulated by fascia. Fascia allows our muscles to lengthen and shorten as they need to and it allows muscles to move freely. When we are injured, ill, or under serious stress, the fascia contracts, sending a message to our bodies to be still to give ourselves time to heal. When part of our fascia is chronically contracted it makes us terribly stiff and can bind with other large areas of fascia to create serious discomfort and muscle stiffness. For this reason, it is important to help the fascia release gently and in such a way that alleviates the overall stiffness. Too aggressive an approach to stretching and exercising after a mastectomy will cause the fascia to tighten even more.

When I was in nursing school twenty-five years ago, the most common of the standard exercises for postmastectomy care was the "wall climbing" exercise. Ten years later, when I had my double mastectomy, the wall climb was still one of the exercises given to postmastectomy patients. When I had my silicone implants removed, I was again given a set of exercises that included the wall climb.

The wall climb exercise involves standing facing the wall and slowly walking your fingers up the wall until you have fully extended your arm. As your arm extends up, you walk in toward the wall to allow full shoulder extension. The idea is that if you do this exercise several times a day you will eventually be able to stretch your arm all the way up over your head.

After both surgeries I tried faithfully to do the wall climb, but I never got very far with it. I concluded I must not be trying hard enough and was left with a sense of failure. I could only go so far up the wall and then reached a point where the **pain** was too acute to continue. I assumed that I didn't have enough "John Wayne" in me to get the job done. This was very disheartening because I had been taught in nursing school that not doing the wall climb exercise would result in a frozen shoulder, for which only surgery offered a possible correction.

Some time ago I had to chuckle when I came across Dr. Susan Love's name for the wall climb. She calls it the "climbing the wall" exercise. I thought how appropriate the name was, since that is exactly the effect the wall climb had on me; it was driving me crazy.

What did help to stretch my arms, shoulders, and chest after my first surgery was swimming. I started out with very little strokes that looked a lot like the dog paddle. As I progressed, the breast stroke and back crawl allowed me to regain full range of motion.

By the time I underwent my second surgery I had learned a lot through my professional work helping others to live less stressfully and more comfortably in their bodies. I had undergone several different forms of treatment for my own musculo-skeletal ailments. These experiences shed some light on why the wall climb did not work and why swimming did work, all of which helped me to develop more effective exercises.

The problem with the wall climb exercise is that it tries to stretch too small a section of the body. We are trying to regain the full range of motion in our arm, and that has to involve more than just stretching and moving the armpit and shoulder. The armpit and chest muscles are the most taut and painful muscles, and the wall climb, since it is done standing up, is an attempt to stretch the most resistant area with the pull of gravity as an added load.

The muscles that make up the armpit and chest area are connected to very long muscles that run down the front and back of the body into the hip, buttock, and front pelvic areas. All the muscles must be worked as they connect with and support each other. Full range of motion for the arm and shoulder entails being able to complete three different movements: extending your arm all the way up, extending your arm up and out to the side and making a circular motion until your arm is arched

"After surgery I thought I would never be able to lift my arm again."

over your head and your fingers are pointing in the direction of your other shoulder; and placing your arm behind your back as you run your fingers up the center of your back, nearly reaching the base of your neck (see Figure 7-1).

"After both surgeries I tried faithfully to do the wall climb exercise but never got very far with it. I concluded that I didn't have enough 'John Wayne' in me to get the job done."

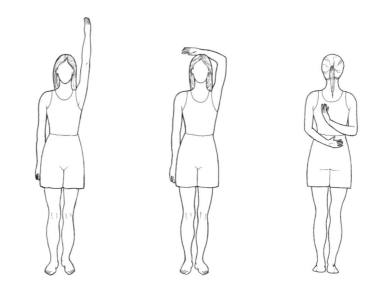

Figure 7-1   Full range of motion

Using the principle of least resistance, your approach to exercising and stretching after your mastectomy should try to identify and use the most flexible part of the body under the easiest conditions, as you try to get movement back into the restricted area. The exercises I have outlined here are all intended to be gentle approaches to regain your flexibility. As I walk you through a number of stretches that I have found effective, keep four things in mind:

- Do the exercises lying down,
- Whenever you feel resistance, stretch from the lower part of your trunk and gradually move up through your armpit, chest, and shoulder region,
- When your extended arm can go no further without causing acute

pain, bend your arm at the elbow. This will allow more flexibility and create less pain.

- Do the exercises on both sides, even if you only have one affected side.

Before You Begin

Before we proceed with the stretches you should be aware that there are two kinds of pain you will experience as you try to regain flexibility in the affected area. The first is acute pain, which is a sharp, hard, alarming sensation that makes you want to stop what you are doing immediately. Acute pain is a loud signal from the mind and body to warn that the body is being damaged. You should never try to override an acute pain signal. Always respect it and immediately stop what you are doing. Acute pain means that you are either trying to force the body to move before the tissue is adequately healed, or you are trying to move your body in a way that is not natural.

The second kind of pain is often referred to as good pain. This is pain that hurts but feels right. Good pain does not have an alarming quality. It feels more like a burning sensation than a stabbing, sharp pain. When you are trying to open up a tight area of the body it will usually feel hot and burn while you are moving it, and afterward it may ache. This pain is necessary if you are going to restore full movement the tight area. The burning, hot sensation comes from blood moving back into muscle as it opens up. Good circulation is an essential part of properly working muscles and is essential for healing damaged tissue. Good pain should be familiar from those times when you have taken up a new sport or done a physical activity that worked a part of your body that hadn't been active in a while.

One of the obstacles to regaining our flexibility after a mastectomy is fear of our bodies. As I mentioned earlier, stress is one of the reasons our fascia contracts and makes us stiff. Cancer is terribly stressful and can have the effect of making us view our bodies as our enemies. Surgery and the changes that our mastectomy brings are also frightening. Many women are not in touch with their bodies and worry that they are not able to accurately interpret the signals their bodies send them when they try

"Once I got my arm over my head, I knew I was on my way."

When you begin to stretch again after your mastectomy, remember that all of your muscles are connected to one another. Try stretching out an area that is less stiff and then moving into the tightest area.

to bring movement back into the surgical area. All these fears are natural but they contribute to our physical, as well as our emotional discomfort. It may help to remember that the more information you have about how a healthy body works and how various treatments and exercises affect the body, the less fearful and powerless you will feel as you work on your physical recovery.

I want to emphasize that if you do not already spend time listening to your body you should start now. Early detection of health problems, not just cancer, depends on our awareness of our bodies. As you tune into the signals and sensations of your body, it will raise questions about what they mean. There are many resources, such as books, documentaries, and professionals that can help answer your questions. And the more attention you pay to your body, the better you will understand the messages it is giving you, and the better your chance of coming to see your body as your friend and ally in your search for health. It can be a very enjoyable and stimulating experience to learn to understand your body.

Practice increasing your awareness of your body as you work on regaining the range of motion in your arm. Listen closely and respond to acute pain by stopping what you are doing. Let your body guide you in knowing when good pain is turning into acute pain because you are overdoing it.

One of the best ways of working through your fear of pain and of your body is to not rush through the stretching and to take slow, deep breaths to calm any panicky feelings. We often respond to fear by holding our breath, which prevents adequate blood flow and leads to tighter muscles. Taking slow, deep breaths, in through your nose and out through your mouth, will increase your circulation and relax your body. The more calm and relaxed you are when you stretch, the less it will hurt.

If you are frightened but breathing properly, you will probably find yourself trembling or shaking. Just as the body cries to release sadness, it shakes to release fear and tension. This is perfectly natural and healthy. As I explained in Chapter 4, you will stop trembling when fear leaves your body, as you continue to breathe and stretch your muscles. Reminding yourself that shaking is one of your body's ways of releasing fear will

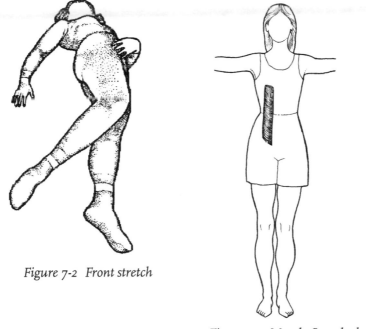

Figure 7-2 Front stretch

Figure 7-3 Muscle Stretched

prevent you from creating fearful interpretations that could keep the fear cycle going. If you feel like crying, don't repress it, let the tears flow. Sadness over the changes in your body frequently surfaces as you work on your physical rehabilitation.

Exercises
EXERCISE 1: LENGTHENING THE TORSO

This exercise can be used right after you get out of surgery. As soon as you have been awake long enough to begin feeling stiff and a bit restless, you are ready to begin stretching and lengthening your torso. This exercise helps with the stiffness that comes from lying and sitting for a long time and it will prepare you to do more extensive stretching when you have healed enough. As well as helping with stiffness, these stretches are a gentle way to build confidence in your ability to regain normal functioning in your body.

Front Side

While lying on your back in bed with no pillows, keep the left leg straight and raise the right knee about halfway. Keeping the right arm extended and behind you so as to brace yourself by keeping your hand on the bed, roll your right leg, hip, and lower back toward your left side as you arch the lower back (see Figure 7-2). The area you are trying to stretch runs from your right groin just inside the crest of your hip bone up into your upper abdominal area, just below the breast region (see Figure 7-3).

The amount of stretch you feel will depend a great deal on what kind of physical condition you were in before surgery. If you regularly stretched and exercised you may not notice much pull from this stretch. If this is the case, the exercise will help you focus on the lower part of your torso in preparation for the next exercises. If you went into surgery with a less flexible body or a very tight body you will notice a pull as you roll and arch your back. If you have a rheumatoid condition that has left you with tight muscles and painful joints, you will easily notice the pull.

Once your back is arched, take a deep breath in through your nose, bringing the air down into your abdomen and letting it expand this area. Hold the breath in this space for about fifteen seconds to continue the stretch. This expansion will help create more of a pull from the lower ab-domen. Giving some resistance to the arch by pushing into the bed with your right hand will also allow for more pull. However, if this is your affected side you will not be able to use that arm and hand, so the rolling, arching, and deep breathing will have to give you the stretch.

Listen closely to your body to make sure you are not feeling any acute pain while you are doing this. If it feels too painful, try shifting around a bit to see if you can ease the pain. If you cannot do it without acute pain, then stop the exercise until you feel you are more ready.

Once you have performed the exercise on one side, switch to the other side. Even if you only had surgery on one side you will still need to stretch both sides of the body. Our musculo-skeletal system operates with a balance between the right and left side. Whenever you make a change in one side of the body it sets off a reaction in the other side. Have you ever noticed how limping can cause stiffness or pain in the opposite

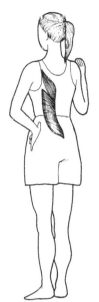

Figure 7-4

hip? By exercising both sides of your body you will maintain proper muscular balance. In addition to balance, working with your unaffected side will prepare it to assist in loosening your tight, affected side. Think of your tight side as bunched material you are trying to thread a drawstring through, and your loose side is where the bunch is going to go as it opens up. By keeping your unaffected side as flexible as possible, it makes that side more available to assist with the "unbunching" of the tight muscle. The tight muscle will be stretched into the open, flexible space. This happens from top to bottom and from side to side of the torso.

Back Side

This is the only stretch that I recommend you do standing up. This stretch is designed to open the muscles in your buttocks and lower back, (see Figure 7-4). Because you are not trying to get movement back into the tight surgical area yet, gravity will not interfere if you stand while doing this. Stand with your legs straight and feet about six to eight inches apart. Keep your arms close to your body and bent all the way up at the elbows. Allow your forearms to cushion and support your chest. Now hike up the right shoulder and drop the left one, as you pull to stretch out the muscle that starts in the outer back buttock area and runs up into your flank or outer lower back area. As you pull up from the right hip your right shoulder may need to come forward and to the left a bit (see Figures 7-5 a & b). Repeat the exercise on the left side of the body. You can also do this exercise lying flat on the bed without a pillow, but you will feel the most stretch if you do it standing up.

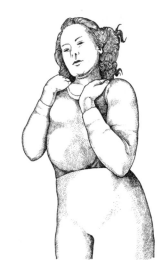

Figure 7-5 a

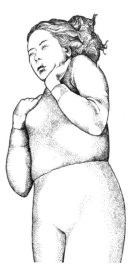

Figure 7-5 b

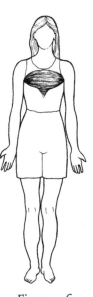

Figure 7-6

EXERCISE 2:
EXPANDING THE CHEST

Not only does the body respond to your mastectomy by tightening your torso from top to bottom but it also tends to tighten the muscles across your chest. You can start this exercise in the hospital and continue it after you get home.

While you are lying down breath deeply enough to expand your chest (see Figure 7-7). Breath in through your *mouth* and exhale through your *mouth*. When you inhale through your nose, the air fills your whole torso and this is the kind of breathing you want to do normally. But for this particular ex-

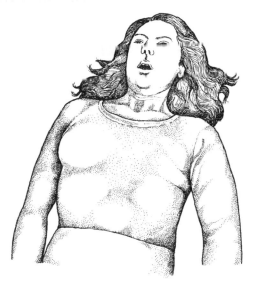

Figure 7-7

ercise you just want the air to fill your chest area to help expand the chest wall (see Figure 7-6).

You will probably find that you experience more resistance to doing this exercise than the last one because it works directly with the trauma-tized part of your body. You may find yourself quite nervous about mak-ing any kind of movement in this painful area because of the stitches and drainage tube. It is very important, however, to begin gently expanding your chest right away so it does not contract inward. Breathing into the area also produces good circulation, which promotes optimum healing. General anesthetic affects the lungs and makes them more prone to in-fection right after surgery but deep breathing into the lungs reverses the effect of the anesthetic.

Remember that your drainage tube has several inches of tubing ex-tending into the incision so it would take a lot to pull out the tube, and your stitches are also quite sturdy. This exercise may cause a slight burn-ing sensation. Exercise 2 can be done while lying, sitting, or standing. If it feels less frightening and more physically comfortable, use your hand or hands to cover and support your surgical area while expanding it. Lengthening the torso and expanding the chest should be done many times a day during the early part of your recovery.

Until you have your stitches and tube removed, limit your stretching to these two exercises. In the meantime, your pain level will dictate how much you can comfortably move your arm. Eating, brushing your teeth, combing your hair, washing, and dressing yourself will provide you with plenty of opportunities to begin getting movement back into your arm and chest.

It is natural to want to curl up into a protective, "hunched over" posture to protect yourself from being bumped and because the hanging tubes and suction bulbs tend to make you lean forward. Try not to hunch over because it will cause your muscles to shorten and you will have more stretching to do later. Try to keep your posture as straight as possible. Prop yourself up in bed in a way that keeps your shoulders up and back.

You can get a protective feeling by placing a hand or small soft pillow over the surgical area to support it. You can also wear something that fits snugly to the area. Binding the area will make it less painful to move around and allow you to maintain good posture and feel comfortable

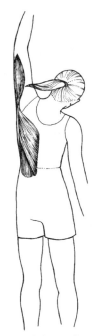

enough to keep breathing into the area in order to expand it. If you have a thin dishtowel or cloth diaper that is long enough to go around your chest you can wrap it around yourself and pin it. This should be tight enough to feel snug but not so tight that it restricts your ability to expand your chest while breathing. A form-fitting, thin-strapped tank top that you can slip on starting at your feet may work, or you may use a one-piece exercise leotard. There is no need to buy something for this purpose; you should be able to come up with something that you already have around the house. You will not need it for very long and you will not

Figure 7-8

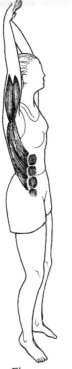

Figure 7-9

be wearing this out in public, so keep it simple.

EXERCISE 3: ARM EXTENSION AND SHOULDER ROTATION

Once your drainage tube and stitches are out, you should be ready to work at getting a full range of motion back into your affected arm and shoulder. The first two exercises will have loosened your muscles, which helps to relieve the tightness in the armpit and chest area. This exercise consists of an arm extension and shoulder rotation.

You may want to practice the arm extension with your unaffected side first. If you have had both breasts removed, you will of course have to begin with one of your affected arms.

Arm Extension

This exercise is intended to replace the wall climb described in the introduction to this chapter. The ultimate goal is to get your arm to fully extend up, which will stretch muscles in your abdomen, side, arm, armpit, and back (see Figures 7-8 and 7-9).

Lie on your back with your arms at your sides and your palms resting on the bed. Initially, you will want to do this exercise on your bed. Later, you may find that doing it on the floor gives you better leverage. If you do this exercise on the bed, you should lie in the middle of the bed with your head at the foot of the bed. Now slowly raise your straight arm up toward your head out from the front of your body. Take your arm up as far as it will go before you begin to experience a lot of pain. When it feels as if moving your arm any further will cause acute pain, bend your arm at the elbow and curl your hand into a loose fist, then bring your forearm and

Know the difference between "good pain" and "bad pain." One means your exercises are helping and the other means stop what you are doing immediately.

hand in toward your shoulder. Once you make a fist, the hand and forearm should rotate in so your fingers can rest close to your body at the front shoulder region (Figure 7-13).

Next, place your other hand on the elbow of the side you are stretching and try to raise the elbow further up toward your head. As you feel more resistance, slide your hand up the arm from the elbow to the place in your armpit where it feels tightest. Now hold this spot and, as you slightly push down on it, continue to raise your elbow. While you are raising your arm and you come to points of resistance, try wiggling the whole arm a bit and see if you can wiggle past a blocked area. Each time you make an adjustment, your tight muscles should give a little more and your arm should extend a little further. The next part of the arm extension exercise is to stretch more of your lower torso by adding Exercise 1 in which you lengthen the front of the torso. Partially bend your knee on the same side you are working with your arm. Raising your bent knee and roll toward your straight leg as you arch your back. The final step is to rotate your elbow, keeping it in the same bent position, around in a circle. You will not be able to do the last step at the beginning of your recovery. This movement can only be done once you can get your bent arm extended up. This rotating action will help loosen the shoulder.

An arm extension done with a bent elbow is just as complete a stretch as one done with a straight arm. In fact, the bent arm gives more of a stretch because it involves more muscles. "No pain, no gain" is not the way you should be thinking. The reason stretching with a bent arm does not hurt as much is because we are using more parts of the body, so the job is more efficiently accomplished. It is no different from using your leg muscles along with your arm muscles to help you lift something heavy.

By combining the abdomen pull with the bent elbow, assistance from the other hand, and wiggling, you will eventually be able to get your arm fully extended up. Regaining full range of motion is going to take weeks to months because you will most likely add movement only an inch at a time. Doing this exercise two or three times a day will speed your recovery, but doing it more than that can fatigue the muscles and bring on muscle spasms, so don't overdo it. Even if you only do this exercise once a day, it will eventually help restore full function to your arm.

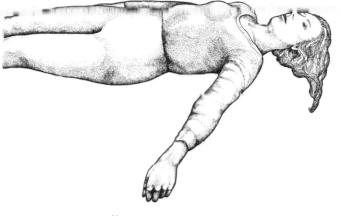

Figure 7-10

Shoulder Rotation

The shoulder rotation exercise works on the circular action of the shoulder and stretches the same muscles as the arm extension (see Figures 7-8 and 7-9). The ultimate goal of the rotation exercise is to be able to bring your arm out from your side and extend it all the way past your head with your fingers pointing toward your opposite shoulder see Figure 7-1). As with the arm extension exercise, the rotation exercise can first be done lying on the bed with your head at the foot of the bed, and later on the floor.

To begin, lie on your back with your arms at your sides. Now slowly move one arm up and out from the side of your body (see Figure 7-10). Move your arm as far up and out as it will go before you begin to experience a lot of pain. When it feels as if moving the arm any further will cause acute pain, bend your arm at the elbow, just as you did in the arm extension exercise (Figure 7-11). Make a loose fist and bring the forearm in close to the top part of your arm with your fingers touching your shoulder, but this time your hand will touch the side of your shoulder in-

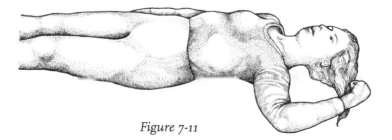

Figure 7-11

stead of the front. Continuing to keep your elbow bent, try to move your arm around at different angles and see where it is most and least flexible. Don't force it. Pay close attention to your body and see where it is able to stretch.

While you are moving your arm at different angles, place your opposite hand on your elbow and use it to raise your arm even further (see Figure 7-12). Then let your hand slide down your arm from your elbow to the tightest place in your armpit. Hold it tightly and slightly pull down and

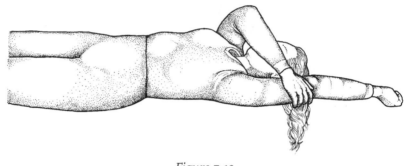

Figure 7-12

try to move your elbow out to the side and up. Once you have worked the area from that angle, move your hand from your armpit further around to your back and pull your back muscle toward your side (see Figure 7-13). Your hand should find your wing bone, which you can open up as you pull it gently toward your side. Depending upon your body and hand size, you may also be able to continue to provide support to part of your armpit with some of your palm (Figure 7-14). Again, you should notice that this allows for even more movement while you try to extend your arm up.

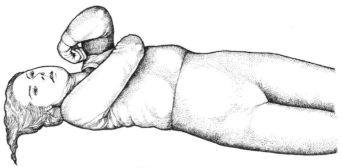

Figure 7-13

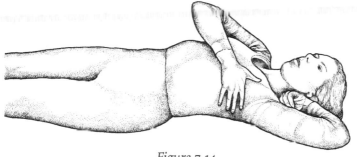

Figure 7-14

Your body will guide
you in how far to
push yourself.

At this point, try to incorporate exercise 1. Partially bend your knee on the same side you are working with your arm (see Figure 7-2). Arch your back a bit as you pull your knee over toward your opposite side. Now at the same time, try to stretch out your front outer pelvic/abdominal area and your back outer buttock and flank area. If you roll slightly to your opposite side when you bend your knee you will be able to get the stretch in both your back and front sides. Focus your attention on pulling or stretching up from the lower part of the torso to achieve the greatest movement in your restricted arm. As with the arm extension, do this exercise consistently one to three times a day, but don't overdo it.

Becoming Physical Again

Doing the exercises described above is the first step in rebuilding a relationship with your body. The next step is to incorporate other forms of physical activity back into your life. For me swimming worked after my first surgery and treadmill walking worked well after my second surgery. Before you are ready to become physically active in a more public way, stretching can be done at home. Stretching is a simple, private, cost-effective way of keeping your body active and feeling alive. You might want to get a stretching guide for use at home and take a class later in your healing process.

Ask yourself what activities you took part in before surgery and incorporate them back into your life as soon as possible. Your doctor or a resource nurse at your clinic can guide you in the timing and type of activities that are safe for you after your mastectomy. Keep in mind the

"Incorporate your old physical activities back into your life as soon as you are able. Try not to favor your affected side. I was forced to use my arm right away if I wanted to eat."

potential risk for lymphedema when you are deciding which activities you will take part in.

As I mentioned, swimming after my first surgery was an excellent form of exercise to regain the use of my shoulders and arms. The strokes I used were very similar to the motions used in the exercises I have described. The water eliminated the pull of gravity and provided a cool environment that helped with inflammation. Swimming is a full body exercise that makes all of our parts work together. Correctly performed, swimming strokes require you to reach out of your abdomen and lower back as you stretch your legs out and extend your arms. It also requires deep breathing that helps circulate the blood, which promotes tissue healing. But swimming did a lot more for me than just get my shoulders and arms working again. It placed an expectation on my body to perform. It required me to rebuild a working relationship with my body and forced me to get out in public.

A friend of mine used Tae Kwon Do (Korean martial art) as part of her recovery. Ginger had a close network of women with whom she practiced and a caring instructor who showed her how to conquer the fear of her cancer by making her body perform. This woman, in her late forties, earned her black belt a little over a year after her surgery. She had seriously considered giving up on testing for her black belt, and was going to be satisfied with the belts she had earned before surgery. Knowing how important the structure of weekly classes, support of good friends, and encouragement from her instructor were to maintaining a positive attitude, she decided to stay with it.

The Susan G. Komen Breast Cancer Foundation truly captures the spirit I am trying to convey in the Race For The Cure. The foundation was established in 1982 by Nancy Brinker to honor the memory of her sister, Susan G. Komen, who died from breast cancer at age thirty-six. The foundation sponsors events in seventy-seven cities throughout the United States. Money earned from the race is donated to help eradicate breast cancer by advancing research, education, screening, and treatment.

On Mother's Day for the last two years, I have taken part in the race-with two friends who have undergone mastectomies, my daughter, and two other friends. The morning consists of a five kilometre wheel/race,

5 kilometre co-ed walk, one-kilometre family fun walk, and kids' 400-metre fun run. All the participants receive a T-shirt and a number and breast cancer survivors wear pink visors. Taking part in the walk I have felt intense emotion in the presence of so many women and families who have been affected by breast cancer. Some people are crying and others are filled with joy. It is an amazing experience to come together with so many people to fight breast cancer, and to share grief.

I want to remind you again to be patient with yourself as you work through these exercises. If you are going to a support group be careful to not compare your progress with others. Each of us begins our exercises with a unique body influenced by things such as genetic structure, age, and activity level before we entered surgery. The size and placement of the tumor, number of nodes removed, extent of silicone leakage, and mastectomy technique your surgeon uses, all affect how quickly you will be able to regain your movement.

Our culture has done women a serious disservice by teaching us to compare and compete with each other rather than embracing our differences and validating and encouraging one another. We can compare to get new ideas to help us in our recovery, but those ideas must be applied realistically to our situation. Comparing can also be constructive if you use it as an assessment tool for goal setting. Ask yourself where you have been, where you are now, and what your particular goal is for recovery from your mastectomy. Looking back at the progress you made in a week or in a month will help you realize how far you have come. If you compare your progress from day to day you may find that you are quite pleased with your commitment to doing your exercises regularly or that you have not been making them enough of a priority to accomplish your goal.

Some women have trouble doing the exercises on their own and feel the need to seek professional help. Asking your doctor for a referral to physical therapy is very appropriate if you feel you are not making enough progress or are having trouble doing the exercises. Just because I have presented some exercises in this book does not mean you have failed if you need assistance to do them. It is extremely common for women who have undergone a mastectomy to require some physical therapy. You can tell the physical therapist what exercises you have been doing and how far you have gotten with them, and then they can further guide you. Physical therapy is an available resource to help you, so assert your needs as you see fit.

Actively working on restoring our range of motion after a mastectomy helps to show us that we are not helpless victims of our circumstances. Psychological recovery from whatever it was that caused us to lose our breast requires that we take some measure of control back over our bodies. Restoring the range of motion in the shoulder and arm is just a beginning in the ultimate goal of accepting our changed bodies. We must regain confidence in our body's ability to function. Cancer and the loss of a breast can make us feel betrayed by our bodies and we can give up on them. Being willing to become physically active is a statement of faith that we are willing to trust our bodies again.

CHAPTER EIGHT

SELF-ESTEEM, BODY IMAGE, AND RETURNING TO LIFE

A mastectomy can be devastating to our self-esteem and body image. Self-esteem refers to how we feel about ourselves, and body image (discussed in Chapter 5) refers to how we feel about our bodies and appearance. Self-esteem and body image are closely connected for most women. For most of us, our self-esteem plays off our body image and both are shaped by the culture we live in, as well as the way we were brought up. As we get ready to return to our lives after a mastectomy we need to take a careful look at whether or not we have healthy regard for ourselves. Good self-esteem is essential to adjusting to and accepting our new bodies. Looking at ourselves for the first time after surgery and returning to work are two important milestones on the path to recovery and full participation in life. They can also be opportunities for growth and change as we re-evaluate our worth as women.

Self-Esteem

In our culture a woman's value is inextricably tied to how she looks. It is common for women to believe that we *are* our bodies, and that our sexual attractiveness is what makes us worthwhile. This attitude is one of the reasons that growing older is so terribly painful for many women. Physical attractiveness in the popular culture is narrowly defined as the almost impossible ideal presented by models and movie stars. The women's movement has worked very hard to attack and change the thinking that places a woman's value on her compatibility with standard

Older women who undergo a mastectomy are presented with the double burden of aging and a surgery that changes a very feminine part of them.

ideas about beauty. This has resulted in many changes. Many of us are raising our children to define people in ways other than their gender-specific traits. And many women think they have shed the legacy of sexist attitudes that their self-esteem is no longer affected by a limited vision of female attractiveness. When we undergo a mastectomy we may be forced to confront the realization that we have not completely left these negative beliefs about our worth and attractiveness behind and they are still affecting the way we feel about ourselves. A deeply personal experience, such as a mastectomy, will really be the test of our self-esteem. Our changed bodies, which no longer measure up to the cultural ideal of the female form, will bring us face to face with our inner attitudes.

Shame

In adjusting to our bodies and assessing our feelings about ourselves after a mastectomy, it is common to discover shame at the root of our discomfort and emotional pain. Shame is the opposite of good self-esteem. Shame is the feeling that we are innately defective and not worthy of receiving love. Shame can be instilled in us in our childhood if we grow up in an abusive family or in one that gives us the message that we are somehow not "good enough" as we are. We can develop shame through our interactions with people who tell us that we are not adequate. Shame can also develop or be accentuated by any experience, such as sexism, illness, or handicaps, that makes us feel as though we are somehow lacking or damaged. The loss of a breast can create a sense of shame and may bring up old feelings of inadequacy. We need to move past any shame we might feel after surgery in order to rebuild self-esteem, which will, in turn, allow us to come to terms with our bodies.

To heal any shame we may be carrying around we need to become aware of our subconscious beliefs about ourselves and our intrinsic value. As we go through life we absorb messages about how we measure up as people. The way our parents behaved toward us, the kinds of relationships we have with friends and partners, and our work performance and environment, all contribute to our self-esteem. These messages help to form our subconscious attitudes toward ourselves. To find out whether shame is holding you back in your recovery after a mastectomy, ask yourself a few basic questions.

1. Do I feel lovable and worthy of good, or do I feel I do not deserve good things? Does my mastectomy seem like just one more thing about myself that I have to hide?

2. Do I know I have a good mind, or do I feel stupid?

3. Do I know I am attractive in my own unique way, or do I feel ugly and unable to measure up to the attractiveness of other women? Do I feel like I can never be attractive to anyone after my mastectomy?

4. Do I have a personality that other people want to be around, or do I feel like a bore? Has my surgery made me unpleasant to be around?

5. Do I have talents and strengths, or do I feel less talented than other people?

6. Do I know that my emotions and feelings since my surgery are normal and natural, or do I think I am weak for feeling sad and afraid? Do I feel guilty for feeling angry?

7. Do I know that I am adequate sexually, or do I feel that I am not as sexual as others? Do I feel that sex is dirty or bad?

8. Do I feel loved by anyone, or do I feel that no one really loves me? Do I feel like no one can ever love me after my mastectomy because I have less to offer?

9. Do I have a sense of self-respect and dignity, or do I feel that I am an embarrassment to myself and others, particularly since my mastectomy?

"I felt like a freak at first. Odd and unbalanced. Now I only feel that way sometimes."

If you answer these questions honestly and discover that you frequently answer in the affirmative to the second half, you are probably burdened with a sense of shame about yourself that predates your mastectomy. That sense of shame will hinder your efforts to come to terms with the changes in your body and to feel good about yourself.

You may discover that overall you have a good self-image, but you have felt unattractive since your surgery. Perhaps your feelings stem back to negative comments you heard as a child about physical disfigurements. Or perhaps your feelings are simply a normal response to having lost part of your natural beauty. These feelings are common and they are

"I know I will never have a youthful body again. That is a hard thing to come to terms with at 29."

not a result of deep shame. If you discover that subconsciously you are operating with a feeling that you are inferior and unworthy, you need to challenge the roots of those beliefs.

Discovering the origin of our negative subconscious beliefs about ourselves allows us to use our rational adult minds to challenge them. Feelings of shame can often be traced to a particular time, place, and incident. Try to think about where you first came to believe that you were unworthy of good things. If, for example, you feel that your body is shameful and should be kept covered, you may remember the way you came to that conclusion. If your mother or father warned you that your body could "get you into trouble" or that your body could tempt people into hurting you, bring that belief out where you can look at it in light of what you know now.

It is important to ask ourselves whether our internal beliefs are serving us well. If they are not, we can change them. A therapist or support group can help with healing deep feelings of shame. (For more information on finding a therapist, see Chapter 13.) Simply bringing hidden beliefs out into the open can help us to change them. When you become aware of a negative subconscious belief at work beneath a behavior or feeling, stop and challenge that belief immediately. As we mature into adults, we become more selective about what we accept as truth. It is never too late to change your core beliefs about your worth as a woman. By healing your false sense of shame you will be able to bring a sense of acceptance and self-love to your recovery from a mastectomy.

Some women turn to an established church for help with these issues. The basic teachings of most of the major religions help us to define our worth in a broader sense than just our physical self. Judaism, Christianity, Buddhism, and Hinduism, to name a few, can all help us to reassess our lives. If you are not comfortable with organized religion, many other helpful approaches emphasize spirituality over religion. There are also many books available whose focus is on healing shame and developing self-acceptance.

After your mastectomy you can begin to ensure that the people around you are life-affirming and make you feel that you are lovable and important to them. If you did not already have such people in your life, you can begin to add them. Support groups and churches are two good places to meet supportive friends.

Coming to terms with our shame and developing our self-esteem can be one of the hidden benefits of having undergone a mastectomy. This may be the first opportunity you have had to learn that you have a worth beyond your body and beyond what you can do for others. A mastectomy can be the catalyst for you to learn to love yourself.

Body Image

Developing a healthy body image after a mastectomy involves gaining an accurate idea of how our bodies look and then developing an attitude of love and acceptance toward our changed bodies. Ideally, our self-esteem is strong enough that our body image feels like a separate issue. Obviously, our physical appearance will affect how we feel, but it should not be the determining factor. We need to appreciate that we are spiritual beings in a physical body. As we age, it will become clear that we are much more than just our physical selves. As our bodies fail, as they eventually will for all of us, we will be forced to look at those parts of ourselves that are separate from appearance. Once you feel sure of your own intrinsic value you are in a better position to begin to work on accepting the changes that a mastectomy has wrought on your body. A sure sign of a healthy self-esteem is the ability to accept and feel love and compassion for ourselves and our less than perfect bodies. Try to remember this as you work with your body image. At the same time, don't be too hard on yourself if you find yourself struggling. Building healthy self-esteem and body acceptance is a process that takes time and work. Women who start with a poor body image continue to bring that body image into their recovery process, which makes acceptance of the changes surgery has brought more difficult.

A lot of descriptive research has been done on how women feel about their bodies after undergoing a mastectomy. I find myself chuckling at the obvious results of such research: that women like their bodies less and find them less attractive after losing a breast. According to these studies, many women still like themselves as people, but don't feel as good about their postmastectomy bodies as they did about their premas-

If you find that you have negative internal beliefs about your body they can be changed. It is possible to accept and love your body again after surgery no matter how you felt about it before or after.

"I looked in the mirror right away. My chest looked like something out of an alien movie. I thought the surgery would be tidier than it was. I really wasn't prepared for how it looked. But I had to go face to face with it."

tectomy bodies. I'm sure this does not come as a surprise to you. It is completely natural to mourn the loss of part of our natural beauty. My second reaction is one of validation. Many of us are such troopers, with such high expectations of ourselves, that we have convinced ourselves that if we were "all together" people we would like our bodies just as much after our mastectomy. It is a relief to know that it is very reasonable and universal not to like one's body as much. That does not mean that we cannot develop a loving attitude toward our bodies, as well as an accurate body image.

Looking at Our New Bodies for the First Time

A healthy body image is an accurate body image. Establishing an accepting, loving new body image after a mastectomy is a two-step process that begins the first time we look at ourselves after surgery. First, we need to allow ourselves the latitude to think and say all of the initial thoughts and feelings we have about how our bodies look to us. Second, we need to develop an attitude of loving care toward our new bodies.

When we look at ourselves for the first time we are likely to be hit with a lot of strong negative feelings about our postmastectomy bodies. It is critical to grieve the changes brought about by our mastectomies (see Chapter 4), and it will not be helpful to suppress the feelings that come up.

The timing of this first step will depend on your individual needs and circumstances. If you live alone and have to change your own dressings after surgery, you will probably be forced to look at your chest sooner than a woman who has someone doing this for her. If you are a person who likes to avoid emotionally difficult tasks as long as possible, you will probably become very good at changing your bandages and draining your tubes without ever having to look at yourself. Some delay is fine, as long as you face the fact that at some point you are going to have to look at your chest. If you find yourself avoiding it for an extended period, ask yourself what would make it easier for you. Would it help to have someone with you? Perhaps you can wait until your first follow-up appointment with your surgeon, or ask a close friend or nurse. If you choose to have someone with you, make sure it is someone who is a good listener and not someone who will try to "fix" your feelings. If your spouse or partner is with you the first time you look at your chest after surgery, it can provide an opportunity to grieve together.

Perhaps you need some time and space for yourself for this private moment? Sometimes our loved ones hover over us in an attempt to spare us any more pain and sadness. If this is the case you might ask for some time alone.

Whatever your initial reactions are when you first look at your naked chest in the mirror, try to respect the feelings and not repress them. Let the feelings surface and don't shut them down by trying to intellectualize how you feel. If you find yourself feeling numb or emotionally blunted, don't worry. This is often a normal part of the grief process. Emotional shock is often experienced as numbness. If you feel as if you look like an eight-year-old now because your chest is flat, you should acknowledge that also.

Common initial reactions to first looking at ourselves after we have had one or both breasts removed are expressed in such words as: "I hate my body," "I look deformed," "I am ugly to look at," "No one will ever want me again." It is common to immediately feel you want to give up and never show yourself to the outside world again. These kinds of negative thoughts may not be very strong or may be accompanied by more accepting thoughts, but nevertheless they should be acknowledged if they exist. These feelings of loss and despair can undermine your self-esteem and recovery if they are not dealt with. They can also fester into a body image that leads you to believe you look much worse than you actually do. The postmastectomy chest, in general, looks more odd than repulsive. Many women are afraid that their chests look terribly ugly. In fact, most of us just look flat chested. We need to sit quietly with ourselves or with someone we trust and acknowledge our negative thoughts.

FORMING A NEW BODY IMAGE

Each time you look at yourself in the mirror you will begin to get more accustomed to your new body and develop an accurate body image. This is important because an accurate body image is closely related to a positive body image. The more you force your mind to see your body accurately,

> Your body is your ally in the fight against breast cancer. Treat it with respect and love.

the more opportunity you give yourself to look at the negative thoughts that surface, which in turn will allow you to turn your attitude into one that is more loving and accepting—the second step in developing a new body image.

After you have, as honestly as possible, taken stock of how you feel about your body after your mastectomy, and have an accurate idea of how you actually look, it is time to try to develop a loving attitude toward your body. If we want to feel good about ourselves as women, we have to deal with our bodies. We can do it with hostility and end up hating our bodies, or we can embrace the experience and open ourselves up to a whole new dimension of womanhood that involves much more than outward appearance.

We need to begin to look at our bodies as something precious rather than something that has tricked or betrayed us. As we make this shift we are building a new positive foundation for a loving, protective attitude toward ourselves. We need to feel bad for all that our poor bodies have gone through and try to relate to our bodies with tenderness and compassion. We need to be grateful for how well our bodies have come through surgery and, in most cases, a battle with cancer. Our body's natural instinct to heal itself has to be honored. Instead of seeing our physical self as scarred and worthless, we need to become its protector and advocate. Instead of being angry and rejecting, we need to learn to embrace our body and befriend it. The more we take a loving attitude toward our body, the harder it will be to think of it as something that has betrayed us, or something that is holding us back in life.

Our scars can become the site at which the battle for our lives was fought and won, as is so powerfully represented in the photograph of writer and breast cancer survivor Deena Metzger. She is shown standing naked with her face to the sun and her arms spread to embrace life. Her scar is tattooed with the life-affirming image of a tree. This poster can be ordered from TREE, Box 186, Topanga, Ca. 90290.

A loving attitude will help us set limits and goals that are good for our bodies. We will want to exercise, eat right, and rest our bodies. Our creative natures will be freed as we develop an attitude of caring and concern toward ourselves. Making the outer self look attractive is one of the ways that love of the body is expressed. If we view ourselves as ugly and shameful, we can create a self-fulfilling prophecy by neglecting ourselves and, indeed, looking very unattractive.

When we are working in a conscious partnership with our body we will discover all kinds of ways to help it look better and move more comfortably. We will become open to exercises that make us feel good, and explore new ways to dress and alter our clothes. This proactive approach puts us in a healthy partnership with our postmastectomy bodies and makes us feel empowered. Treating our bodies with love and compassion offers us the opportunity to change old behaviors. If you were prone to ignoring or abusing your body, through such things as eating disorders, or compulsive exercising, or as a result of sexual abuse, your mastectomy can be an opportunity for positive change.

Returning to Work

Returning to work will be one of the biggest emotional steps in your recovery after a mastectomy. It will be a test of your self-esteem and your body image and a major hurdle in your return to life. Most of us have three concerns foremost in our minds when we prepare to go back. First, you may be wondering whether you are ready. Second, you may be concerned about how you will relate to your co-workers after your illness and surgery. And third, you may be worried about how you look.

Recovering at home probably seems easy in comparison, as your family, if you have one, has been with you from the beginning. Going back to work means that we have to face people for the first time with our postmastectomy bodies.

WHEN TO GO BACK TO WORK

The timing of your return to work will depend on how quickly your chest heals, as well as your overall recovery in terms of energy and emotional wellness. The type of work you do will also influence how soon you are able to return. If you do a lot of heavy lifting, unless there is some way to go back to light duty, you will have to wait longer than someone with a desk job. If your work is very mentally or emotionally taxing, you may need extra time to gather your strength and concentration. If you are undergoing cancer treatment, the timing of that may also affect your return to your job.

Before your surgery the doctor may be able to give you a general approximation of when you can expect to be able to return, but that can only be determined afterwards. Your doctor will give you a release form to indicate what return date is appropriate for your health, but it will be up to you to decide if that date is right for you. Hopefully, the amount of sick time you have available will not influence your return date, but very often it is a deciding factor. If a medical release from your doctor determines how much time off you are allowed, make sure your doctor is aware of your emotional needs. Sometimes supervisors are able to help with financial concerns and make informal, temporary adjustments to your schedule so you can come back to work without jeopardizing your health. Don't hesitate to ask for some kind of compromise, such as reduced hours or a modified job description, if that is what you need.

You may want to ask the people close to you if it looks to them like you are ready to return to work. They may be able to help you make a better informed decision, but remember the final decision about when to return is up to you.

Relating to Co-workers

It can be very difficult to know how to deal with your co-workers when you return to work after a mastectomy. The experience of undergoing a mastectomy is a very private and painful one, and for many of us it is not something we want to be particularly public about. Perhaps you have a few people at work to whom you are quite close. They will probably already be familiar with your situation and will make your transition back to work as easy as possible for you. On the other hand, you may not be close to your co-workers and returning to work after a mastectomy and, very likely, breast cancer will be awkward. Your co-workers may want to express support but don't know how. They may not want to upset you or pry and so they behave as though nothing happened. Some co-workers may not be able to understand your need for privacy and will be overly solicitous or ask questions that make you feel uncomfortable. You need to determine what is comfortable for you. How much about your mastectomy do you want to share and with whom? You need only reveal as much as feels right to you about your health and your operation.

Because of the magnitude of your health situation, it is likely that the people in your workplace will be aware that you had a mastectomy. If they sent a group card or gift they have already had a chance to reach out from a safe distance and that can act as an icebreaker when you first return. You can acknowledge their gesture and say as much or as little as you wish about your health. It is often the initial silence when you first come back that creates tension. If you choose to tell just a few people at work how you are doing and give them an idea of how you would like others to behave, they can tell the rest of the people in your workplace how to approach you. If you find people avoiding you entirely, remember that it is because of their own fears and discomfort.

If you had a co-worker you did not get along with before your surgery, don't be surprised if that person begins to treat you better. Although you may be tempted to interpret the improved behavior as phony, it may be that your operation has led the person to see your relationship differently. Even the most bitter and resentful people often live by a code of ethics that dictates they not kick someone who is down. I encourage you to enjoy the break from previous negative feelings and power struggles and use it to help keep your stress level down while you focus on your recovery.

If you have been the instigator of your troubles with a co-worker, the emotional trauma of your mastectomy may give you a different perspective and you may want to rid yourself of negative energy in your relationships. Perhaps you will find yourself letting go of anger and resentment about a lot of little details that used to bother you. Improved relations with others in your workplace can be another of the hidden benefits that come from your mastectomy.

If you have a work situation in which you deal with a lot of clients and departments who are aware that you have been on a medical leave of absence but not aware why, you can tell them as much or as little as you wish. If you do not want to talk about your mastectomy you can say, "I was not well for a while, but I am feeling much better now. Thank you for asking," or something to that effect. Very few people would push past an

"Having a mastectomy has affected my self-esteem in a positive way. I feel like a warrior princess, like I can conquer anything!"

answer like that. If someone does press the issue and ask you what exactly was wrong, you can simply say, "It feels really good to be back at work and to not have to think about my health all the time."

Of course, you may want to talk about your condition, but be aware that in these early stages we can get quite emotional and it may not take much to send us into a fit of weepiness. We need breaks from thinking and talking about our mastectomy. Someone's gentle, caring questions can feel wonderfully supportive but can also open the floodgates of our sorrow, which at some workplaces can be inappropriate and uncomfortable. You may feel differently from day to day about how open you wish to be, and that is your prerogative.

DO I LOOK OKAY?

Trying to get ready for our first days back to work can be emotionally draining and very frustrating. We are usually ready to return to work long before our chests are completely healed or we have gotten comfortable wearing our prosthesis. Going back to work forces us to confront the realities of our situation, including changes to how we can dress, long before we are emotionally prepared. (See Chapters 9 and 10 for prosthesis and clothing tips.) When we go back to work we are often still struggling with grief and self-conscious about how we look. If you find your co-workers staring at your chest, remember that they are probably just curious, and that clothed, it is virtually impossible to tell that you have had a mastectomy. You can be certain that they will soon forget. Part of your emotional healing requires that you focus on the loss of your breast, but that does not mean everyone else is as fixated on how you look. Most people are only going to be concerned with how you feel and your health.

I strongly suggest that you go out into public a few times before you return to work. Even if you do not have the strength to buy groceries on your own, go with someone else so you have practice dressing in different clothes and spending time in the world. Try to get to a shop that carries postmastectomy items before you return to work. There are helpful early recovery clothes and other items that will be invaluable for your confidence and self-esteem. The fitter can also be extremely helpful in talking about your appearance and showing you some ways to accom-

"The first time I went out in public I felt like everyone was looking at me. After a couple of months, when I had my clothing and underclothes sorted out, I felt better."

modate your missing breast in attractive clothing. Talking about your appearance concerns with someone who understands will help you to feel less self-conscious as you return to public life.

I went through the experience of returning to work after breast surgery twice. The first time was after I had my elective mastectomies and immediate reconstruction. I had just completed my master's degree the month before and was working at two part-time jobs. I was the director of mental health services in a four-hundred bed, long-term facility where I had worked for four years. I was quite close to my staff and had let people know ahead of time about my upcoming surgery. Because I had immediate reconstruction with implants I did not have to deal with prostheses or clothing alterations. I had been in contact with my staff while I was on medical leave to let them know how I was doing. My first day back I was greeted with a lot of consoling smiles. People's biggest concern was whether or not they should hug me, or if that would hurt. I started back to work slowly, just a couple of days a week. My other job was in a very small mental health clinic where I was working as a psychotherapist. I had only been at the clinic for a month and had very few clients. I worked for a warm, sensitive psychiatrist who seemed to know just how to act, and I was not in a position to tell my clients about my surgery. Before I returned to either of those jobs I worried about how I looked but in both situations the openness of my co-workers, taken from my lead, made it more comfortable for all of us. In fact, I found going back to work easier than waiting for surgery.

Unsurprisingly, it was much more difficult to return to work after my second surgery when my ruptured implants were removed and I had to begin using external prostheses. I was working in a private psychotherapy practice with my husband, so I had no co-workers, just clients. I handed out a notice to all of my clients before my surgery explaining what kind of surgery I was having and why. I knew that my first patient would be the hardest and expected that it would get easier with each additional person. I worried about being in such close proximity with them in my small office, where they could see up close how I looked. I knew it was my job to attend to their emotional needs, and didn't want them to feel as though they had to take care of me, but I did want to allow them to

"Now I put out the garbage in a T-shirt without my prosthesis. I was worried that I would always be too self-conscious to do that sort of thing."

express their caring. I was also worried that my clients would be "too nice" to me, and that I might begin to sob. In spite of my depression, I quickly showed myself that I could cope. I was able to exchange a few words about my condition and then refocus my attention on my client's problems. One woman, about my age, greeted me by saying, "You look beautiful." My eyes became misty as I was deeply touched by her kind, accepting words, and I simply said, "Thanks." It was as if my clients knew how much I needed to focus on them to regain my confidence. My work helped tremendously to get me out of my house and back into a constructive, positive activity. It took me about two weeks to get beyond the intensity of facing clients for the first time after my surgery, but my concern about how I looked lasted longer. As my chest healed, and I went from fiber-filled to foam-filled and then to silicone prostheses, each new form made dressing easier and helped me feel more confident and comfortable. I believe I would have gone through these feelings of fear and sadness regardless of when I returned to work.

Two close friends of mine had similar experiences in their return to work after undergoing mastectomies. Getting comfortable with their co-workers again did not take long, and they both felt supported and cared for, but it took longer for them to feel comfortable about their appearances. One woman approached the situation with a lot of humor, which made it easier for her to talk about her struggles. Knowing that her co-workers felt comfortable enough to tease her again made her feel she was being treated the same as she had been before her surgery. People were not overly protective of her, which allowed her to focus attention away from her changed body. Both women found that the love and acceptance with which they were treated at work was good for their self-esteem and body image.

If You Are Not Returning To Work

Women who do not return to work often face special challenges as they do not have to reenter public life the way women who work outside the home do. Retired women and those who work at home need to make sure they do not become "shut-ins."

One woman I know is making tremendous changes in her life and particularly her work life that reflect a greater sense of self worth, as she goes through her struggle with breast cancer. Beth has challenged herself about how she spends money on herself. Her friends helped her to realize she had put money in a savings account for a rainy day but was not using it. It dawned on her to use some of her savings so she could have a longer medical leave. She held a belief that she always had to earn her worthiness, and battled with feelings of shame about not working, but she let her friends help her find a new attitude that was gentler with herself. Beth gave herself permission to not return to her private practice as an attorney because the stress was too great and she had been unhappy for several years before she was diagnosed with cancer. She decided it would serve her better to find a salaried part-time position in a law office and supplement her income by refinishing furniture, which she loves to do. Beth has made many changes in her diet and exercise routine as well as her work that have made her feel more positive and in control of her life. She has added meditation and Tai Chi as part of her spiritual life, which help her to stay connected to her body as well as build and maintain good self-esteem. Regardless of whether you return to an old job, change your job, or don't return to work at all, it is important to make sure you get back into the swing of life.

CHAPTER NINE

CHOOSING YOUR PROSTHESIS

A prosthesis is a fabricated substitute for a missing body part. A breast prosthesis is shaped like a breast and made of substances that are intended to feel and look like a real breast. Breast prostheses were first introduced in the 1950s. They come in different shapes, sizes, and skin tones to match your body features.

I have been advised by people in the business of marketing breast replacements not to refer to them as prostheses. Instead I have been told to call them breast forms. Calling a prosthesis a breast form is supposed to soften the sound and not put the postmastectomy woman in the same category as an amputee. I object to this approach because I believe it reflects a discriminatory attitude toward handicapped people and I also object to the suggestion that I have to be protected from the hard reality of my situation. I am not emotionally fragile and I want full credit for my loss. I lost both breasts, which were a very important part of my body, and I now wear two prostheses. As a result I use the terms prosthesis and breast form interchangeably.

There are three basic kinds of prostheses. The first is the fiber-filled nylon type that is used immediately after surgery. The second is a soft foam style, and the third is a weighted gel type, either silicone or some other type of synthetic material.

Fiber-Filled Prostheses

Fiber-filled prostheses are beige, nylon shells shaped like breasts that open in the back (the side that goes next to your chest) and are filled with a fiber-fill material similar to the material used as pillow stuffing. The opening in the back allows you to put in as much or as little of the fiber-fill as you want. The American and Canadian Cancer Societies provide them free as part of a visit from the Reach for Recovery volunteer which will usually take place during your hospital stay. Your doctor has to write an order before someone from Reach for Recovery can visit you. If you want to be visited make sure to tell your doctor. If you are no longer hospitalized, you can call the Cancer Society and they will arrange a visit for you at home. The fiber-filled prosthesis is not sold in specialty shops. If there is no Cancer Society chapter in your town call their central number before your surgery and they will mail you a fiber-filled prosthesis (see resources listed in the back of the book).

The fiber-filled prosthesis is very soft and comfortable against healing tissue but does not look or feel as natural as the other types. Because it is so soft and light it does not hold much shape or contour to your body like the other styles. Fiber-filled prostheses do allow you to experiment with size before you invest in a more permanent and expensive type. This is particularly helpful for women who have had a double mastectomy. Fiber-filled prostheses can also be very helpful when trying to alter lingerie, which will be covered in detail in Chapter 10. The extreme lightness of the fiber-fill prosthesis is a good match with the light materials used to make lingerie.

It is possible to experiment with different materials for your first prosthesis. I didn't particularly care for the fiber-filled prostheses so I experimented to make them more workable. I tried to find something that provided some shape but was also soft enough. Then I realized why I had saved all those spare shoulder pads over the years. Little did I know I would be able to use them after my mastectomies. I ended up cutting some shoulder pads to the same shape as the nylon prosthesis shell, and found that they worked very well combined with some of the filler material. I put the shoulder pad into the pocket first, then added the fiber-fill, so the shoulder pad was on the side that went next to my clothes. The shoulder pads were stiffer than the fiber-fill that came with the prostheses, so the prostheses had more form. They presented a smoother surface under my clothes and looked more natural.

Fiber-filled prostheses are the type most commonly used right after surgery.

"One day my sister
pointed out that I
was bouncing on one
side and not the
other. Once I got the
silicone prosthesis I
was more balanced."

Foam-Filled Prostheses

The second type of prosthesis is a foam-filled type. These are relatively inexpensive, costing approximately $30 to $70 U.S. for one breast form. Some insurance plans consider a foam-filled prosthesis an accessory rather than a prosthesis. Most insurance plans set a limit for the number of prostheses they will reimburse and an additional dollar figure for clothing and accessories. Because the foam-filled prostheses are inexpensive and insurance companies realize this type of prosthesis is often purchased in addition to a silicone prosthesis, they designate them as accessories to allow you to purchase both, while keeping the cost down by limiting the number of the more expensive silicone breast forms allowed.

Foam-filled prostheses generally come in an oval or butterfly shape. They are light and soft and can take a lot more wear and tear than the silicone type, as there is no concern about them bursting or rupturing. They are particularly convenient for doing such sports as volleyball or basketball, where you may be hit in the chest. Foam-filled prostheses work well in a tight-fitting sports bra. Foam breathes and will not trap perspiration between the prosthesis and your skin, so it is lighter and cooler to wear in the summer than a silicone type prosthesis.

Foam prostheses can be used for swimming but should not be used in a hot tub because they will shrink and become progressively stiffer and harder. They can be pinned into place with a tiny safety pin. However, repeated pinning will ultimately cause a deterioration where they are pinned and cause the foam to lose its fullness and shape, which might be noticeable under tight-fitting clothes and a sheer bra. Foam-filled prostheses are quite easy to care for. They can be washed by hand with a gentle soap. I use dish detergent or plain shampoo for mine. After I wear my foam prostheses in chlorine water I wash them out with a chlorine-removing shampoo. Because they can shrink they should always be washed in cool water. After washing them, roll them tightly into a tube shape to squeeze out the water. Then use a clothespin to hang them on a clothesline if they have a flap or lay them on a flat surface with the full, front side down. They will dry faster with the front down because gravity will pull the water to the peak in the breast and allow better drainage. It usually takes about eight to twelve hours to completely dry them out. Don't put your foam prosthesis in the dryer unless you use only the air setting with no heat.

I started using foam prostheses about two weeks after my surgery. My drainage tubes were out and I had healed enough to wear the slightly heavier forms. They made me feel more like my old self. I used them in a postmastectomy "undershirt" that came with fiber-filled prostheses and in bras that I had used before surgery. I was able to pin them in place so I did not yet have to concern myself with altering any of my clothing. Going back to work had been very difficult at first because I only had the fiber-fill prostheses. They felt like a wadded-up ball of tissue and I was worried about what people would think. I didn't want to put my clients in an awkward position. After all, they were coming to me for counseling. My role as a therapist, along with my weakened body, vulnerable emotional state, and lack of adequate clothing options, made this a very difficult time. When I began wearing the foam prostheses they really helped give me confidence that I could get back to a normal life again.

Experimenting with clothes and fillers helped me to feel that I had some control over my situation. I felt restless, bored, and scared all at the same time. Creating new methods to make myself feel presentable helped me feel less like a helpless victim. A big part of me just wanted to collapse into a ball and give up, but I knew that really wasn't an option. Every new little idea, such as using shoulder pads with my first fiber-filled prostheses, made me feel as though I was winning the fight to regain my power.

Silicone-Filled Prostheses

Silicone-filled prostheses are very soft and feel much like a natural breast. They contain silicone gell and are covered with a translucent film. Silicone prostheses are often referred to as permanent prostheses, which gives the impression that they will last forever. They are quite expensive, ranging from $180 to $450 U.S. per form. My bilateral set cost me $700. Unfortunately, they are not at all permanent. They usually come with a two-year warranty and can last between two and ten years. Three to five years is a more realistic life expectancy. Since women are getting and sur-

In some areas the Cancer Society or various postmastectomy shops donate prostheses to women who cannot afford them.

Wash your silicone
prosthesis using the
same soap you use
on yourself or
your hair.

viving breast cancer at ever younger ages, we need our prostheses for many years. This means we will probably purchase several over the remainder of our lives.

A postmastectomy specialty shop manager explained that there are two types of silicone used to make the prostheses. The silicone prostheses costing about $300 to $400 U.S. are made of top-grade silicone in a thick gell that holds its shape. The silicone prostheses that sell for about $180 U.S. are made of a lower grade silicone that has a more liquid consistency. The less expensive type comes with a permanent cloth covering that is used to hold the shape, since the silicone is not thick enough to do that on its own. The less expensive one is harder to wash because of the cover, and it will not last as long as the more expensive one. Even with the cover, the lower grade of silicone prostheses does not offer as firm and consistent a shape as the more expensive ones.

Silicone prostheses are used after the surgical area is essentially healed. They are made to contour to your chest and to match your body shape and size. They come in many different shapes, such as oval, triangular, and butterfly (see Figure 9-1). The classic asymmetrical (triangular) style can be used interchangeably on either side. But many styles of silicone breast forms are made to be worn on either the right or the left and have a tail designed to give more fullness to the side of your chest. Your healing must be complete because, if you are fitted for a silicone prosthesis before all the swelling is gone, you may end up with the wrong shape or size.

Silicone-filled prostheses come in different skin tones. Typically they are made in three shades: ivory, blush, and tonie. Ivory is meant for very light-skinned women, tonie is a very dark tone intended for African American women, and the blush tone falls between the other two shades. Sandra, an African American who owns a postmastectomy specialty shop, told me that she sees the industry making an effort to accommodate all women, but admits they have a long way to go. She was asked by one company representative what new products were most needed and she told them more options in the darker tones should be available. Shortly after she provided her input, she received a new sili-

Figure 9-1 Common prostheses shapes

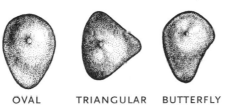

OVAL   TRIANGULAR   BUTTERFLY

cone prosthesis that was completely black. She laughed remembering it because, of course, there is no human being on this earth who has truly black skin just as there is no person with totally white skin. She said the prosthesis was made by a small company in a small town and she could only assume they had not seen many black people. She was able to tolerate their ignorance because she recognized that they were making an attempt to serve all women. Another specialty shop fitter told me that choices in breast forms all boil down to money. Because there is a smaller dark-skinned population to serve, it is not profitable to offer many options in darker skin tones. I can guess at the pain and anger many women must have felt when there was only the ivory breast form available. It is painful enough to have cancer and lose a breast without being faced with a prosthesis that does not recognize one's racial uniqueness. This frustration still exists for women of color as of this writing because only two manufacturers produce prostheses in darker skin tones and they only offer one shape and no attachment nipple.

The first time I held a silicone prosthesis in my hand it felt very strange. I had a difficult time trying to imagine wearing one, let alone two. It struck me as heavy and burdensome. When I began wearing the foam forms I thought they would be just fine. They were cheap, soft, light, and, most importantly, they felt like just another clothing item. The way the silicone prosthesis felt reminded me of a chicken breast. This makes sense, since the prosthesis attempts to replicate the feel and weight of flesh. The fitter I was working with said I would eventually want a silicone form because they feel more natural and stay in place. My resistance to having to deal with breast replacement made it easy for me

"What the specialty shops have to offer is pretty limited. There is no way to get an exact fit, so I have had to come up with some alterations on my own."

to be skeptical and think that the emphasis on silicone prostheses was a way to sell the most expensive product. I was also afraid of having anything to do with silicone again, since my implants had made me so ill.

As time passed and I physically healed and began to adjust emotionally, I could start to see the truth in what the fitter had told me. The foam form was so light that it kept riding up on me. This is less of a problem for women with one breast remaining, but it can still be annoying for them. The foam form was stiff, whereas the silicone one actually has a little bounce to it like a normal breast. I asked my surgeon and he felt the silicone wouldn't cause a health problem because the silicone was completely encased and was being used externally. He couldn't tell whether I would have an allergic reaction to the prostheses because I was already hypersensitive to the chemical compound from my ruptured implants. But, he added, if I didn't feel comfortable I could switch back to the foam-filled ones, especially during the hot summer months.

I took my questions about the silicone prostheses back to the fitter. She had the most experience watching women's reactions to these products. She told me that prostheses cause skin irritation for some women but it is extremely rare. She also pointed out that the silicone breast forms were sold with a cloth cover for women who were not comfortable wearing them directly against their skin. The cover is a cotton pocket the breast form slips into before putting it into a bra.

I was concerned about spending such a large amount of money and then finding out I could not tolerate the silicone forms, but the fitter explained that the prostheses came with a warranty and the shop would allow me to return them if there was a problem with the fit or they caused a skin reaction. Because the shop absorbed the cost of those returns, they worked hard to achieve a correct fit from the beginning. The returned prostheses were donated to the American Cancer Society for women who could not afford to buy them. Not every place that sells postmastectomy products provides the same service, so find out what your dealers offer and use this knowledge to decide which dealer or shop to give your business to. The more we postmastectomy women assert ourselves as a group, the more the industry will have to become competitive and work to accommodate us.

By the time my body had healed enough to be fitted for the silicone breast form, my psyche was also ready. They felt much more natural than my foam prostheses. Without a cover they can feel cold when you first put them on, but they soon adjust to your body temperature, which also makes them feel a part of you. They usually come with at least a partially hollowed out back to accommodate all kinds of surgery. Once I had my silicone prostheses I became much more comfortable giving and receiving hugs because I knew I felt more natural. I also had a greater sense of balance. The feeling of balance that silicone prostheses provide is especially appreciated and valuable for women who still have one breast.

CARE OF YOUR SILICONE PROSTHESIS

There are a number of simple things you will need to do to take care of your silicone prosthesis. First of all, the prosthesis will need to be washed. If you are wearing it against your skin, you should wash it daily to prevent oil buildup from affecting the outer casing. If you are wearing the form completely covered, and have not perspired much, you will not need to wash it as often. Since mine are covered and I don't wear them during physical exercise, I wash them about once a week, except during very hot spells in the summer months. Wash the prosthesis using mild soap, such as the soap you use on your face or in the shower. Gently soap it and rinse it with warm water, then pat it dry with a towel.

Silicone prostheses have to be worn and handled carefully to keep them from being punctured. They should never be worn around pins or stored near sharp objects. Some women pin the cloth cover that comes with the form to other garments to hold it in place. Be very careful that the pin does not open and puncture the prosthesis. Also be careful when someone is pinning a corsage on you, or when you add a decorative pin to your outfit.

If you store your silicone prosthesis properly it will last much longer. The breast form comes packaged in a box with a mold inside to hold it. It is strongly recommended that you store the form in this box when you aren't wearing it. However, there are a few suitable alternatives for storage. Don't lay the form on a flat surface because it will lose its shape and deteriorate from pressure on certain points of the prosthesis. Your pros-

Your silicone prostheses can be safely stored face down in a drawer of clothes that has been arranged to support its shape.

thesis should be stored with the full, front part facing down into something that will support the shape. The prosthesis is intended to be removed from your bra every time you are not wearing it and placed in its original box. If you are not using a pocket in your bra and need to wash the prosthesis daily, placing it in its box will not be a problem. However, a lot of women want to be able to leave their prosthesis in their altered or pocketed bra until the bra needs to be washed. Storage, too, can be a problem if you have limited space in your bedroom, especially if you have two prostheses boxes.

A handy alternative is to place your prosthesis (in or out of your bra) face down into a drawer of clothes. Make an indentation in the pile of clothing to support the full part of your form. As long as the prosthesis is not resting on a flat surface, and the full part is supported while placed face down, it should be fine. Your underwear drawer will most likely work best, because it holds clothes that are soft, small, and movable, which makes it easy to create an indentation for the form. I find it convenient to keep my prostheses in my bra and leave them in my underwear drawer. Even if I have changed my bra, at the end of the day I will put my prostheses in a fresh bra and leave them in the drawer overnight because I am always short of time in the mornings and don't want to fool with one more detail when I am getting dressed. I store the original boxes under my bed in case I wish to use them some day.

It was recommended to me that I should carry those boxes to store my prostheses when I travel. This wasn't a practical suggestion because the boxes are quite large, even for small breast forms. Like most people, I try to keep my luggage to a minimum and I don't have room for two large boxes. I always wear my silicone prostheses when traveling because they are too expensive to risk losing or being damaged in the baggage handling process. What a panic it would be to lose a breast form! It isn't as though you can go to the nearest drug store or department store and pick one up. Once you have reached your destination, your prosthesis will keep very nicely in a suitcase full of clothes, just as they do in your underwear drawer.

The silicone breast form is made to withstand exposure to salt water and chlorine. I was told by my fitter that the silicone form could be used in a hot tub because it was manufactured under very high temperatures, but the catalogs that display these products specifically say they are not recommended for hot tubs. I spoke to a consultant from one of the leading breast form manufacturers and she confirmed that they are not recommended for use in a hot tub. She said the only forms recommended for hot tub use are the foam prostheses. Even though the foam-filled forms shrink and become hard from the hot water, I still wear them in the hot tub instead of my silicone forms because the foam-filled forms are less expensive to replace.

I want to stress the importance of checking your form regularly for defects, especially while it is still under warranty. We all want to believe that once we get fitted we won't have to worry about our forms again for a long time, and because they are so expensive we expect them to hold up. My fitter had suggested I bring them in to have her inspect them every six months during the warranty period. I followed her advice for the first year and a half and then felt I didn't need to do it that one last time. About one week before the warranty was up I looked closely at them and found some little bubbles. I immediately took them into the specialty shop and had them replaced with a new set. Both prostheses were starting to break down. The warranty usually states that a prosthesis will be replaced if found to be defective within the two-year period, but replacement forms will not be covered under a new warranty.

When inspecting your prosthesis, look for tiny bubbles. Because many of you will purchase your form through the mail or from a dealer who is not close to home, you will need to rely on yourself to do the inspecting. Bubbles will usually start to form close to the seam or edge, on the lower part. You should inspect for bubbles along the entire edge of the seam on both sides. Another way to check for bubbles is to place the form in your flat, firmly held hand with the full front side down. Then let the form gently relax into your hand while you keep your hand firm and straight. This position should allow the center of the form to be more exposed while the sides relax. Now look for any little bubbles in the center of the form. Some prostheses have little indentations in the center of the back for comfort and to help keep their shape. When you hold the form in your palm, the little holes or indentations should not fill up with gel.

Silicone prostheses give the closest weight and feel to a natural breast.

Look out for tiny
bubbles in your
silicone prostheses
as they indicate that
the gel is breaking
down.

You can also gently push the gel up through these holes from the other side to look for bubbles. If you have to push the gel through the hole, and it does not show bubbles, it is not deteriorating.

Bubbles mean that the gel is starting to breakdown into a more liquid form. Without the gel consistency the form will lose its shape because it will not have enough density. The outer casing will help to give shape but it will not be as good as it was before the breakdown. Your prosthesis will develop large air bubbles as the gel liquifies, which will push on the back of the breast form, making it change in size and shape. Once your prosthesis shows a few little bubbles, it will take between two and six months before it will completely liquify and look much different.

In chapter 10 I discourage the use of underwire bras; this should help you appreciate why. The constant rubbing against such a hard surface can cause the chemical breakdown to take place, making your prosthesis watery.

Attachable Silicone Breast Forms

One manufacturer offers a silicone breast form that can be attached to the chest with an adhesive strip called the "adhesive skin support." In essence, the breast form is velcroed to your chest. The adhesive strip is about an inch wide and is shaped something like a triangle (see Figure 9-2). The strip lines the outer edges of the back of the prosthesis. One half of the strip is permanently attached to the back of the prosthesis and the other half comes with a very strong adhesive on the back to attach to your chest. The strip is intended to be worn all the time and the adhesive is supposed to last for a week. In actuality, the strips last anywhere from three days to three weeks, but three to seven days is typical. This will vary according to lifestyle, and body and skin type. Higher activity levels, frequent bathing, swimming, and perspiring may decrease the length of time an adhesive strip will remain attached to your skin.

Each attachable silicone breast form costs about $450 U.S. The strips are $5 U.S. each and come in packages of five. The cost of this breast form is likely to exceed the amount that your insurance plan will reimburse and the strips are often not covered by insurance. You should be

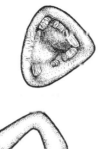

Figure 9-2 Attachable silicone breast form

able to order the strips from the same place you purchase your prosthesis.

When you are not wearing your breast form attached to your chest, you should wear it in the cotton cover it comes with, so the other side of the strip does not rub against your skin. When you do have your prosthesis attached to your chest, you can use regular bras without pockets, go without a bra, or wear a strapless bra. The most desirable feature of the attachable silicone prosthesis is that it allows you to wear more styles of clothing, such as backless sundresses or strapless evening gowns.

There are a few drawbacks to attachable prostheses. The adhesive strip cannot be put on or taken off at will. You need to wait until the adhesive wears off before removing it because the adhesive is so strong that if you try to take it off before the adhesive has worn off, it will cause a skin irritation. You will have to be comfortable with the strip as a regular part of you. You will wear it in the shower and to bed every night, as well as during lovemaking.

Many women love this style of prosthesis because fashion was a big part of their life before surgery and they like the increased clothing options the attachable breast form provides.

I recommend that you ask for a sample of the adhesive strip and go home and try it before actually buying an attachable silicone prosthesis.

The postmastectomy industry has a long way to go to address the prostheses needs of women of color.

It sounded wonderful. For a bit more money I could have more clothing choices. I wanted to know that I was still an attractive woman who could still dress to look sexy. A little voice in my head reminded me that I had never really dressed that way before, so why would I start in my early forties? I also realized that I would have to have two sets of bras, one with pockets for when I didn't use the adhesive strip and another set of regular bras to be used with the adhesive strip. I pushed my concerns aside and decided to order the attachable forms.

I went home with a sample adhesive strip to try on my chest while I waited for my prostheses to be delivered. I put the strip on, wore it to bed and through the next day, and realized that it was not going to work for me. Because I am naturally a very kinesthetic person who relates to life through the feel of my body, I was overly aware of and bothered by the presence of the strip on my body. It reinforced my sense of loss. I felt ashamed and defective with the strip on and wanted to hide my body from my husband. I did not like bumping into a rough thing on my chest while showering and could not imagine having my husband experience the same thing during lovemaking. I did not anticipate wearing my prostheses during lovemaking, which would leave the rough, velcro-like strip exposed. I figured if I was having this kind of reaction while wearing only one strip it would be much worse wearing two. It seemed ridiculous to put myself through this just so I could wear a certain kind of evening dress maybe once every five years. Because I did not want to wear the strip anymore I pulled it off before the adhesive had worn off, leaving a raised, inflamed, slightly painful red mark that took several days to heal. I called my fitter back and had her stop the order and replace it with the same prostheses without the adhesive strip.

If you decide on the attachable breast form, keep in mind that you will probably also want to purchase a foam-filled prosthesis to use when you are extremely physical. The adhesive strip is supposed to keep your form on securely for most activities, especially when the strip is new, but I wouldn't count on it holding the prosthesis in place during vigorous athletic activity. You may be very comfortable dancing in an evening dress at a wedding, but I would not recommend playing volleyball on the beach in a bathing suit and expecting the strip to hold. A new adhesive strip has just come out that has an even stronger bonding property for more active women and women who perspire heavily. If your skin is not sensitive and you don't have skin problems from radiation treatments, you may want to try the stronger adhesive strips.

Non-Silicone Prostheses

Some companies also sell breast forms made out of other types of syn thetic material which is supposed to feel like natural tissue. They are weighted in much the same way as the silicone prostheses. They only come in one shape and one skin tone (beige) and do not have an attachable style with the adhesive strip. They are less expensive than silicone prostheses, about $200 U.S. per prosthesis. These are a good choice for those who are allergic to the materials used to make the silicone prosthesis. The non-silicone weighted breast forms are puncture proof and can be worn in chlorine and salt water. They also come with a cloth cover.

I consider the non-silicone prostheses somewhere between the foam-filled and the silicone type based on how natural they feel and how long they wear. They come with a one-year warranty. The material does not feel as much like normal tissue as a silicone prosthesis, but is much closer to flesh than a foam-filled one. The extra weight helps them to stay in place, but they don't have the bounce of silicone forms. When they begin to deteriorate, the synthetic material becomes lumpy, similar to an old, overused, foam-rubber couch pillow.

This prosthesis may be a practical option for athletic activities. You care for it by hand washing it. It can be used in a regular or a postmastectomy bra.

It is also possible to make your own weighted breast form. One woman I met made her own prosthesis using a bean bag, which seemed to have just the right weight. The key is to assume that if you are persistent enough you will find a way to reshape an attractive breast and achieve a comfortable sense of balance.

The important thing we need to ask ourselves when choosing a prosthesis is what is going to be the best match for us. Really listen to your own needs and don't allow yourself to be talked into buying something that just isn't right for you. Buying a prosthesis is an emotionally vulner-

Your fitter is in a
position to answer
almost all of your
questions about
breast forms. Be sure
that you make up
your own mind about
the products that
best suit you and
your lifestyle.

able time and even the strongest and most assertive woman can find herself being talked into something by a fitter. We may feel that the fitter can help us become normal again, so we tend to listen to them more than to ourselves. Our job is to take in the information about our prosthesis options, then give ourselves enough time to process all of it to reach the best decision. Fitters often don't realize the power of influence they have over us at that time in our lives. I was fortunate to have a fitter who repeatedly told me that if I got home and had second thoughts, I could change my decision. If you do not feel comfortable with your fitter, take your business elsewhere.

Matching a Mate

One of the most difficult and frustrating problems faced by women who only have one breast removed is trying to match a standard-size prosthesis to their remaining breast. Just as it can be a challenge to make standard-size bras fit body shapes which come in all shapes and sizes, making a prosthesis match a natural breast poses the same type of problem.

The difficulty might be discovered when it is time to be fitted for your first silicone prosthesis, or it might become a problem later if you should gain or lose a lot of weight. As you probably know from past experience, your breasts are one of the first places to show weight changes. When we have both natural breasts, weight changes just mean having to go up or down a cup size in a bra. But when you must match your remaining breast with a very expensive fixed-sized prosthesis, size changes become a much bigger issue.

This is such a common problem that products have been invented to remedy the situation where the natural breast has become larger than the prosthesis. You may hear them referred to as breast enhancers, equalizers, or accessories. Enhancer and equalizer are interchangeable terms. They come in cloth, foam, or silicone gel. A silicone enhancer costs between $45 and $175 U.S. and the foam and cloth varieties cost between $6 and $20 U.S. per enhancer. Your insurance company may require a doctor's order for the most expensive silicone equalizer before they will reimburse the cost. An enhancer is a thin cup that is placed in the prosthesis pocket of your bra before the prosthesis is inserted. The weight of the breast form holds the enhancer in place. Breast enhancers have been available for years, mainly from major department store catalogs, in the lingerie section. Now breast enhancers come in specialty catalogs for postmastectomy wear and are carried by the same businesses who sell prostheses. Their care is the same as for foam-filled and silicone prostheses.

It can be a challenge to match a prosthesis to a natural breast.

If your remaining breast changes size and no longer matches your prosthesis, or a standard-size prosthesis does not match your natural breast, you can temporarily improvise with shoulder pads.

Of course the best way to keep evenly-sized breasts is to maintain a steady body weight. If you start to put on a few pounds, reduce your calories and the number of grams of fat in your daily diet, and increase your level of exercise. It will be a lot easier if you watch your weight closely and do not let your weight go up more than three to five pounds before taking it off. It takes a long time to take off ten pounds and many people give up halfway so that they put on a few extra pounds every year like clockwork. This weight gain is not healthy and can take a real toll on your self-esteem.

It is important to acknowledge, however, that maintaining a stable weight is not always possible and you should not mentally beat yourself up for gaining weight. In addition, women going through chemotherapy are told to increase their caloric intake to strengthen the body's reserve with added nutrients and at the same time many experience nausea that prevents them from regular exercise. On the other hand, some women have trouble eating enough during chemotherapy because of their nausea and they lose weight. If this is the case for you, when your treatment finishes your weight will probably stabilize to where it was before your surgery.

If you are serious about wanting to lose weight I encourage you to talk to your doctor about how and when it would be safe for you to attempt weight loss. There are also many excellent weight loss clinics. When selecting a weight loss program make sure the staff includes a physician and requires an initial physical exam. Weight Watchers offers a medically sound, self-help weight loss program that you can use after your doctor has given you the go-ahead to diet.

Modified mastectomies and lumpectomies can also pose a problem when you are trying to even out breast size and shape. The missing portion of the breast can leave a noticeable indentation through fitted clothing. Most companies that supply postmastectomy products offer accessories just for this purpose. A selection of cloth and silicone products (which are referred to as accessories), made to fill in the portion of the breast that was surgically removed, are now available. An equalizer is often used when a significant amount of tissue has been removed. The price can range from a few dollars up to about $175 U.S., depending on the size and the material from which they are made.

If your lump was located in the lower part of your breast, the accessory or enhancer will be held in place by the weight of your breast, so a pocket to hold the additional piece in place is not needed. But tissue missing from the top portion of the breast is more difficult to fill in because there is no breast covering the piece to anchor it. A foam or cloth accessory will work best if you are missing tissue from the top of the breast because you can pin or sew it to your bra. The silicone equalizers do not work well on the top because they cannot be pinned or sewn.

Some women have a significant collapse in the chest wall after a mastectomy. This will affect how well a prosthesis matches the remaining breast or a second prosthesis worn on the side without the collapse matches the other side. I have quite a bit of caving in on one side but it does not affect how my prosthesis sits because the collapse falls primarily in the center of the back of my prosthesis, leaving enough tissue for the prosthesis to rest on. But for many women this collapse or caving in can be large enough or in a location of your chest that makes your prosthesis sink in and appear smaller than the other breast. If using a larger prosthesis does not achieve a balanced look, you can purchase pads that are designed to fill in the chest wall. The pad sits between your chest and your prosthesis and the weight of your prosthesis should hold it in place. These pads are also called accessories and cost only a few dollars. A breast enhancer may also solve this problem by adding more fullness to the collapsed side.

Nipples

Most silicone breast forms either have a slight bump that looks like a nipple when seen through clothing or a more defined, natural-looking nipple. However, there are some silicone forms that come without a nipple, or with a nipple that does not match the one on the remaining natural breast. The prosthesis nipple may be a different size or in a different location from the nipple on the remaining breast.

In this case you may want to purchase a prosthesis without a nipple and use an attachable nipple. The attachable nipple is attached to the polyurethane skin that covers the silicone prosthesis. An adhesive cannot be used to secure the nipple because it would cause the coating of your silicone prosthesis to break down. It attaches through the suction that is created between the two surfaces, which only works with silicone prostheses. Nipples come in two sizes, small and large, and only in blush and ivory skin tones. They are easy to care for. You just hand wash and towel them dry.

My fitter said most women do not use them because they do not stay on very securely and most women find that the nipple on the silicone prosthesis is adequate. If you are going to use an attachable nipple you need to keep in mind that the artificial nipple will not become erect in response to temperature changes, so it will still look different than your remaining nipple under certain circumstances.

Developing a Relationship with Your Prosthesis

Your prosthesis needs to become a part of you if you are going to become comfortable about how your prosthesis fits into your daily life. Building a working relationship with your prosthesis will take away the sense that it is a burden. It will become instead, a desirable means of helping you feel attractive.

Developing a relationship with your prosthesis builds off the exercises to treat phantom pain. If you have not been bothered with phantom pain, I recommend that you spend some time reading the material from Chapter 5. You should also review the body image section in Chapter 5.

Initially, a prosthesis can feel like a burdensome thing that we hang on our bodies and carry around. This can create a heavy mood and make

Try to get comfortable seeing your prosthesis as a part of you. The more you incorporate it into your life the less you will resent it.

us feel depressed or resentful. If we develop a relationship with our prosthesis, we can see it as something that serves us. We need to befriend it instead of being embarrassed about it or resenting it. The prosthesis offers us a way to feel more normal and feminine. It is tempting to pretend that the prosthesis does not exist or devalue it and hide it. After all, this is a breast replacement, and the breast is still a private part of our body. But feeling private about our prosthesis is quite different from feeling that it is a shameful secret.

So not only do we have to see our existing body in an accurate way, we also need to create a mental picture of ourselves that includes our prosthesis. We need to allow ourselves to see how the prosthesis makes us look. We also need to know how we experience wearing the prosthesis. Most of us wear a prosthesis many hours of every day so it behooves us to think about what the prosthesis means to us and what role we want it to play in our lives.

The importance you attach to your prosthesis will probably be similar to the importance you placed on your breasts before you had one or both removed. If your breasts were something you just took for granted and did not pay much attention to, you are likely to also down play the importance of your prosthesis. However, if you were the kind of woman who really liked your breasts, enjoyed shopping for them, and made them a special part of your appearance, you are likely to give the same kind of attention to how you choose and wear your prosthesis. Your previous selection of bras is a good indicator of how you related to your breasts before surgery. If you preferred a soft, simple, casual style of bra, then comfort is probably a high priority for you and you are probably more inclined to want a natural look. If you liked fancy, lacy, sexier styles of bras, then you are probably more inclined to go for a particular look than to be concerned about comfort. And of course, many of us fit into both categories. We have our natural, casual times and we also have our sexy, pretty times which are reflected in our clothes, including our undergarments.

Achieving awareness about how you thought and felt about your breasts before your mastectomy allows you to think about what you wish to achieve with your prosthesis. You may want to reread the section in Chapter 1, What Our Breasts Have Meant to Us. Have you ever asked yourself what it feels like to have breasts? Do you know what sensations they bring to you through touch? And what does it feel like to walk around with breasts? For instance, how much do your breasts bounce when you walk? When does bouncing pose a problem? Does it hurt when you are jogging but feel fine when you are casually walking in a swimsuit along the beach?

Your prosthesis needs to become a part of you in order for you to not feel physically fragmented or lacking. This is the time to make some choices about what makes you feel most like the kind of woman you wish to be. You may achieve this by trying to re-create a feel and appearance that matches how you were before your surgery, or you may want to develop somewhat of a different you. Some women are sick of very large breasts and enjoy wearing smaller prostheses after a bilateral mastectomy. They have fun wearing a variety of clothes they could never wear before because they were too large-breasted. They find a sense of freedom they never had after they hit puberty. On the other hand, some women have felt cheated with their small breasts and wear larger prostheses. They are likewise able to wear new styles of clothes that were not an option before. This is a possibility for women who have had both breasts removed as well as for women with just one breast gone. Breast enhancers make it possible to add to your smaller remaining breast if you wish to purchase a larger prosthesis.

If you have had a bilateral mastectomy, you have the option of going bigger some of the time and smaller at other times. You may choose a larger silicone prosthesis that is worn most of the time but a smaller foam style for athletic activities. Having a bounce is usually not desirable when you are trying to play tennis or run bases on a baseball diamond. For rigorous athletic activities a smaller, lighter breast that does not move around will work best. Having no breasts during sports is often what women wish for because breasts tend to get in the way. Now you can choose the size of your breasts during various activities.

Once you have explored and defined how you want your body to look

A hidden benefit of a double mastectomy is the opportunity to wear larger or smaller breasts at will.

Accessories and
enhancers are items
used to keep breasts
looking evenly
matched and to fill in
space left after a
lumpectomy.

and feel, you are ready to start experimenting with different ways of bringing life to your prosthesis. I found that I compartmentalized my brain with regard to my body image. In one compartment I deal with my body image and my phantom sensations. I have a clear image of my body as it looks now and I limit my breast sensations to my remaining flesh. If I have a tickle or an itch, I feel it only on my actual chest wall, where my breasts used to be.

My second mental compartment contains my body image as it incorporates my prosthesis. The more I have worn my different prostheses, the more I feel as though they are part of me. When I had my silicone implants put in, I did not have to change where my brain sent messages of sensation because I did not have a missing space, but I did have to relate to how the implants felt to my hand and how it felt to have them in my body and in my clothes. They felt different than my natural breasts when I walked, ran, washed myself, and made love. Initially I did not like the unnatural feel of them and I had to get used to how they looked. Eventually my implants felt like a part of me, and I developed an accepting attitude toward them and learned to like and appreciate their positive aspects. My breasts were finally even in size and fit into a standard-size bra cup. I would grow old without having sagging breasts. In fact, I would have the best-looking breasts in the whole nursing home. And most importantly, my implants had enabled me to avoid breast cancer.

When I first got my prostheses I was faced with the same situation. The prostheses felt as if they just hung off me, yet I did not want to wear a heavy, harness type of bra. In time I realized the problem was not with the type of prostheses I had purchased or with the style of bra I was wearing; instead it had to do with developing a working relationship between my body and my prostheses. I needed to extend a sense of my living body to my prostheses. I found myself taking more interest in how the prostheses felt during various activities. I could not extend a sense of nerve impulses to the prostheses, but I could make them feel more like a part of me. The attachment seemed to happen from the outside in, rather than from the inside out. It was as if I saw myself willfully adding my prostheses to my body as I discovered how they could serve me. This made them feel more alive to me, rather than being things I had to lug around. Of course, I do not really think my prostheses contain my life energy or life force and, I know that they are not living tissue. This is merely a symbolic way of thinking and picturing how my prostheses fit with my body, so I can accept their presence in my life without resenting them. Also, by picturing my prostheses as a part of me I feel more confident and natural wearing them.

CHAPTER TEN

MAKING CLOTHES
WORK AGAIN

Our society is set up to accommodate women with breasts. We need breasts to fill out those bras the manufacturers make, as well as the darts and extra space in the chest area of most of our clothes. So the big question is, how do we acceptably fit into the world of clothing again when we are missing a breast or breasts?

Clothing During Recovery

It would be wonderful if there were just one simple solution for replacing a breast and clothing ourselves after a mastectomy, but unfortunately it isn't that easy. First, you have to find clothes for the first few weeks after your surgery. Immediately after surgery you will probably find that all those bulky bandages will be sufficient to fill in some of the empty space under an oversized shirt or pajama top. If you have only lost one breast, you might be able to wear a T-shirt if it is very large and you begin by putting it over the arm on your affected side so you don't have to stretch the arm up very far. However, most of us find a button-down blouse or shirt the most comfortable in the beginning of our healing process.

The most helpful garment I found for those early days of my recovery, before I was healed enough to wear a bra, was a little knit "undershirt" that came with an extra panel in the breast area, sewn to the outside. It reminded me of a little girl's undershirt because it had small straps and a form-fitting cotton body. The panel opened at the bottom and fastened with velcro. The one I used was called Vitali-Tee and it now sells for $80 U.S. I found the Vitali Tee at a specialty postmastectomy shop. My insurance paid for 80% of the cost. One of my friends received her care through a women's breast clinic and they provided her with one of these undershirts as part of their routine post-surgery packets. My undershirt came with two fiber-filled prostheses covered in a white cotton material and designed as a pocket with a panel in the back, so fiber could be added or subtracted as desired. The shirt had a velcro strip inside the panel and on the prostheses so the prostheses could be attached. In addition, the American Cancer Society provided me with another temporary set of prostheses, much like the one that came with the "undershirt." They could be pinned to the inside of a shirt without the undershirt, but putting them in the undershirt first made them much more comfortable and secure.

I really want to encourage you to find comfortable clothing for that initial healing period. We go through enough misery after a mastectomy without having to suffer from returning to a bra too soon. There are lots of tank tops, undershirts, and camisoles that can easily be altered by adding a front panel, if you don't have access to ready-made products or if they are too expensive for your budget and not covered by insurance.

"Since my surgery, I find that what I wear and how I wear it has become really important."

Bras

After your drainage tubes are out and your surgical area has healed, you will probably feel that you can tolerate wearing a bra for a few hours. You won't be ready for your permanent prosthesis yet, but wearing a bra will give you more clothing options. Your first bra should have a wide enough band around your ribs so it will not cut into your incision if your incision is below your breasts. The softer the bra material, the better. Your nerve endings will be so raw at this point they will not need further irritation from scratchy lace. This is the time to really listen to your body. If a bra is uncomfortable, wait a bit longer or try another style.

You have three basic options when it comes to bra types. There are ready-made postmastectomy bras with pockets sewn into them, standard bras without alterations, and standard bras with alterations. One type of bra is not better than another, it is purely a matter of personal

Postmastectomy
bras tend to be quite
heavy duty and may
not suit women who
were used to a
light style.

preference. Your previous way of dressing, body and breast size, financial resources, availability of products, and comfort level will all play a part in the choices you make. You may end up using several different bra styles to accommodate your different activities.

Think of the bras you chose before surgery. You most likely have a drawer full of different kinds of bras in varying colors, textures, and styles. In some ways, adjusting our bras to our postmastectomy bodies reminds me of when we first developed breasts. Most of us began with a simple little bra and gradually added new styles as our bodies changed and we entered into new activities. Before we knew it we had a lacy bra, a black bra, a strapless bra, and a sporting bra. Think of your new body as a chance to relive a bit of your adolescence as you grow into a new kind of woman again.

Many women find that they are quite happy using ordinary store-bought bras. They don't have to bother with expensive specialty products. They appreciate being able to just slip in their prosthesis without having to fuss with a pocket, and like knowing their bras can be thrown in the dryer without worrying too much about how often they have to replace them.

STANDARD BRAS

Women who use regular bras may have already been using an adequately styled bra or may have changed their style to one that has enough support to hold the prosthesis.

One woman I spoke with said she wears regular bras but had to change the V-cut style she wore before her surgery. She found that she had to go to a bra with more support in the center between the cups. In order to use a regular bra, the cup has to completely cover the prosthesis; otherwise the breast form can slip out or move around, giving the breast a strange shape. V-cut bras do not have enough fabric in the center to completely cover a prosthesis, and if your prosthesis extends beyond the cup it will cause a bulge or unsightly line which will be noticeable through form-fitting clothes. I have found that bras with a curved shape in the center, and at least one inch of material between the cups extending up from the rib band, work best.

Ready-made postmastectomy bras come with sewn-in pockets in the cups. The pocket is usually left open on the top part with a flap that folds back to allow you to slip your prosthesis into the pocket. The flap may or may not have a snap to keep the pocket closed. The flap should stay in place once it is resting between your chest and the prosthesis. Sometimes the opening is on the outer side of the cup instead of on the top. Netting, stretchy nylon, or a stretchy polyester/cotton blend are used for the pocket.

Postmastectomy bras tend to be full-support bras with a wide rib band, closed at the back with three hooks. The center piece of material between the cups usually extends $1^1/_2$ – 2 inches up from the rib band. They come in nylon, polyester, and cotton. Some are smooth and simple while others are quite lacy. Postmastectomy bras are generally only available in beige, white, and black. These specialty bras are very well made and should hold up a long time, especially if they aren't put in the dryer. These bras are excellent for larger-breasted women.

One of the reasons postmastectomy bras are most often made in the heavier, more secure style is because breast cancer occurs most frequently in women over age fifty. Many older women come from a generation that was taught to conceal their bodies, so the industry has been trying to provide postmastectomy products that suit women in their fifties, sixties, and seventies. However, many of us have had mastectomies at a much younger age, and we want different options. Hopefully the medical supply industry will soon to take note and provide a wider range of styles.

Many postmastectomy bras have a pocket made with the same sort of net material used to make a bridal veil. I personally could not imagine wearing such an abrasive material against delicate skin. The breast skin is naturally very sensitive, and after a mastectomy the remaining skin is usually even more sensitive because of nerve damage. I have to wonder whether the person who decided to use netting for the pocket was a man with very thick skin. This type of bra pocket is best avoided.

A postmastectomy bra bought through a medical supply store or specialty shop will probably cost between $35 and $60 U.S. Many insurance

One option if you do not care for standard postmastectomy bras is to alter standard bras.

Find out how much
your insurance will
cover towards
postmastectomy
products, including
bras, before you buy.

plans specify a set amount of money that can be used each year toward bras, but others may set an actual number of garments and a "usual and customary" price. You can find out by calling the customer service number of your insurance company, usually listed on the back of your insurance card. Some medical supply companies and specialty shops are service providers for insurance companies, which means they will submit your bill for you and accept the price set by your insurance company. Often they will be willing to call your insurance company for you to find out about your benefits. Being fitted for your first bra after surgery is an emotional time and it can be very difficult to talk to the insurance company without crying. Don't hesitate to ask the specialty shop owners if they will talk to your insurance company. If the shop won't call for you, perhaps you have a partner or a good friend who will be more than glad to help.

I am very familiar with how insurance plans work and how to access the information I need, yet when I tried to find out about my benefits I found myself overwhelmed, frustrated, and confused about what I was hearing. I found my customer service representative cold and insensitive and unwilling to take the time to help me understand. I ended up in tears, and terminated the call without getting the information I needed. My husband phoned for me the next day and got the same woman. He too found her difficult and unhelpful, but because he had more objectivity and emotional strength at that time he was able to get the information. I am a mental health professional and I couldn't handle the situation, so don't be hard on yourself if you need help with some of these details. Needing help does not make you weak or less worthy as a person. It simply means you are a normal human being going through the grief process.

ALTERING STANDARD BRAS

The cost of specialty bras is high and if your insurance benefits are limited or not available, altering standard store-bought bras is a good alternative. Another reason to alter your own bras might be convenience. If the nearest specialty shop or medical supply company is far away or even

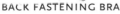 *Figures 10-1 a & b Suitable bras for altering*

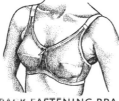

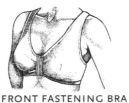

BACK FASTENING BRA   FRONT FASTENING BRA

out of town, or has hours that conflict with your schedule, you may find it easier to alter your bras yourself.

In addition, smaller-breasted women are often not comfortable with the style of specialty bras. They may be used to wearing slimmer-cut bras with smaller straps and rib band, and cups made of such materials as stretch nylon or knit cotton.

I was used to a simple, light bra because I was not very large-breasted. When I was shown what was available in specialty postmastectomy bras I felt my mood drop. Some of those bras reminded me of corsets. I was still a young woman and didn't want to feel like a woman from a different era. When I asked if there were any more delicate styles I was told I was no longer going to be able to wear the kind of bra I had worn in the past. I was informed that I would need much more support, hence a bra with a lot more material. I reacted the way most people do when they are told what to do. I decided to do it my own way.

I tried using a bra without a pocket but found that I was worried about my prostheses falling out, so I learned to alter all my bras and have never had to purchase a ready-made mastectomy bra.

Before you begin, make sure your bra is suitable for altering (see Figures 10-1 a & b). It must have a cup shape that will completely cover the prosthesis. You need a bra that will adequately hold the prosthesis in place and give a smooth, attractive appearance through your clothing. If the prosthesis extends beyond the bra cup or is squished in too small a cup it will create a bulge or unattractive line through fitted clothes. In addition, squishing the prosthesis will eventually make it lose its natural shape and deteriorate, shortening its lifespan.

In order to be
suitable for altering,
your bra must have a
cup shape that will
completely cover
your prosthesis.

The bra you intend to alter should have a minimum of a half-inch rib band. If you choose a bra without a wide enough band under the cups and around the back, your prosthesis will sag. The band should push up the prosthesis in the same way that an underwire works with a natural breast. An underwire should *not* be used with a silicone prosthesis because the constant rubbing of the prosthesis against the hard surface can cause the silicone to break down. If you really prefer an underwire, and replacing your prosthesis frequently is not of concern to you, make sure the top of the wire on the side is well covered so it will not puncture your prosthesis.

The center front of the bra should have a piece of material that extends at least an inch above the rib band between the cups. It does not matter if you use a front- or back-fastening bra as long as the rest of the style is suitable. V-cut bras with only one hook in the center front will not work, however. I tried several bras of this style because I wore them before my surgery, but repeatedly found that they didn't work well. The V-cut did not cover my prostheses and the single hook in the front didn't offer enough support.

Bras made with nylon, cotton, stretch knit cotton or any kind of cotton/polyester blend seem to work fine in either a smooth or a lacy material. Sheer stretch nylon does not work. It sags badly with the weight of the prostheses. Prostheses in a size 2 or less are well supported by the stretch cotton or cotton blend bras.

The piece you add to the cup to make the prosthesis pocket can be nylon, cotton, or cotton blend, but should be stretchy. The pocket piece does not have to be made out of the same material as the bra. I usually use stretch knit cotton or a cotton blend fabric because they are easiest to work with and they absorb perspiration well. (For those of you who are not seamstresses, stretch knit cotton is T-shirt material.)

One of my friends told me about ready-made pocket pieces. I have never used them but they would be another good option to simplify altering bras and certain swimsuits. The pocket pieces are sold individually or in pairs and cost $3 to $5 U.S. each. Since I had already taught myself how to make and sew in a pocket I found that starting from scratch was just as easy for me and a lot less expensive. I could buy a yard of jersey cotton knit for about $5 or $6 U.S., which would be enough material to alter both cups in eight to twelve bras, depending on the width of the fabric.

If the bra you want to alter is of good quality it should last one to two years, depending on how often you wear it, what you wear it for, and how you wash and dry it. It will only take you twenty to forty-five minutes to alter both sides once you know how, so altering is a worthwhile time investment.

Standard Back-Hooking Bras

Start by making a rough pattern piece using a piece of paper.

1. To make the pattern, lay down the paper and place the bra on top of it, facing down.
2. Trace the outside shape of the front of the bra about an inch extending beyond the bra (see Figure 10-2). The pattern should include the straps, so that about an inch extends above the top of the cup. The side should also extend another inch beyond where the cup ends.
3. If you are altering for one side only, find the center by first folding the front of the bra in half. Then leave an inch to hold over for a finished, folded, center edge. (Figure 10-3)
4. If you are sewing two pockets you can make one piece that fits across both sides. I usually try to be generous with my material allowance since I can always trim, but can't fix it if I have not allowed for enough material in the pattern.
5. Take the paper pattern, pin it onto the material, and cut it as indicated. (Figure 10-4)
6. Once you have cut the material, begin attaching it at the top of the bra. Fold over and hem the pocket piece by hemming each seam just prior to attaching it to the bra (see Figure 10-5).
7. Then attach it to the top of the bra with the pocket's right side up, again using a zigzag stitch (see Figure 10-6).
8. If you are making one pocket, before you attach the top center you will also need to fold over and stitch the center seam (see Figure 10-7). You can attach both the top and center at the same time. When you attach the center do not sew all the way down. You will need to leave enough room to turn the bottom hem under before you attach it.

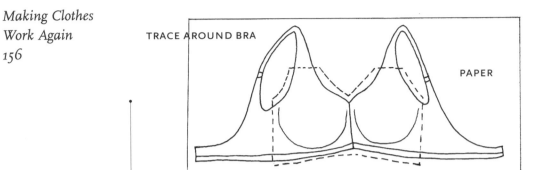

TRACE AROUND BRA

PAPER

Figure 10-2 Making a pattern for a back-fastening bra

9. Next, turn under and stitch the bottom and then the bottom side seams.
10. When you are attaching the bottom seam, make sure your material is even with the bra bottom so there is no ridge. Use a large enough zigzag stitch so the bottom is securely and smoothly attached to the bottom of the bra. This will be especially important for women whose incisions are in this area, but it is also important for others, because the area carries a lot of weight and can be easily irritated. (Figure 10-8)
11. The remaining upper side seam is attached only slightly at the strap level and a little way up from the area under the armpit, leaving an opening between those two points to insert your prosthesis (see Fig-

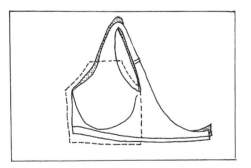

Figure 10-3 Pattern for altering one side

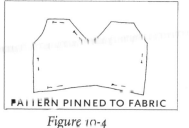

PATTERN PINNED TO FABRIC

Figure 10-4

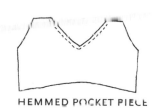

HEMMED POCKET PIECE

Figure 10-5

ure 10-9). Don't close the very end scam on the outer sides. Most prostheses are made with a wing that extends off to the side to give a more complete, full shape. This wing has to have room so it is not cramped.

12. Finally, sew a seam down the middle to secure the prosthesis.

Sports Bras

Another type of bra that I have found suitable for altering is the tight-fitting sports bra that does not open in the back or front. This style is so snug that you may feel it doesn't require a pocket to hold the prosthesis, depending upon what kind of activities you plan to do in it. The more

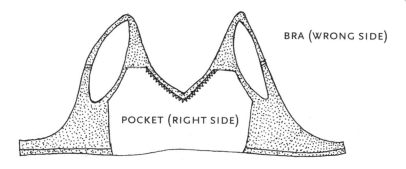

BRA (WRONG SIDE)

POCKET (RIGHT SIDE)

Figure 10-6

physical a sport is, the more a pocket is needed to keep the bra and prosthesis from moving around. I want to be able to stay focused on the activity at hand without worrying that my prostheses are migrating. Skin irritation from a sweaty prosthesis is another concern in a bra without a pocket to absorb perspiration.

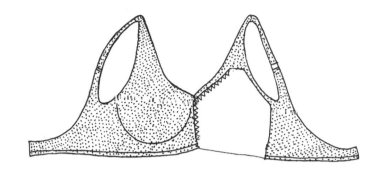

Figure 10-7 One pocket alteration

METHOD ONE

Alterations to a sports bra are a bit harder to sew because the bras do not open so they don't give you much maneuvering space. To alter a sports bra, use the same techniques as with a standard bra with a few changes.

1. Start making your pattern from the bottom and side seams and proceed to the center top. Sports bras are made large enough across the bottom that an opening does not have to be left on the lower sides for the wings. (Figure 10-10)

BOTTOM SEAM ZIG ZAGGED

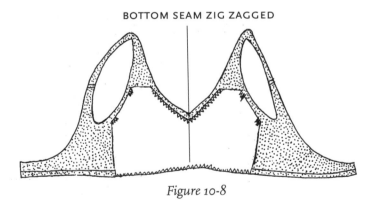

Figure 10-8

2. Cut the material so it is wide enough to extend across the bottom from one side seam of the bra to the other side seam, plus add an inch on all edges for hemming.
3. Use the instructions for altering a standard bra to complete the alterations.

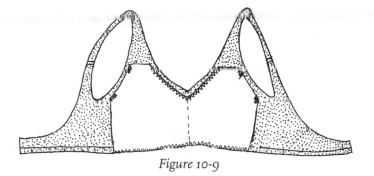

Figure 10-9

METHOD TWO

Although I have altered a few sports bras as described above, I have stumbled onto another method using the back upper piece of a pair of cotton underpants that produces a better outcome for a double–sided alteration. I have never tried it on a one-pocket alteration but I assume that this approach would also work for that.

This approach differs from the standard bra method in two ways. When using this approach to alter a tight sports bra I do not cut the material to extend as high on the straps because I leave the top open to insert my prostheses, rather than leaving an opening on the upper side of the cup area. I also work from the bottom up when sewing a sports bra this way.

1. To make your pattern, turn the bra inside out and tuck the back of the bra behind the front material so the back is out of the way for tracing. (Figure 10-11)
2. Place the bottom of your bra across the back of the elastic waist of the panties, matching up the edges.
3. Cut the material wide enough to extend one inch beyond the side seams of the bra and long enough to cover the entire breast area along with the widest portion of the straps.
4. You will notice that when you try to fit the material to match up at the center after you have stitched the sides it leaves an excess of material in the cup area.
5. Begin sewing by hemming the sides all the way up.
6. Attach the elastic to the rib band, making sure the two edges are even, then stitch the sides to the side seams of the bra only up to where the outer side starts to narrow into a strap. (Figure 10-12)

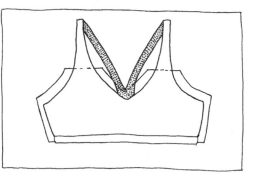

Figure 10-10 Making a pattern for a sports bra

7. Pull the material up and turn it under to make a hem so it matches with the center top of the bra and stitch it just to where the bra begins to narrow to make the strap. If you are only making one pocket, you can stitch the center seam at the same time as you sew the top center seam.

8. After you have fitted the pocket piece and sewn the top V-center, make a dart from inside the pocket that will take up the extra material before you sew the outer, upper side and strap portion (see Figure 10-13). It does not have to be exact; in fact, a bit of a gap in the upper cup

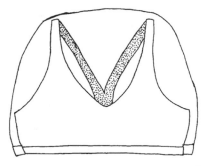

Figure 10-11 Making a pattern for a sports bra using cotton underwear

area makes it easier to insert your prosthesis. Because you are using a soft material any extra fabric should not cause skin irritation.

9. Stitch the rest of the side seam.
10. Next stitch across the top of the rib band with a zigzag stitch.
11. And lastly, stitch up the center of the bra to separate the cups, using a straight stitch.

Front-Hooking Bras

As I mentioned before, bras that hook in the front will only work if they have at least two hooks and no V-cut between the cups. Your front-hooking bra should have a cup that is curved and full enough to completely cover your prosthesis (Figure 10-1b). If you are sewing pockets on both sides you will have to cut and sew two separate pockets. A back-hooking bra is much less work because you can use one piece of material for both sides. However, if you prefer a front-hooking bra and you need a pocket on both sides, it will be worth your time to do the alteration. If you are only adding one pocket, altering a front-hooking bra is no more difficult than a back-hooking bra.

Sewing a front-hooking bra will be the same as a back-hooking bra except that your center seam will be sewn to the center edge of the cup. Get-

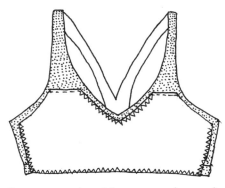

Figure 10-12 Attaching a sports bra pocket

ting the center pocket seam exactly even with the edge of the cup will not be as important as with the rib band seam because the pressure points are different in the center of the bra than on the bottom, so it should not cause an uncomfortable skin irritation.

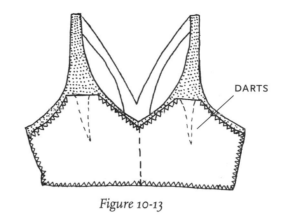

Figure 10-13

ALTERATIONS AFTER A LUMPECTOMY

As I mentioned in Chapter 9, a pocket is not necessary to hold an enhancer or accessory in place if the tissue has been removed from the lower portion of the breast, but when the tissue is from the upper part of the breast keeping the accessory in place can be a problem. There are two ways to go about securing the piece you are using to fill in the missing breast tissue after your lumpectomy.

If you are using a silicone enhancer to fill in a fairly large indentation, I suggest you sew a slip pocket into the inside of your bra to secure it, using a cotton or cotton blend stretch material. You can use this pocket for most types of accessory.

1. To begin, place the enhancer on a piece of paper and trace about three-quarters of the way around it, adding an extra inch to allow for enough material to stitch the piece to your bra and still leave enough "give" so the enhancer can be inserted into the pocket (see Figure 10-14). The remaining quarter should be drawn with a flat edge.

2. Pin your pattern to the material and cut it out. Hem the top of one side.

3. Hem the top straight edge (Figure 10-15).

4. Now turn your bra inside out and put it on with the enhancer against your breast to fill in the space where you are missing tissue.

5. Take a pencil and make a few marks to indicate where you need to sew your pocket. The flat edge will go on the top or slightly off to the

outer side at the top, depending on which location seems to work best with your body and your surgery.

6. Last, place your pocket piece on the inside of the bra cup where you have made pencil marks and stitch the unfinished edges with a zigzag stitch. Do not hem the edges that are attached to the bra because it will show through. (Figure 10-16)

The second approach to filling in a space left after a lumpectomy is to sew a cloth accessory to the inside of your bra. Since many of the cloth accessories are inexpensive, it is feasible to consider purchasing one for each bra and stitching it right into your bra. Wash your altered bra in cool water and line dry it to prevent the accessory from shrinking, which can lead to puckering and unsightly lines through your clothes.

Here again, shoulder pads come into play. As an alternative to a purchased accessory, you can cut out a piece of a shoulder pad that will fill the space left by your lumpectomy. You can recover the pad in a cotton stretch material if the original material is not a good color for your alterations. Attach the pad to the inside of your bra or insert it into a pocket as described above.

Swimsuits

Wearing a swimsuit and swimming can still be a part of your life after a mastectomy. You may have to make a few modifications to your suit style, but I think you will be surprised, as I was, to discover how many swimwear options are still available.

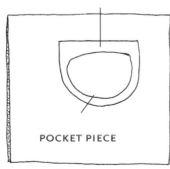

Figure 10-14

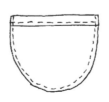

Figure 10-15 Enhancer pocket

Buying a swimsuit is
a traumatic
experience for many
women even before a
mastectomy.

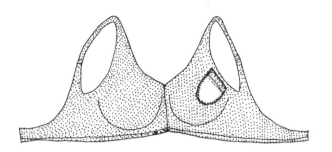

Figure 10-16 Attaching enhancer pocket to bra

You will no longer be able to wear a bikini with a small top that shows cleavage, or a swim top that leaves the upper part of your breast exposed, and even if your scars are on the sides or the bottom of your breast area, you will still need more upper coverage. Before surgery many of us enjoyed wearing little bikinis. For those of you who fit this category, you will feel the loss the most. Don't try to deny your feelings or tell yourself that you are being vain or petty because you feel bad about not being able to wear a bikini any more. Your feelings are completely natural. Finding a swimsuit that feels comfortable and attractive is a problem for many women in our culture and adding the burden of finding the right suit after a mastectomy is particularly difficult. Be gentle and patient with yourself through this process.

A bikini top will not work because it won't cover your scars or your prosthesis adequately. As with your bra, your swimsuit needs to completely cover your prosthesis. In addition, the top of your swimsuit should come up far enough so that when you bend over, your prosthesis is not visible. Otherwise, there will be a visible space between your chest and your prosthesis because the prosthesis will fall forward, leaving your chest area exposed. Many swimsuits have a wide piece of fabric inside that lines the breast area and blends into the straps. This fabric, combined with the tautness of the swimsuit material, will cover the upper part of your chest and hold the material and prosthesis close to your body.

When choosing a swimsuit you will want to take into account the placement of your scars, the visibility of your prosthesis, and how active you will be while wearing a swimsuit. You may want to sun bathe, go in the whirlpool, do vigorous lap swimming or some other type of water sport. A lot of women become very emotional when they approach the swimsuit issue after a mastectomy, which can make them feel more confused. Breaking the problem down can pull you back to a rational, problem-solving mode.

The simplest way to find a swimsuit is to get one from the same place you purchased your other postmastectomy products. The shop will generally carry a selection of altered swimsuits. Some women's department stores that carry postmastectomy products may also carry swimsuits or be able to order you one out of a catalog. These one-piece suits with pockets sewn into both sides are usually very well constructed but are quite expensive. Because they have pockets on both sides, the pockets are usually made with a netting material which is left very loose so that the natural breast has room to fit into the cup. All of the special postmastectomy suits I have seen come with built-in foam cups.

I found the pre-altered suits too conservative for my taste. Many of them had skirts, which I don't like, and I didn't want anything to do with that scratchy net material, and I had never liked swimsuits with foam cups. However, I tried to be open-minded and set aside my preferences. I did find a few swimsuits that were more my style but they were sold out in my size. The woman in the shop told me that the manufacturers don't make very many in the smaller sizes and that they sell out immediately. Obviously, if the smaller sizes are selling immediately there is a demand for them. In time I hope that people who make postmastectomy products will realize that women are not all the same size and not all want the same kind of product. Breast cancer is striking ever younger women, who often want different styles from those often preferred by older women. One of my motivations in writing this book was to help women address their unique clothing needs after a mastectomy. The medical supply industry changes only very slowly and we should not be limited by that in our clothing selection.

I left the postmastectomy supply shop without buying a swimsuit to give myself some time to decide how I would handle the situation. When

The ideal swimsuit
for altering is one
with a loose hanging
lining on the top.

I began to experiment with swimsuits I was pleasantly surprised to discover many options for altering a wide range of suits. And after helping two friends alter suits, I have learned even more about the possibilities.

Swimsuits can be altered with or without a foam cup. Even a tank-style, lap-swimming suit can be altered. Probably any one-piece swimsuit you already have at home can be altered. The more the breast area is defined with foam cups, lining, and rib elastic, the easier the swimsuit will be to alter and the more secure it will feel. If you want to alter a two-piece suit, the top will need to cover most of your upper chest. There are suits available in a two-piece style that have a large, maximum-coverage sports bra top. As long as the top does not ride up easily, these too can be altered.

Altering Swimsuits

To begin, you can try altering a favorite one-piece swimsuit that you already have at home. Once you have the suit on, insert the prosthesis to determine how to add a pocket that would hold the prosthesis securely. Look at the lines and seams of the suit first from the outside and then the inside. If, after trying on the suit, you have determined that the suit is not cut properly to cover your chest and scars, you can use that suit to get a better idea of what kind of swimsuit you need to look for. It is generally more comfortable to experiment with swimsuits in the privacy of your own home. Take your time, and if you get hit with a wave of sadness during the process, you can take time out for a few healing tears.

If you have more than one kind of breast form, let yourself see the differences in the suit between a foam-filled prosthesis and one made of silicone. For those with a natural breast remaining, you will need to determine where the prosthesis should sit in order to be at the same level as your other breast. Picture in your mind the swimsuit sewn and being used in activity. Being able to visualize the process and the end product which will help you to identify how to go about altering the suit.

To alter your swimsuit, you will need swimsuit lining material. This is a stretch fabric, which is usually a blend of Antron and Lycra. The cost is about $6 U.S. per yard and is usually 44 to 60 inches wide, and comes in black, white, and beige. If you look inside regular swimsuits, most of the linings are made with either the white or beige color. I have bought a yard each of the beige and the white and with them I have already altered six suits in the last three years and have plenty of material left. I recommend buying a yard because it is convenient to have the material on hand for the next time you want to alter a suit.

Swimsuits with Foam Cups

It is a simple matter to secure a panel to swimsuits that come with foam cups. The material around the cups is usually thick and the cups will give you a defined and secure shape to hold your prosthesis. When altering a swimsuit with foam cups, remember that the breast form may fill more space than is provided in the cups. The cup usually supports and defines only the front part of the breast and so the cup will only completely support the breast on a small breasted woman. I mention this because it is tempting to try and put a small piece of material just across the back opening of the foam cup to hold the prosthesis. Unfortunately, this won't provide enough room for a prosthesis. The panel should extend beyond the cup. Using a full panel rather than just covering the back of the cup will give you enough room to shift your prosthesis around as necessary so it is at the same level as your other breast. Try on your suit with the prosthesis before you alter it to get the best sense of how big the panel should be and where it should be attached to the suit (see Figure 10-17).

Making a Pattern

If you have already altered a bra you will have begun to get a feel for how to gauge the size and shape of your pattern pieces.

1. Start by making a trial pattern piece out of paper. The type of pocket you make and the way you attach it will be determined by the lining if any already exists in your swimsuit. If your swimsuit fabric is thin, make a pattern piece to cover both sides of your chest, even if you only need one prosthesis pocket. Look at the inside of the breast cup area to determine how far down your pattern piece will need to extend to make a large enough pocket, then turn the suit over, place it on top of the paper and trace (see Figure 10-18). You should work from top to bottom when making a pattern.

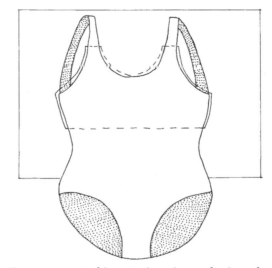

Figure 10-17 Making a swimsuit prosthesis pocket

2. Cut out your pattern and pin it to your lining material. Remember that your lining fabric has more stretch going one direction than the other. The greater stretch should be from side to side, not from top to bottom, to accommodate your natural movement. More tautness from top to bottom will not confine you and will help to hold your prosthesis more snugly against you.

3. Cut around your pattern piece into your fabric. Make sure that your panel has enough material that you can hem the edges at least 1/4" around the top and sides with a zig zag stitch to prevent fraying. Do not hem the bottom of your panel until after you have attached the top of the piece to your swimsuit. This will allow you to get a better fit from top to bottom.

Swimsuits with a Loose Chest Lining

Swimsuits with loose hanging (bottoms unattached) linings in the chest area only are the simplest to add a pocket to. Simply slip stitch your panel piece to the neck of the suit and across the top of the straps. Leave the panel free along the arm curves so your prosthesis can be inserted and either hand or machine stitch the panel sides to the existing lining at the sides. Finally, hem the bottom of the panel to the elastic or bottom of the lining and sew two seams up the middle, approximately 1 to 1¹/₂" apart to prevent your prosthesis from slipping around. The final step is to sew a small snap at the center edge of your pocket opening (Figure 10-18).

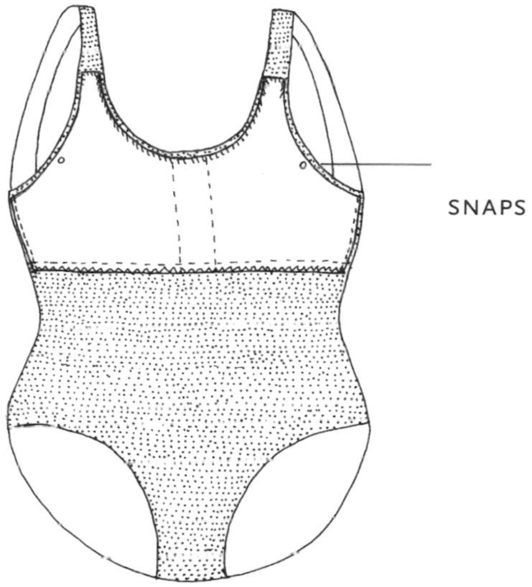

SNAPS

Figure 10-18

Altering Unlined Swimsuits

To alter an unlined swimsuit the procedure is similar to altering a swim-suit with a loose hanging chest lining, only you will be making both pieces of the pocket with your panel piece.

1. To begin, cut two pieces of lining fabric with your pattern piece. Hem both panel pieces.
2. You should place one finished panel side against the inside of your suit, and the other with the finished side against your skin and sew the two together using a straight stitch at the very edge of the fabric pieces. (Figure 10-19) The two pieces create a pocket in which to place your prosthesis.
3. Attach the pocket piece to your swimsuit as you would do with a loose chest lining (described above).

Try taking the lining
from one swimsuit
and sewing it into
another suit.

Sewing One Pocket

If you are only sewing in a pocket on one side of your swimsuit the center should be stitched before the sides. If you are attaching a one-sided pocket to a full, straight lining without cups you will need to do it by hand. I do not recommend sewing one-sided pockets to a full lining without cups because the stitching and pocket are likely to show through the front of the suit and the pocket will likely not be very secure. Even though it takes more material, you will get a smoother look and a more secure pocket if it extends across both sides.

Altering Fully Lined Swimsuits

If your swimsuit is fully lined you will need to attach the panel piece to the lining by hand.

1. Hem your panel piece using a zig zag stitch and then attach it to the lining by hand. Be careful not to catch any of the actual swimsuit fabric in your stitching or it will show through the suit.
2. The two center seams that keep the prosthesis in place should also be stitched by hand, making sure to keep the swimsuit fabric free.
3. Attach the panel in the same manner as on the other varieties of suits, leaving a hole at the underarm to insert your breast form.

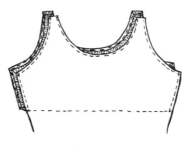

Figure 10-19

Simple Tips

You may find that the lining from one suit could be used for altering another suit. If you cut out the upper lining of an old swimsuit, you may be able to use it for a pattern piece by just adding a little on each edge to hem. You may also be able to use the lining from the top of an old two-piece suit to make pockets in a one-piece suit. Cut the lining as close as possible to the edges of the suit where it is attached. If the one-piece suit is fully lined, cut down just far enough to cover the chest area.

If you have altered a suit, when it wears out you might be able to re-move the panel and use it again on a new swimsuit. Be creative and have fun seeing how many ways you can do your alterations.

Sleepwear

Sleepwear wouldn't be an issue if it were just for sleeping. We could slip on a long T-shirt in the summer and flannels in the winter and be done with it. But as you know, our nightclothes mean more than that. Many women enjoy changing into feminine and sexy clothes because they en-joy dressing for their partners as a part of their sexual expression, or they simply want to feel feminine and sexually attractive again.

The majority of women become comfortable enough with their changed bodies that most nights they allow themselves to be seen by their partner in a way that makes it apparent one or both breasts are gone. Most nights they are not concerned with how they look, but are more focused on comfort. Not many women wear a sexy nightie to bed every night. Most women save those kinds of garments for a special, ro-mantic evening with a sexual mood. Few women are going to wear a prosthesis to bed or try to disguise the missing breast; they usually wear the same kind of pajamas they wore before their surgery. Many women enjoyed sleeping in the nude before surgery, and after a certain amount of adjustment time, they resume sleeping without clothes.

Some women who are very private with their bodies and have kept it covered, even in front of their husbands, wear their modified bra to bed every night. If you are going to do this, don't sleep in your silicone pros-thesis because it will put too much pressure on it and distort the shape when you roll over and lie on it. Use a foam-filled or fiber-filled breast form.

Most women, however, find it uncomfortable to wear a bra to bed. Af-ter-effects from surgery often make it even more uncomfortable to wear binding clothing for a long period of time. If you don't want to wear a bra to bed but it is important to you to have the appearance of having two breasts, you will need to alter your own clothes.

The postmastectomy industry does not make sleepwear because there is too much variance in what women want, which makes it unprofitable. Because of the start-up production and marketing costs associated with a new product, it is only profitable when a particular item will be purchased by many people, . I don't expect this to change, but you can keep checking with your supplier or fitter to see if any sleepwear has become available.

T-shirts, button-down pajamas, or anything without a defined breast area cannot be altered. This type of nightwear will have to be worn with a bra or without any alteration. During the colder part of the year you could use the Vitali-Tee undershirt that holds the fiber-filled form. These are not as binding as a bra and still allow you to have a breast form under your garment.

If you want to do alterations, your choice in gowns, babydolls, and chemises will be determined by your surgery and the look you are trying to achieve. If you have had both breasts removed, you may want to pad both sides or change to a style that looks nice without any padding. If you have a remaining breast, matching it will be your main objective.

If you have had both breasts removed and want to wear something feminine and sexy, I encourage you to try a gown, chemise, or babydoll that is designed without a defined breast area. Even a sheer material will look very nice without any prostheses, as long as the garment does not have breast areas that are left unfilled. You can also choose a babydoll outfit with a matching sheer robe for a bit more coverage.

Altering Sleepwear

If you prefer the appearance of breasts but do not want to wear a bra, you will have to alter a garment that has a defined breast area such as a teddy or nightgown.

1. You will need to find a matching piece of fabric that will be sewn into the breast cups. Chiffon, stretch Lycra, and nylon work well for this. If you cannot find the same color, consider a contrasting color.

2. Cut the piece to fit the cup and then attach it to the inside of the cups with a zigzag stitch, by sewing it to the edge of the cup that is closest to your chest.

3. To make the lining fit the cup, you may need to make a dart or two to create a rounder piece that sits deeper in the cup

4. After you have lined the inside of the cup, using the same fabric make a pocket similar to that which you would make to alter a bra. You can use this approach to alter one or both sides.

5. If you have one breast remaining, line the cup on the side that still has a breast.

6. For the side(s) that do not have a breast, you can either leave the pocket open to insert a prosthesis or you can fill it with fiber-fill material and close it off completely, making it a permanent form in the garment. Since you are using fiber-fill, you will be able to hand wash the garment with the breast area filled.

If You Do Not Sew

The American and Canadian Cancer Societies provide a list of places that sell postmastectomy products, including people and places who do alterations for mastectomies. This is a good place to start looking for resources in your community. Many dry cleaners who offer alteration services are quite familiar with mastectomy alterations. In a major metropolitan area, it typically costs about $5 U.S. per cup to have a bra altered. You will need to provide the bra and the fabric. Swimsuit alterations would cost a little more, depending on the alteration required. Recently I learned of a major department store that sells a full line of postmastectomy products and that will sew a pocket into any other regular bra they sell for only $4 U.S. per cup.

You may be surprised to find out how much help is available through people you know. Many people feel helpless and don't know how to show us that they care after our mastectomy. When we can give them a way to help, it makes them feel better too. If you do not have a sewing machine, don't know how to sew, or are physically unable to manage the task, ask yourself whether you know someone who could do some sewing for you. Most likely they will be delighted to do it.

Altering your own bras, and sleepwear and swim wear offers you the chance to get creative and to take control of your fashion needs.

It is a great idea to reach out to someone who you know has already been through a mastectomy. I have had the opportunity to help a couple of friends alter their swimsuits. I felt honored to help. Not only did I have something to offer from my experience, but I was also able to learn more about altering swimsuits for women who had different needs and wanted different styles from me, adding to my experience and knowledge. We learned from each other and working together brought us closer and opened the door to talk more freely about our mastectomy experiences and how we were coping with them.

Be Creative

The key to successfully altering your clothes is to draw from your creativity and not get hung up by perfectionism. Remember, you are the only one who is going to see the inside of your garment. The stitching does not have to look like it was done by a professional tailor, so whether you do it by hand or by machine it doesn't matter, as long as it is secure. The pocket pieces do not have to be exact. Each time you alter a bra it may look slightly different from the last one.

When I was getting started with altering, I used catalogs and flyer ads to stimulate ideas. I looked at pages of bras and quizzed myself about which bras would or would not work. I also looked very closely at specialty postmastectomy clothes. At the specialty shop I would study the different kinds of clothes to see how they were altered, the types of fabric used, and how the pockets were shaped and attached.

The next step was to try on clothes I had at home to see what I could use as it was, and which ones had possibilities for alterations. My final step was to venture out to the stores and look around for new types of clothes that would serve my new needs, as well as clothes that I could easily alter.

My favorite sports bras are the ones I make with the underpants because they turn out so comfortable and they remind me of my creative, clever side, which I did not realize I had until after my mastectomy. I hope you also allow yourself the opportunity to discover your special, creative nature.

CHAPTER ELEVEN

SEX AND INTIMACY

Becoming sexual again may be the biggest hurdle you go through or it may seem quite an insignificant part of your recovery after a mastectomy. Since our breasts play such an important part in our sexuality, it is natural to worry about how we are going to reconnect with our sexuality now that we don't have a breast—or breasts. We fear that we are unattractive to our partner and worry about whether we can have a full and satisfying sexual experience after our mastectomy. We worry that we will be so uncomfortable in our changed body we will become inhibited in the way we dress and conduct ourselves sexually. Many women who have had both breasts removed are concerned that they will not be able to replace the erotic sensations and sexual pleasure that their breasts provided. Most of us also worry about initiating sex. Should we initiate sex, or will that put our partner on the spot of having to make love before feeling ready or, worst of all, will our partner think that we are now ugly and untouchable? Our rational mind may know better, but our fears are not always based on rational thinking, so we can create some pretty big worries.

Be careful when comparing how you approach sex after losing one or both of your breasts to how other women approach it. It won't be helpful to listen to other women's reactions and decide that there is something wrong with you if your experience is different. As with other aspects of our recovery process, how we become sexual again and how we feel about our sexuality and sex life will be greatly influenced by our personal history. The role sexuality plays in our life before and after a mastectomy is shaped by attitudes and behaviors we learned as we grew up and by our adult sexual experiences. Take the time to consider your sexual life before surgery and your feelings about yourself as a sexual being.

Many women were comfortable with their sexuality, and their sexual education and experiences have been positive, so for them it is a matter of applying the attitudes they had before your surgery to their new situation. But for many women who have mastectomies, sexuality was not a comfortable aspect of their lives before surgery and they bring that discomfort to their current sex life. Carefully assessing your sexual attitudes will help you to work through the issues that may surface after your mastectomy.

Growing up, many of us picked up a lot of inaccurate ideas about sex. If you are still carrying beliefs that hold you back sexually, this is a good time to identify and change them. Feelings of shame about sex are common. Many women were taught early that girls are not supposed to like sex, that sex is for their husband's needs, or for procreation, not for their own pleasure. They were told that thinking or talking about sex is a sin, that their own sexual parts are dirty and should not be touched. Some girls were taught that a woman's body should be kept covered so her parts are not a temptation to men, and that if a man goes "too far" it is the fault of the woman. At the same time, our culture has implied that women are only valuable as bodies.

These are a few of the myths and negative attitudes about sex that can hold us back from pursuing a safe, emotionally comfortable, satisfying sex life. The women's movement has opened a lot of doors for us to challenge these ideas. However, I think it is important to say them out loud once again, because after a mastectomy we may find that the remains of these sexual beliefs we thought we had dealt with come up again. We may not realize that we still carry some of these beliefs in our subconscious.

If your subconscious belief is that girls are not supposed to like sex, it doesn't leave much room for you to grieve the loss of the erotic sensations that used to come from your breast. If you consider your genitals dirty and don't believe that you should think or talk about sex, then exploring new ways to enhance your sexual experience is going to be very difficult. It is hard enough to reveal our changed bodies to an intimate partner without the added burden of the belief that showing our body is

Getting sexual again after a mastectomy is likely to bring you face to face with a lot of your hidden ideas and assumptions about sex.

wrong. Whatever negative attitudes you may be operating with will inevitably restrict your sexuality.

Childhood sexual abuse or rape may have influenced your feelings about your sexuality. The way you have coped with such experiences will affect the way you will cope with losing a breast. Some women with histories of abuse have repressed their feelings and use the same avoidant approach with their sexuality after a mastectomy. A woman who has repressed her feelings about past abuse is likely to not be in touch with her own sexuality. She may take her sexual leads from her partner and do whatever her partner wishes so she doesn't have to face her thoughts and feelings about sex. Or she may resist sex as much as possible, again, to keep from stirring up repressed emotions. But many women with traumatic sexual histories have done remarkable work on themselves and their sexuality and are much more in touch with, and often more comfortable thinking and talking about, their sexuality than the average woman.

One common reaction of a sexual abuse survivor to the loss of a breast is anger and a huge sense of injustice. They feel they have worked hard to come to peace with their past and have embraced their sexuality, and now they have to face another sexual loss and go through the whole issue again. This might be the initial reaction but, because many abuse survivors have learned to move beyond a victim posture, they are usually able to use their anger to energize them enough to move out of the victim role and take charge of their recovery.

The re-examination of a woman's sex life can also unleash repressed memories of childhood sexual abuse. Sexual abuse memories can come out at any age. They usually surface under two different circumstances. The first occurs when the abuse victim is in a stable and secure enough situation to support her as she faces the truth. The second circumstance that can lead to the release of sexual abuse memories is when an experience triggers the memories. Sexual abuse victims frequently fear being physically harmed, and especially fear mutilation. Having a sexual part of your body removed can trigger the fear of mutilation and make you feel as if the abuse is happening again. If a mastectomy raises new issues

Is your old sex life
enough or do you
need more? After a
mastectomy is the
right time to
reevaluate how you
approach sex and
what you want
from it.

of sexual abuse, it is very important for you to seek out a good therapist to help you heal.

As you begin to re-evaluate your sexual needs and expectations after a mastectomy, you may be faced with other issues. A woman who has a mastectomy may realize that she has always been a lesbian but has never admitted it. Because the loss of a breast is partly about sexuality, it automatically causes us to re-evaluate our sexuality. If a woman has been repressing her true sexual identity, it is likely to come to the surface. Breast cancer often occurs about the same time that we are facing our middle-aged introspection time. It can be a tremendous emotional burden to have to face the reality of your sexual preference at the same time as the rest of your losses, but on the other hand, it can be incredibly freeing to finally come to know and accept yourself. If you find yourself questioning your sexual preference, I recommend that you find a therapist who can help you sort out your thoughts and feelings. A good therapist will help you define your sexual preference without trying to influence you. It is my belief that people are born with a sexual preference, not shaped into one. So be wary of a therapist who has an agenda for deciding your sexual preference. I also encourage you to educate yourself by reading about the subject of sexual orientation. There are many good books written by lesbians who share their process of developing a sexual identity.

A woman's age will often make a difference in how she and her partner cope with sexuality and the loss of her breast. Many older women were taught that sex is a private matter that should not be discussed. As well, older women may have physical conditions not related to their mastectomies that have already forced them to change or limit their sexuality. Chronic pain, joint problems, heart conditions, fatigue, and many other health problems may affect how women approach sex. In addition, older couples tend to emphasize intimacy rather than intense sexual pleasure. Comfortable, warm, and tender holding of each other that allows for physical limitations can play a much bigger part in an older couple's sex life than a younger couple's. Elderly couples may not talk about sex as much or as openly, but often they have gone through so much together that incorporating the loss of a breast into their sex life is done quite easily. This does not mean that elderly couples never have intercourse or do not care about the loss of a breast. It is a significant loss for them too.

Older single or widowed women may be less likely to take on new sexual partners, but that does not mean they never do. And they also have to deal with their changed appearance and desire to appear feminine and attractive. For older single women who may become physically intimate, the approach will be the same as it is for any single woman. (See Sex and the Single Woman, later in this chapter.)

Reclaiming Your Sexuality

There are two ways to go about returning to your sex life. You can go back to your old style or you can build an entirely new ideal for your sex life. Women with comfortable, safe, satisfying ways of relating sexually are able to return to this solid foundation as they become sexual again. Women who have open communication and deep understanding with their partners can make the adjustment from sex before surgery to sex after surgery fairly easily. Such women know they are loved first as a person, and that sex is just one way in which the love is expressed in a relationship. This foundation of love will support the couple during the insecure time they go through as they adjust to the loss of a breast. Of course, both people will need reassurances. The woman will need to know that she is still sexually desirable even though her body is changed. Partners will need reassurances that they are being considerate and supportive enough. Most partners are extremely concerned about not adding to our pain in any way, and need to know when and how to physically touch our body as it is healing and when and how to touch to express sexual desire. A strong relationship built on a foundation of love will support a couple as they struggle together to regain physical intimacy.

Unfortunately, some women do not have secure, loving relationships. However, they too may return to using their old, familiar sexual approach. Many women have never had fulfilling sexual relationships but still manage. Perhaps other areas in their relationship mean a great deal to them, and outweigh what is lacking in the sexual area. We all do

"It hasn't affected our sex life. We are so used to the change that I don't think we really notice anymore."

what we feel we must in order to get through life. We make trade-offs that make sense to us even if they do not seem to make sense to others. There are times when we feel we cannot tolerate any more change, so we hold on tightly to the status quo. If you find yourself confronted with the realization that your relationship is not sexually sound or supportive, but you don't feel strong enough to change it, don't be hard on yourself. Remember that there is no time limit on making healthy changes.

The second approach to returning to your sex life is to build a new structure. You may have considered your sexual life and decided you are tired of the status quo. Instead of finding the "old and usual" sexual routines a comfort, you may find that they make you angry and impatient. You may decide after coming through the trauma of breast cancer and surgery that you deserve more out of life, and that you need to balance out some of the pain with more pleasure, and sex is one of the ways to try to even the scale.

Feeling in control of your sexuality can help you to avoid feelings of despair and thoughts that you are a trapped and helpless victim. Because losing a breast affects our sexuality, any way we can compensate for this loss will make us feel that we have some control. Maybe your mastectomy will be the catalyst that leads you to expand your sexual expectations.

There are many women who have been married for twenty years yet have never had an orgasm. If this is your situation, you may decide it is time to include your needs as well as your partner's. Any negative attitudes you may still be holding will come into play now. Having identified some of your limiting sexual attitudes, you can work on replacing them with new attitudes or statements. Repeating these new ideas often to yourself will help to reinforce them. This may be the time to start telling yourself that sex is a pleasurable part of life that you deserve to experience fully. You will also need to remind yourself that a good sexual relationship requires open communication.

Masturbation is one way to explore and discover how your body works and what it likes in preparation for changing your sex life. There are positive ways and destructive ways to use masturbation. If you are masturbating to learn more about your body so you can build a better normal connection with your partner, that is important and healthy. However, if you are masturbating in order to avoid having sex with your partner, you can lose the opportunity to grow together sexually after surgery and remain stuck in an unfulfilling sex life. It is important to ask yourself if your masturbation is enhancing your sex life or taking something from it. If you and/or your partner are avoiding the subject of sex, masturbation can make it easier to avoid facing it. It can be much easier to masturbate than go to your partner and try to talk openly about sex. Of course, if you are single or in an unsatisfying relationship that you know is not going to change, masturbation is a valuable way of releasing sexual tension.

> Open communication is essential to good sex, especially after a mastectomy.

The longer we go without dealing with our sexual wishes, the more likely we are to become discouraged and resigned about our chances for a fulfilling sex life. We may cope with our despair either by masturbating alone or sexually shutting down altogether. Both partners can do this. Even if you have a history of talking about sex and working out problems, the changes from the mastectomy may be bigger than either of you have had to face and you may not know where to start.

COMMUNICATION

As women we need reassurance that we are still attractive and sexually desirable. We may feel very timid about the changes to our bodies and fear that we will not be enough for our partner in this new lacking body. We may feel we have less to offer sexually. If we reach out to initiate sex, we may be afraid of putting our partner in the impossible situation of having to be sexual with us when they really are not attracted to us any more. We do not want to be pitied, and we don't want our partner to make love to us just to make us feel better. Our need to know that we can still be desirable puts us in an uncomfortable situation: if we initiate sex or try to talk about it, we may fear our partner will conceal his true feelings to avoid hurting us.

And our partners experience a similar kind of bind. They too struggle to deal with the changes in us and in themselves and feel a lot of confusion and uncertainty. Men are often thought of as sex-hungry and insensitive to the needs of women. It is true that a healthy male is interested in sex but most men are not driven by it, and are sensitive to the needs of women. This sensitivity, in fact, makes it very tricky for men. They are supposed to support us and accept us with our new bodies, and still be attracted to us, but they do not want to be accused of "only caring about one thing." They want us to know that they love us for more than our bodies and care about what we are going through. Our partners are often acutely aware of how close they came to losing us and are still dealing with their fears. Most men long for a schedule to follow with the right time frame for all these steps back to health and sex. But, of course, that is not possible because each of us is a unique individual with our own history, set of needs, and time frame.

Once our partners get past the point of initiating sex, they still face a lot of new territory. Your partner has seen you go through a great deal of physical pain, and the last thing he wants is to cause you any more. How and where can he touch you? He wonders what feelings of insecurity or grief he will unleash in you if he touches any part of your chest. If he totally avoids your chest, will you interpret that as a sign that your chest is ugly and repulsive to him? Often, one of his greatest initial fears is that, in fact, he will think your chest is repulsive and will not be able to relate to you sexually any more. He knows how important it will be to you that he accept and like your changed body. He may fear that maybe he is one of those superficial men who cannot be there for you. He thinks he has more depth than that, but worries about failing you and adding to your tremendous pain.

It is important to remember that our partners also go through a loss when we lose a breast. Through their sexual expression of their love for us, they develop their own relationship to our breasts. When one or both of our breasts is gone, they also mourn. New ways of relating sexually can be established with time, but for now, the routines that you have both relied on have been broken. Sexual routines can be experienced as a special ritual that belongs exclusively to you as a couple, and having to let go of familiar sexual patterns can feel sad and threatening. Couples find that certain positions just don't work any more, and certain parts of the body are no longer available for sexual pleasure because they are literally gone or because tissue and nerve damage makes touch painful.

You are probably wondering how you and your partner are ever going to get beyond these terrible binds. When we are close to a problem and the subject is emotionally loaded, it is easy to feel overwhelmed and confused. Ask yourself what advice you might offer someone else if they were bringing the problem to you. When we take an objective viewpoint it is amazing how easily we become able to identify our problems and generate ideas about how to rectify them.

Pretending you are giving someone advice will probably give you insights into beliefs or internalized rules you have that are hindering you. Of course, the most common advice you are likely to offer someone in your situation is to talk to their partner openly and honestly. Then you may hear yourself respond with, "I couldn't do that because I do not know how to talk about sex," "I do not want to hurt his feelings," "Maybe I will embarrass him or put him on the spot and just make it worse," or "What if we open up all this pain and then get stuck in it?"

It is true that communicating can be very uncomfortable at first when you have unspoken rules against talking about sex or feelings, but that does not mean you cannot master it. The biggest obstacle to good communication is that people often give up in the middle. They try a few words, stir up some discomfort, and take this to mean their efforts are not working, so they panic and give up. Good communication often requires several attempts before the job gets done. If you tell a person something and you want to make sure you have been understood correctly, ask them what they heard you say. This will give you an opportunity to clarify and reassure the other person if there were any misunderstandings.

Sex is about tenderness and vulnerability. It is a time when we should be able to let our guard down and open up our hearts to give and receive love and acceptance with our partner. Communicating about a loaded issue, such as sex, will go much better if both partners start from the premise that you each want what is best for the other and that you love each other. In that case, if the conversation becomes painful it will be easier to realize that you are having a breakdown in communication, rather than thinking that your partner is intentionally trying to be hurtful. As

Both partners are likely to experience fear when they become sexual again.

Sex is about
tenderness,
vulnerability and
intimacy. None of
those things require
a breast.

you try to discuss your losses and your needs, try to draw on the trust you have in your love for each other.

The first step to communicating with your partner is to share what you have been discovering about your old attitudes, and if those beliefs are negative, how you intend to replace them with new ones. Letting your partner know your new attitudes and sexual goals should lead to a positive discussion.

At this point it is helpful to check to see how your partner is feeling about what you are saying. Your partner may react with delight, or with feelings of insecurity and inadequacy and may feel somewhat threatened. If your partner seems threatened, try to convey that the change you desire is more about you than about your partner. Explain that your surgery has created a new desire to want more from life, or a desire to add to what you already have. Try not to fall into blaming each other about the problems in your old sex life. Instead of blaming, it will be more productive to assess what has and has not been working for each of you and come to an agreement on a new approach that will enhance what has been good in the past. This general talk about sex should be done at a time when you are not going to be sexual. You can then use this talk as a reference point for further communication during actual lovemaking.

Your partner may not be as ready as you are to begin discussing changes. Filling in the blanks for your partner can be a great set up for hurt feelings. Most of us have a strong tendency to fill in moments of silence with our own insecurities. Remember that silence can mean the other person has not yet found the words to express what he or she is feeling or is not yet emotionally ready to share those feelings. If the timing is not right, ask for reassurance that the issues you want to discuss will be brought up later. Coming right out and asking your partner what he thinks and feels may spur him to formulate his own thoughts about the surgery and your sex life.

Changing Perceptions
Sex and sexual intimacy do not start in bed. Open communication of sharing our feelings and listening closely to our partner's feelings is the building block for being able to please and be pleased emotionally and

sexually. Revealing our preferences does not just refer to how we like to be sexually touched. It also includes preferences in such things as styles of clothes, fragrances, music, alcoholic beverages, and atmosphere. Learning to think about these things and share them with our partner allows for a special, close connection.

I have come to realize that I am getting older and some of my feelings about getting older and my sexuality were mixed up with the imposed changes from my mastectomies. I am not able to wear a lot of dresses because I am a middle-aged woman who no longer wears a size seven. I wear a size ten because my hips are wider and I have a middle-aged belly and thicker thighs. I really hate this fact, but so do all the other middle-aged women I talk to. As we get older our bodies change and we find that we no longer look as good in certain clothes. Having to be limited in my clothing choices by my age and my surgery feels like a double whammie. But it is helpful for me to realize that all my disappointment does not come from my surgery, and it is just a normal part of aging.

This is a natural time to begin to reassess the meaning of sex and reshape it to fit our gradually aging bodies. As I mentioned before, intimacy typically takes on more importance in an older couple's sex life, and the change is a subtle progression that occurs over many years. Going through the loss of a breast can make this subtle shift a more conscious process as we are faced with rethinking our sexuality after the mastectomy.

There are several ways to make up for the lost pleasurable sensation after a breast is removed.

RESUMING YOUR SEXUAL RELATIONSHIP

A primary aspect of regaining your sexuality is the issue of when and how your partner looks at you without clothes. I give my husband full credit for us being able to get through this one. My husband was the first person beyond the surgical staff to see my chest. He saw my chest even before I did because I was sent home the same day I had both of my implants removed, and the dressings had to be changed and the drainage tubes drained that same evening. The hospital staff taught him how to do all this in about five minutes, just before I was discharged. He did it like a trooper without a word about how I looked. Neither of us was ready to think about how I looked, let alone talk about it. I was in shock and totally

The better you feel in
your clothes, the
more attractive you
will feel, and hence,
the sexier you will
feel.

removed from myself, and my husband was completely focused on my needs and was not ready to look at his own reaction to the changes in my body.

So, although Jim had seen what my chest looked like, we still had not really considered my chest as it related to our lovemaking. We did not even get close to dealing with how my surgery would affect our sex life until my drainage tubes were out and my chest had healed enough to tolerate a fair amount of touch. It was very important to me to have my husband initiate sex again. I needed him to ask if we could make love. Normally, we both felt comfortable initiating sex, but after surgery I felt far too vulnerable. We made love for the first time a couple of weeks after my surgery. His initiation reassured me that he did not find me disgustingly ugly and that we could still be sexual together. I couldn't have cared less how good or bad the sex was that night; all I needed to know was that it would still be part of our lives.

It was a while later that we faced looking at my chest as part of our sexual experience. I had begun to wear babydoll outfits on occasion to try to feel more sexual and attractive. One night, while making love, Jim stopped what we were doing and sat me up facing him, and took off my top. He looked directly at my chest and just held me as I cried. Neither of us spoke a word. Our actions and the loving, acceptance that filled the room said it better than any words could have. This is one area in which no one can write a script for you. We all have our own ways of feeling sexy and desirable, and have our own levels of comfort with regard to initiating sex and revealing our body. You need to trust that the love between you and your partner will pave the way for both of you to accept how your body looks and be able to return to pleasurable lovemaking.

I still do not like to sit up in bed reading in the nude on a hot summer night without something covering my chest. Jim has told me to not worry about it and has reassured me that he has no trouble looking at my chest. But I do not like how it looks so I usually cover myself with a light, feminine top. This is for my own comfort and goes beyond what my husband needs. However, being fully exposed during love-making is not a problem for me. When I am making love I am coming from an inner place of sensuality.

We need to have a positive mental attitude about sex that is translated into action through our body. We need to believe that our sexual passion is a natural, normal way to express our love and desire to be closely connected to our partner. The greatest turn-on to a healthy male is when a woman desires sex and can communicate that openly. We should be able to feel the passion and desires of our body and use them to make a deep connection with our partners.

I recommend a twenty-minute videotape produced by the Minnesota chapter of the American Cancer Society entitled *A Significant Journey: Breast Cancer Survivors and the Men Who Love Them*. Several couples share their journey of putting sex and intimacy back into their relationship after the loss of a breast. The film offers input from other couples who have shared your struggle, and covers the issues of both partners in a sensitive and realistic manner. Watching this tape in the privacy of your own home with your partner can be an excellent way of opening up communication about the effects of your mastectomy on your sex life and how to go about coping with it. You just need to call 1-800-582-5152 in the U.S. to request a tape and they will mail you one free of charge.

I also very much liked a booklet published by the American Cancer Society entitled *Sexuality & Cancer: For the Woman Who Has Cancer, and Her Partner*. Reading this booklet together would be another excellent way to begin communicating about sex. As well as short discussions about issues that relate to sexuality, the booklet includes illustrations of intercourse positions that are more comfortable during the physical healing process. You can receive a free copy of this booklet by calling 1-800-ACS-2345.

HONESTY AND TACT

Tact is a very important part of building and preserving good interpersonal relationships. We all know that sometimes concealing our thoughts and feelings or telling little white lies is the kindest way to go. But if we take it to an extreme and use tact to avoid sharing our feelings, we are merely avoiding having to deal with emotionally difficult issues. None of us wants to hear our partners tell us they think our chest is unattractive and would prefer that we keep it covered. But do we really want

> Books and tapes can help you to become sexual again after a mastectomy if you and your partner find you are stuck.

our partner turned off to spare us bad feelings? Or do we really want to know what is or is not attractive to our partner? There is no correct answer to this question. It is a matter of personal integrity and how we as individuals define that. The strength of your relationship, your communication skills as a couple, and your partner's ability to use tact are all going to influence how much you want to open up this issue. I personally appreciate some sense of protectiveness from my husband, but do not want him to be overly careful with me about potentially hurtful realities because I think it limits our relationship by putting tight, unspoken rules into play that can create tension or, at least, guardedness. This guardedness can lead to less emotional connection and leave both of you feeling less loved and understood.

Dressing as it relates to your sexuality is one very important aspect of reclaiming your sex life. In this area I have greatly appreciated my husband's honesty. About nine months after my second surgery, I had to buy a formal dress for a black tie wedding. The first day I went out shopping, it was extremely painful and I did not buy anything. The whole experience felt designed to make me realize my days of looking attractive and sexy were over. I tried to be strong and positive when I started out, but by the time I was done I was physically and emotionally exhausted and I still had no dress. I finally found a long black dress, cut quite low in the front, that made me feel sexy. When I got home and tried the new dress on, my husband and daughter said they liked it. After much searching I found a black bra that I could alter and wear under my long dress. I wore this dress to the wedding and to the neighborhood Christmas party.

A year later when I was trying to select a dress from my closet to wear to my husband's company Christmas party, he confessed that he thought my long dress was inappropriate for me after my surgery. He told me that he hadn't wanted to hurt my feelings or discourage me when I first bought it, because he knew it was my attempt to overcome my surgery. It matters to me that I like what I wear, and that I feel good in it, but I also feel as if my husband had this mastectomy right along with me and I care about what he thinks. I needed his frankness. I was not angry with him for not telling me right away, though, because I knew he loved me and was just trying to support me and help me adjust to all the changes.

Recently, my husband and I went shopping together for a dress for me for our anniversary. This time we did a good job of communicating. He asked questions about which styles worked and which did not work after my surgery. I felt some sadness as I had to say no to many styles but I was able to communicate that to him. Yet the pain did not stop us. We seemed to share the pain as we moved forward. We ended up buying two new dresses that we both liked.

PHYSICAL CHANGES AND NEW POSSIBILITIES

Whether you have lost one or both breasts, after surgery there are some changes to your body that will have to be compensated for sexually. A woman's nipples and breast skin have a lot of sexual nerve endings. The nipples are set up neurologically so that when they are stimulated they send sexual pleasure sensations to the genitals. Some women have such significant sensation in their breasts that with enough stimulation they are able to achieve an orgasm without being touched genitally. When the breast is removed, this powerful sexual source no longer exists. This can be experienced as a great loss to the woman for her own pleasure, as well as her partner's. When breast arousal is no longer available or is less available because one breast is gone, your partner will also feel the loss.

Breast sensation can be lost even if the nipples and skin have not been removed. I lost all sexual sensation in my breasts after I had my breasts removed and implants put in. This was unexpected because my incisions were below my breasts and none of the outside skin and nipples had been cut. Women who have had implants for enlargement reasons also frequently lose breast and nipple sensation. They still have their original breast tissue inside, but the incision made to insert the implants and the disturbance of the breast tissue from inserting the implant can damage the nerves that regulate sexual sensation.

Some women lose not only sexual sensation in the breast area, but are also left with skin pain that makes the area very uncomfortable to touch. The nerve endings in the breast and surrounding area may feel raw. This painful sensation tends to decrease gradually over many years, but it can come and go from day to day. This pain makes it very difficult for your partner to know whether or not to involve your chest during

Make sure you communicate what touch is painful after surgery so you don't end up focused on avoiding pain rather than gaining pleasure.

lovemaking. You are not able to provide one simple rule about what is or is not comfortable and pleasurable because it can change constantly.

This is another reason that open communication is so important. You need to be able to talk about the changes in your body's sensations. Accepting pain rather than discussing the matter can lead to a whole new set of problems. Sex is supposed to be a time when you share bodily pleasures, not a time to endure misery. If you try to disguise pain instead of telling your partner what you need, you will find yourself stiffening your body as a way to brace against anticipated pain. Stiffening your body is exactly the opposite of what you should be doing to achieve full sexual pleasure. You need to be able to relax and give your body over to the sensations, instead of controlling what is happening with your mind. When we use our mind too much during sex we complicate the experience and cheat ourselves and our partner.

If you find that you have lost sexual sensation and/or have a painful sensation in your chest area, ask yourself what other things you and your partner can do to make up for the lost chest pleasure. Your lips are also an erotic part of your body that have a neurological connection to your genitals just as your nipples did, but the connection is usually not as intense. Pay attention to your body and it will tell you what it likes. This is an important time to explore your senses and discover how they can enhance your lovemaking. Your senses of taste, touch, sight, smell, and hearing can all add to your sexual pleasure. Good wine, warm baths, soft materials, romantic movies, incense, perfume, and music are all examples of how we can open our senses to increase our enjoyment of sex.

One sex therapy technique used by Masters and Johnson is called "sensate focus."[16] This approach helps with performance pressures, as well as building sexual body awareness. If you are trying to learn how to compensate for the lost erotic sensations from your breast or either of you is experiencing a lot of stress about sex, you may want to try all or some of the sensate focus exercises.

In the first stage of the sensate focus exercises, the couple is instructed to have two sessions in which they will each have a turn touching their partner's body but are to exclude touching the breasts and genitals. The purpose of the touch is not to be sexual but to establish greater awareness of touch sensations by noticing textures, contours, temperatures, and contrasts while doing the touching, or to simply be aware of the sensations of being touched by their partner. The person doing the touching is told to do so on the basis of what interests him or her, not on any guesses about what his or her partner likes or dislikes. The touch should not be a massage or an attempt to arouse the partner sexually. Talking should be minimal during this first stage because talking detracts from awareness of physical sensation, but the person being touched must let his or her partner know through words or body language if the touch is uncomfortable.

In the second stage of the sensate focus exercises the breasts and genitals are included in the touch. Continuing to focus on awareness of physical sensations, the person doing the touching is instructed to begin with general body touching before adding touch to the genitals. Again, sexual arousal is not the goal at this stage. A "hand-riding" technique is used at this stage as a more direct means of nonverbal communication. The person who is being touched places her hand on top of her partner's hand and gives signals to her partner through the movement of her hand. Signals can be given to indicate that she wants more pressure, a lighter touch, faster or slower stroking, or a change to another spot.

The third stage of the sensate exercises consists of the couple practicing mutual or simultaneous touching, but still not engaging in sexual intercourse.

The fourth stage is a continuation of stage three. At some point the woman assumes a position of sitting on top of her partner, but does not insert his penis into her vagina. In this position, the woman can play with the penis, rubbing it against her clitoris, vulva, and vaginal opening whether or not there is an erection. She can go back to nongenital touch or cuddling if she wishes. The focus at this stage is still to build awareness of body sensations.

Once the couple feels they have developed a greater sense of body awareness, overcome their performance fears, and feel comfortable with each other again, they will find themselves naturally resuming intercourse.

Try to keep an open mind as you experiment. You and your partner

Sex for the single
woman can be
enriched by
establishing a
relationship first.

will create a tremendous amount of intimacy and sensuality as you explore new ideas about sexual activities. Maybe there are sex positions that
one or both of you have wanted to try but were too shy to suggest. Or
maybe you have wanted to buy a vibrator or watch an X-rated adult
movie. Instead of having your mastectomy limit your sex life, you can actually use it to go further than you have in the past.

Sex and the Single Woman

Facing sexuality again after a mastectomy can be a particularly fearful
and despairing time for a single woman. Many single women feel as
though no one will ever want them sexually or be attracted to them after
learning they are missing a breast. While this is a common feeling, it
does not mean it is true. Women with a partner suffer from the same
kinds of thoughts. These fears should be considered a normal initial reaction to having a mastectomy. You will be able to work through your
fears, and as time goes on you will find your attitude has changed.

Just like women in relationships, single women struggle with all
kinds of sexual issues. In addition, there is a perception that single
women are free and easy about sex. Of course, this is not generally true.
But single women often feel pressure even before surgery to always be
on the go to prove to others and to themselves that they have full lives. After surgery, they can feel very isolated because their image as a swinging
single has been altered by the loss of a breast.

If sex for you has been a series of one-night stands and you continue
to approach sex in the same way, you are more likely to experience sexual
rejection than women who first develop a relationship. Sex without a relationship misses the emotional intimacy that makes it more than just a
physical experience. When a sexual part of your body is missing there is
less to fill the encounter. Most men and women who are having one-
night stands are not relating to each other from a place of sensitivity and
depth, which puts the woman with a mastectomy at greater risk of feeling rejected because it does not allow for the reassurance that she is
more important than her body. I am not saying that people who have
one-night stands are not capable of intimacy, emotional depth, and sen-

sitivity. I am saying that the experience of the one-night stand does not allow for more than a superficial connection.

If you become extremely comfortable with your new body and feel secure enough to be able to shake off any rejection you may encounter, you will not have to change your sexual style. But if you conclude that it is time for a change, your surgery can open the door to reshaping a new sex life. You may decide that you wish to build more of a relationship before becoming sexual. You may find that you have been running from a fear of commitment or intimacy in your past relationships. Your mastectomy may be the turning point in your life to rework your relationship with sex and intimacy.

There is no correct time to tell a new partner about your mastectomy. My advice on dating is the same regardless of the age of the person. Take the relationship in small steps as you share about yourself and get to know the other person. Practice healthy, open communication. Don't try to create an impressive image. Just be yourself. Remember, when you decide to go on a date you are only agreeing to spend a few hours with a new person. At the end of those few hours you will make a decision as to whether you consider it worth your while to spend more time with this person.

Each time you are together you should be getting to know the interests, behaviors, attitudes, and emotional development of this person. As you spend more time with each other you should find that this person has demonstrated enough emotional maturity and sensitivity to earn your trust. If not, it is probably not in your interest to continue this relationship.

At some point, you will want to share your history of breast cancer and mastectomy. Open communication does not mean you have to reveal everything immediately. It means you use clear, direct words to convey your message. Telling someone you have had a mastectomy is not a confession. There is a big difference between hiding a dirty secret and preserving your right to privacy. I think of sharing my personal history as a privilege that people have to earn. They earn it by showing me they will handle my vulnerable side with acceptance, gentleness, and sensitivity.

"It is reassuring that I have had a relationship since my surgery. It doesn't affect him at all and that has made me less self-conscious."

A mastectomy is a
difficult thing for
a couple to go
through, but it
cannot turn a good
relationship bad.

Many single women feel they do not have a choice as to whether or not they have reconstructive surgery. They often feel that it is a "must" to try to replace the lost breast. I strongly want to encourage you to take your time to make this decision. You can have reconstructive surgery done at any point in your life, but you can't completely undo it once it's done. You may want to seek counseling, and bring the issue to a post-mastectomy support group to help you sort this out. See Chapter 12 for the pros and cons of reconstructive surgery.

All women run the risk of giving up on their sexuality after having a mastectomy because of their despair from the loss and their fear of rejection. Single women are especially prone to giving up. I strongly encourage you to accept the challenge and not let this happen to you. I hope that you will allow yourself to work through your loss and emerge with a sex life that is physically and emotionally satisfying regardless of whether you have reconstructive surgery or use prostheses.

The Unsatisfying Relationship

On top of the trauma of having to deal with breast cancer and the loss of a breast, you may find yourself in a bad or nonsupportive relationship. It may be very painful for you to read portions of this book because it reminds you how much your relationship is lacking. You may find yourself doing additional grieving over not having a supportive partner. If you are not in the position to do anything about it right now, it is still important to not deny your feelings. You do not have to take immediate action and leave your partner, but you don't have to play a pretend game with yourself by repressing these thoughts and feelings. It is all right to quietly admit to yourself that you feel sad and angry that you do not have a better relationship. It may help to share your feelings with a close friend or therapist so you don't have to carry the burden alone.

If you do not have a particularly good relationship, it did not turn bad just because you had a mastectomy. A mastectomy is a difficult thing for a couple to go through, but it cannot turn a good relationship into a bad one. If your relationship seemed to get bad after your mastectomy, perhaps the whole experience has opened your eyes to what you have been living with all along. You may have been using certain defenses, such as putting on blinders and channeling most of your energy into your kids, work, or outside friendships, to cope with the situation. After surgery, you will either return to redirecting your focus or, as you strengthen, you may decide that you have had enough and being alone would be better than living with your partner.

Before you give up on your relationship I strongly encourage you to consider your contribution to the problems in the relationship. Ask yourself how you could change to make things better. Do you need to speak up about your needs so your partner has a chance to address them? Do you play the wounded martyr when your partner doesn't read your mind? Have you ever suggested couples' counseling to try to give your relationship new tools?

If you have tried all these things and still find yourself unhappy, angry, or hurt, you need to ask yourself whether you are doing yourself an injustice by remaining in the relationship. A breast cancer diagnosis does not automatically mean that you are going to die soon or have a shortened life. Once you have finished the treatment for your cancer and the healing after your mastectomy, it is time to care about creating the best quality life you can have. If you remain in your relationship, at least know why you are still there. You will feel better about yourself if you feel that you have at least made a choice about your relationship. This can be a very confusing time and it is a good idea to seek counseling before taking any action.

CHAPTER TWELVE

BREAST RECONSTRUCTION

Breast reconstruction, or creating an artificial breast, is an option available to most women who wish to replace the breast(s) they have lost. There are two basic methods of breast reconstruction. The first method creates a new breast using an implant. The second method uses your own tissue from another part of your body to create a breast.

Making the Decision To Have a Breast Reconstruction

There are many reasons why women choose to have a breast reconstruction.

Some women have a tougher time than others accepting the change that a mastectomy has brought to their body. They feel ashamed and find that they are hiding themselves away. Some women report feeling ugly and deformed, while others feel sickly and can only imagine being able to feel whole, healthy, and rid of their cancer when they no longer have to look down and see a chest without a breast. For such women reconstruction represents a renewed state of health.

For some women the decision to undergo reconstruction has little to do with poor self-image but rather is centered more around the issue of lifestyle. They do not like being limited in clothing selection. They want to be able to go to regular clothing stores and buy what they like without having to be very selective or concerned about alterations. Women who choose reconstruction may want the freedom to wear sexy nightwear without any more limitations than they had before their surgery. And many women resent or feel financially burdened by having to buy special postmastectomy products, and find using an external prosthesis too much of a hassle. Women who are extremely physically active may also find that an external prosthesis gets in their way.

The desire to return to their old sex life is another reason some women opt to have a breast reconstruction. Even though the artificial breast cannot restore the lost sexual sensation, just having two breasts makes many women feel more sexual. Most women have reconstruction not because of pressure from their partner, but because of their need for self-acceptance as a sexual partner. Younger women often feel they have more years during which to experience life and want to be able to do that with an intact body, and single women may not want to complicate new romantic relationships with the fact that they are missing a breast. Bringing up cancer and a missing breast in the earlier part of a relationship can seem to start off the relationship with too much intensity. Of course, even with reconstruction the issue will come up eventually, but many women feel the reconstruction buys them time and makes the disclosure more natural.

These are just a few of the reasons why women choose reconstruction and I am sure there are many more. If reconstruction makes sense to you and you think it will help you feel more at peace with your body, your self image, and your life, then it is probably the best option for you, and I encourage you to explore a breast reconstruction with your surgeon.

Reconstruction can be performed at the same time as the mastectomy or at a later time. If you get implants later, they will be inserted either through your mastectomy scar or through a fine incision under the breast area where the lower breast tissue meets the chest wall.

There are many surgeons who are very skilled at performing mastectomies but that does not mean they are also trained and skilled at doing breast reconstructions. The most important thing to look for in the surgeon who is going to do your reconstruction is how well the surgeon has kept up on the latest procedures and how much experience the surgeon has had with reconstruction. Your oncologist and primary care physician can provide you with names of surgeons. Another resource is the nursing staff at an oncology clinic or hospital oncology station. The nurses

Reconstruction can be done at the same time as you have your mastectomy or any time afterwards.

usually have a good feel for the personality and competency level of the various surgeons who work with them and will be glad to share their impressions.

It is essential that you feel you can talk to the surgeon and that the surgeon take the time to explain all the options and the risks associated with each type of reconstruction procedure, and answer your questions. Expect your surgeon to be able to describe what your body will look and feel like after the reconstruction. Ask to see pictures of the anticipated outcome of each type of reconstruction, ideally pictures of the work that your surgeon has performed. Do not let yourself be pressured into making a decision on the spot. Go for the consultation, gather information, and take it home to think about.

Types of Breast Reconstruction
IMPLANTS

The two basic types of breast implants are silicone and saline. Some silicone implants were made with a polyurethane coating but because polyurethane may cause cancer and also get into breast milk and negatively affect infants, it is no longer manufactured. A more recent form of silicone implant is called a double lumen implant. It is made of a silicone gel sac surrounded with a layer of saline and covered with a solid silicone shell. The idea is that if the silicone gel starts to leak it will seep into the saline instead of directly into the chest. Most silicone implants are made with a solid silicone shell containing silicone gel.

Saline implants are filled with saline, which is sterile salt water, and covered with a solid silicone shell. The amount of salt in the saline is made to match the salt level of our bloodstream.

For reconstructions, breast implants are generally placed under the pectoralis major muscle to create a breast shape. The implant could be placed on top of the muscle, but this is not recommended with breast cancer because some breast cells remain in the muscle. Having the muscle closer to the surface allows for better detection of a lump. Sometimes the implant alone is enough to build a breast that matches the natural breast. Often there is tissue in the surgical area that can be used to help pad the implant to form a full-sized breast.

For saline implants the surgeon will either use a standard or an expander type of implant. Standard implants are already filled at the time they are inserted. The chest muscle and remaining tissue settle into a breast shape as the implant pushes out against the taut chest wall. Expander implants are empty sacks with a valve which are surgically inserted under the muscle and gradually, over several months, filled with saline by the surgeon to stretch the chest area to make more room for the implant. The saline is added in the doctor's office. When the chest has reached the desired size, the expander is surgically removed and a permanent implant is inserted. Expanders may create a more natural appearance and fuller breast, and some surgeons feel that they reduce the risk of capsular contracture (See some Cautions About Implants, below).

Implants require less extensive surgery than tissue transfer reconstruction, hence, the recovery time is considerably less. Implants are a particularly good choice for smaller-breasted women who do not have to create a large matching breast, or for smaller-breasted women who are having a bilateral mastectomy and want to replace both small breasts. Implants generally do not work for larger-breasted women because there is not enough space under the chest muscle to expand the tissue into a large breast.

SOME CAUTIONS ABOUT IMPLANTS

Remember that implants only come in a few sizes, so if there is not enough surrounding tissue left after your mastectomy to help build the breast, matching your remaining breast may be a problem. Also, your implant will not change size as you gain or lose weight but your natural breast will, so maintaining a matched pair of breasts can be tricky if you experience significant fluctuations in your weight. Your implant will not sag with time but your natural breast will droop as you age, so you may need to wear a bra more often to compensate for this difference.

Some people find that silicone implants have a more natural, flesh-like feel than saline implants. The saline implants feel more like water in a balloon than like soft, moving breast tissue. But other women don't notice the difference in feel. The skill level of your surgeon will play a part in how the saline implant feels and looks. If the shell is not filled with the

Ask your surgeon for pictures of their work, both successful and less successful outcomes, so you can get an idea of how you might look after reconstruction.

Silicone and saline
are the two basic
types of implants.
Silicone implants
have been at the
center of a lot of
controversy and are
now available only to
women undergoing
reconstruction who
also agree to be a
part of a study.

correct amount of saline, it may have a sloshing sound or feel. If it is not filled enough, it can also create ripples under the skin.

You should also know that implants may not last forever. Implants can be an excellent option for older women because they will not need them to last for as many years. But younger women should not expect their implants to last for a lifetime. The longer your implants are in, the greater the chance of complications. Both silicone and saline implants can rupture upon sudden impact, such as a car accident. You cannot expect to have a great deal of pressure applied to your chest without risking your implant developing a leak. A small child throwing her full weight onto your chest could create a rupture or weaken the implant shell, leading to future leaks. Regular impact sports are not advisable if you are trying to preserve your implants.

One common problem with implants is capsular contracture, which is scar tissue that shrinks around the implant, making the breast feel hard. This is a way that the body deals with the foreign object. Contractures are estimated to happen anywhere from 10% to 75% of the time.[17] Contractures are particularly common with silicone implants. Contractures can cause pain and also distort the shape of the implant, making it hard and in extreme cases, deforming the breast. Capsular contracture can be treated with further surgery, in a capsulectomy, or by the removal of the implant followed by using an external prosthesis, or having reconstructive surgery using your own tissue.

Silicone implants can rupture and cause bruising inside the chest. The silicone gel can also bleed through the implant shell, and this leakage can put tremendous strain on the immune system as it tries to deal with what the body interprets as a dangerous intrusion. Some women have become very ill from leaking silicone and there are cases where it is suspected that women have died from complications from silicone leakage. Autoimmune system and connective tissue diseases are also cited as suspected silicone-related complications. Lupus, multiple sclerosis, and arthritic conditions are examples. Silicone implants were banned by the FDA in 1993 for cosmetic use and are now only available for women who need reconstruction after a mastectomy or deforming accident and who are willing to be a part of a study.

Saline implants have less risk than silicone because only their shell is made of silicone, but for women who are hypersensitive to silicone the shell alone may cause problems. Saline implants also carry a lower risk of capsular contraction. As well, if they deflate or rupture, they will lose their shape but the body will be able to absorb the salt water.

The first study of women with silicone breast implants, carried out by the Mayo Clinic in 1994, indicated that there was no significant correlation between the use of breast implants and autoimmune and connective tissue diseases.[18] I consider this to be a very poorly conducted study because it merely compared the medical records of women who had implants with women who did not have implants. The women themselves were never examined or interviewed. If you have ever had a chance to read your medical record, you will see that very little is recorded from your visit. A brief summary of your chief complaints and the treatment used is all that will be recorded. All the other little questions you bring to the doctor that are addressed verbally without treatment will not be included. Women with implant complications often have long lists of minor to major complaints. The numerous, vague, and varied symptoms are often deemed not worth mentioning to the doctor by the patient. Many women feel like hypochondriacs and do not want to burden their busy doctor with minor problems. Unless these women were asked if they had all the symptoms that seem to go along with breast implant complications and the full response was entered into the record, there is no way their records could have produced a reliable profile of the complications.

Three years after this first study the Mayo Clinic did further research into silicone implants.[19] This more recent research showed that women having reconstruction after mastectomies were almost three times more likely to need additional surgeries than those who had implants for cosmetic reasons. More than 24% of all women who undergo breast implant surgery have complications severe enough to require a second operation within five years. 30–50% of women who have mastectomies receive breast implants. The most common complication for these women was contracture and the next most common problems were ruptures and inside bruising. Women who had implants after cancer

Contractures occur in between 10%–75% of the time and are particularly common with silicone implants.

The exact relation
between silicone
implants and
autoimmune
disorders is still
unknown.

surgery had a 34% chance of requiring a second or third operation, compared with 12% who had implants to enlarge their breasts. Women who received implants after preventive mastectomies also often had to undergo a second surgery. It is speculated that postmastectomy implants are more likely to result in complications because of the trauma of surgery and radiation therapy. What is still unknown is the exact relationship between silicone implants and autoimmune and connective tissue disorders.

All this suggests to me that if you are a healthy person without a heavy demand on your immune system from excessive stress or disease and your implants do not rupture, you will probably tolerate implants well. But if you have a long history of a lot of stress, other immune system conditions such as chronic allergies, or your immune system has had to fight something like cancer, then you may have problems down the road. Some surgeons, such as Dr. Randolph Guthrie, author of *The Truth About Breast Implants,* believe most women will tolerate the implants best if their bodies have had a period of time to recover from the mastectomy and cancer treatment. Waiting until chemotherapy and radiation are over and your body is in a stronger state may be very beneficial in the long run.

So far, there is no definitive research to tell us what the body does in the presence of silicone and under what conditions the body is likely to have a negative response. Research is now underway on substances other than silicone that can be used to fill implants. So far saline implants seem to be the safest bet. With the huge lawsuits and the heightened awareness of the possible dangers of implants, we can be assured that pharmaceutical companies are not going to be so quick to put a product on the market without having it thoroughly tested first. The FDA now has authority over the approval of the use of implants. When implants first came on the market the FDA did not have to approve them. The implants were not adequately tested and some companies ignored negative test results. Women's health is finally starting to be taken seriously and we can hope that in the future companies will be more cautious about using potentially unsafe products in our bodies.

My sister and I are both nurses who underwent preventive bilateral mastectomies with silicone implants that later ruptured, but our reaction to the ruptured implants was completely different. My sister has worked in surgery, so she was very used to and comfortable with surgery. She considered saline implants to be safer than the silicone implants. Since there was a surgical procedure to allow her to have breasts it seemed reasonable to avail herself of that option. And she figures that when her saline implants wear out they can be replaced with new ones.

I have worked in mental health nursing so my orientation has been to look at the psychological impact of having implants and further surgery. I consider surgery to be very invasive, and emotionally and physically traumatic, and believe it should only be used when deemed absolutely necessary. I knew I would be able to deal with the change by working through my feelings. There was no question for my sister that surgery was her best option, and there was no question for me that removing the ruptured implants and then leaving my poor body alone was my best option. I had many more health problems than my sister after my silicone implants ruptured, but she has also had some similar health problems.

My sister has told me she could not imagine herself without breasts and considers me to be very brave to go without them, and I consider her very brave to be able to face surgery with such ease, which is something I cannot do. Intellectually we know that there are strengths and weaknesses inherent in our own different methods of coping. We seem to accept each other's way as merely a statement about how we best cope and do not judge or try to change the other one. Both of us have remained comfortable and satisfied with our decisions.

> "I think that my reconstruction problems were a matter of bad timing."

RECONSTRUCTION USING YOUR OWN TISSUE

Because breast implants tend to work best only for smaller-breasted women, and because of the increasing awareness of health complications from implants, surgeons have been successful at developing forms of plastic surgery that make a breast out of a woman's own tissue. Extra fat, muscle, and skin is taken from various parts of the body to create a new breast and fill in collapsed areas of the chest. In rare cases where a radical mastectomy has removed the pectoralis major muscle along with a significant amount of tissue from under the armpit, this new approach can fill in the hollow areas. Implants cannot fill in all the space that is left after a radical mastectomy. Providing a woman is still in good health and less than age sixty-five, tissue transfer surgery can finally offer a woman who had a radical mastectomy years ago the option of reconstruction. Age is a factor because this type of surgery requires a good blood supply to the chest and the circulatory system weakens with age.

Creating a breast to match the other one is easier with tissue transfer procedures because you are having a breast custom made instead of depending on standard implant sizes. How many times have you heard a woman say, "If I could only take this and put it up here," referring to removing her excess abdominal fat and using it to make bigger breasts? Well, now it can be done. In fact, the tissue can be taken from wherever there is extra; the unsightly can now be put to good use.

There are two ways to transfer tissue. The oldest method is called the "tunnel" approach, which takes skin, muscle, and fat from either the back or the abdomen and pulls the tissue under the skin into the new desired location. The blood vessels are not cut, so the blood supply remains intact; the tissue and blood vessels are just stretched to the new area.

Latissimus Dorsi Muscle Transfer

This surgical procedure transfers skin, muscle, and fat and the blood vessels that nourish them from the back to the breast area. A flap made of skin, fat, and the latissimus dorsi muscle is tunneled inside the body from the back to the front of the chest. The latissimus dorsi muscle is a triangular-shaped back muscle that moves the arm, draws the shoulder back and down, and pulls the body up when climbing. The skin and muscle remain partly attached to the blood and nerve supply. This procedure is sometimes done with the addition of an implant depending on the tissue available and the size of the breast to be created.

The latissimus dorsi transfer should take about three hours to perform, and you will be hospitalized for three to six days, and will not be able to return to normal activities for about four to six weeks. This procedure leaves a significant scar in the back where the tissue has been removed. There is a risk that the blood vessels feeding the flap could become blocked or twisted, causing the tissue to die. The loss of the back muscle may cause the shoulder to drag and hinder you in activities that entail reaching, pulling, and pushing, such as swimming, tennis, overhead scrubbing, pushing up from a sitting position, rowing, and climbing.

TRAM Flap

TRAM stands for transverse rectus abdominis muscle, which is a pair of muscles (one from each side) that extend down the front of the torso into the abdomen. These muscles support the spine, lower back muscles, stomach, and intestines, and stimulate the stomach and intestines for digestion. An incision is made, extending from one hip bone to the other across the abdomen. The skin, muscle, and fat are tunneled up through the torso to the chest.

Breast reconstruction using your own tissue is a more complicated surgery than Implants and will require a longer period for recuperation.

This procedure is fairly limited because the tissue can only be moved so far from its original location. It is also not an option for women who have had other surgery that has already cut across the areas where the tissue needs to travel through the tunnel, such as a caesarean section. Even though the blood supply is not changed, there can be complications from dragging the tissue through the tunnel, leaving problems in the surrounding area. Hernias are a fairly common complication that can show up down the road. Sometimes plastic mesh is sewn into the abdomen to make up for the missing muscle. But according to Dr. Guthrie in his book, *The Truth About Breast Implants,* the mesh deteriorates with time and can make hernia repair even more difficult. He also points out that this type of surgery is usually chosen to avoid having a foreign object used in the body, yet the mesh is exactly that.

A fifty-two-year old woman I spoke with said she had one breast removed as a result of breast cancer and had asked about having a reconstruction done with her own tissue. The surgeon had told her she was too old to have that kind of surgery, as her skin was not youthful and elastic enough for good results. She was forty at the time. A few years later she had her surgeon put in a silicone implant. She had the implant for about three to four years but, in looking back, she knows the implant ruptured fairly soon after it was inserted, because it started to lose shape within the first year. She used an external prosthesis to fill out her bra because

"It is much better
when it is all your
own fat. It looks
more natural and it
feels more natural."

her implant had lost so much of its shape so quickly. No one mentioned the possibility that her implant had ruptured; she was told that that was the way her implant had settled and there was nothing that could be done about it.

Finally, she insisted on having an MRI (magnetic resonance imaging) done which determined that her implant had ruptured. She had the implant removed and a TRAM flap performed. Magically, her skin became youthful enough by her late forties to make her a candidate for the reconstruction using her own tissue. The abdominal tissue was tunneled up to her chest and shaped into a breast. No implant was required to complete the job. She was in the hospital for about four days and was out of work for a month from a sit-down job that required only light lifting. She has had no complications from her TRAM flap, which was performed four years ago. She said she has had no back problems, and was told a mesh was sewn into her abdomen where the flap was removed to help support the area. She is very pleased with how her breast looks but weight gain has caused her natural breast to become larger, so she has sewn pads into her bras to make even-sized breasts.

Gluteal Free Flap

The second surgical approach that moves skin, muscle, and fat from one place to another is called the "free flap" technique. This procedure completely detaches the fat, muscle, and skin from the original spot and moves it externally to the new location. The blood vessels are cut and then reconnected after the tissue has been put in place to form the new breast. Because the tissue does not have to stretch to the new location it can be taken from any part of the body that has enough muscle, fat, and a good blood supply, such as the buttocks, abdomen, thigh, or back.

The gluteal free flap was the first free flap procedure. The upper or lower portion of the gluteus maximus (buttocks) is used for the flap. The tissue and blood vessels are completely detached, and then reattached to the chest. The blood supply is hooked up to the blood vessels in the armpit. Sometimes an implant is added if the flap alone does not produce the desired outcome. If the flap is taken from the top of the buttocks, it will leave a gap in the upper part of the buttocks that can be seen through tight-fitting clothes and a scar that will show with a low-cut two-piece swimsuit. If the flap is taken from the lower portion of the buttocks, it will flatten that part of the buttocks, as well as leave a scar. Regardless of where the flap is taken from, one side of your buttocks will be different than the other side, which can also be noticeable through clothes, unless of course you have both breasts done in which case your buttocks will match.

Free TRAM Flap

The free TRAM flap procedure uses the same muscles as the TRAM flap, but the flap is completely detached from the abdomen and reattached to the chest instead of tunneled up to the chest. The abdominal free TRAM flap is more frequently used than the gluteal free flap because it leaves fewer cosmetic problems. Clothes can more easily disguise the missing tissue on the abdomen than on the buttocks.

There are drawbacks to the free TRAM flap procedure, however. The loss of abdominal muscle will make it difficult to keep the remainder of your abdomen pulled firmly in place. The abdominal muscle is critical for supporting your lower back. If you do not have a strong, well-functioning abdominal muscle, it can lead to lower back pain. One of the most common ways of treating lower back pain is to strengthen the abdominal muscle through situps. Doing situps can be very difficult or even impossible after this type of surgery.

In addition, in any free flap procedures the tissue used to make the breast can die if the blood supply is not adequate. Even if the surgery is done with a great deal of skill and the blood supply is initially sufficient, circulation is one of the things that decreases with age, which would put you at greater risk of having the tissue die from lack of blood. People who have smoked heavily or currently smoke are not good candidates for this surgery, since smoking decreases circulation. People with diabetes, heart disease, and other conditions that prevent good circulation should not have this surgery.

The free flap procedures have many pluses. They make a more complete reconstruction possible by allowing as much tissue as needed. Free flap procedures allow for a good match to the other breast and for creat-

Reconstruction with your own tissue makes it easier to match a breast the same size and shape as your remaining breast.

ing larger breasts. The tissue is soft and normal right from the start and will not become hard the way an implant is prone to do. The tissue will hang naturally like your other breast so it will look more normal right away, as well as over the rest of your aging process.

The free flap procedures takes longer to perform than the tunnel approach and requires the skill of a vascular surgeon along with a plastic surgeon. The longer you are under anesthetic the greater risk there is for developing blood clots, which can cause a stroke or even be life-threatening. Some plastic surgeons are very good at doing both surgeries but many do not have enough experience with these procedures. Ask your surgeon how long it takes to complete the surgery. If the answer is between three to five hours, it indicates a fairly experienced surgeon. If the answer is eight to twelve hours, I suggest you find a different surgeon. If you live in a smaller community, you may need to travel to a larger facility in order to make this surgery an option for you.

One woman who had the free TRAM flap has been very pleased with the result of her reconstruction except for not being able to have even-sized breasts. During chemotherapy treatment she gained thirty pounds, and because the tissue flap contained so much fatty tissue her reconstructed side gained much more weight than her natural side. She found this extremely frustrating because the great discrepancy was very difficult to compensate for and the whole purpose of having the reconstruction was to not have to bother with external prostheses and accessories.

> Most reconstructive surgeries will be done in pieces. It may take a few tries to get the results you want.

Nipple Reconstructions

Regardless of what kind of reconstructive surgery you have, if you wish to have a nipple, it will have to be added at a later time. As I mentioned in Chapter 2, the ducts lead into the nipple and, because breast cancer usually occurs in the breast ducts, the nipple is routinely removed in the attempt to cut out all the existing cancer. If you only want to fill out a bra without having to use an external prosthesis, a nipple may not seem necessary. But if you want to be as close as possible to your pre-surgery breast, you will want to add a nipple.

Nipples are added later because the new breast will be very swollen right after reconstructive surgery. You will have to wait until the inflammation goes away and the tissue settles into its new place, or the swelling from the implant has receded, to know where the nipple should go. After a few months the breast will have settled into its permanent shape and size, so the nipple can be lined up to match the location of the other nipple.

The nipple is made with a flap of skin, usually from the inside of the thigh, chest, groin, or vagina. If it is done well, the nipple should match your other nipple in shape and color. You can have just a nipple made out of a flap and then the skin around it, called the areola, can be tattooed on, or the nipple and areola can both be made out of the grafted skin. This procedure is considered a minor surgery and can often be done under local anesthetic in an outpatient department.

Some women have a second surgery done at the same time as the nipple is being attached to make adjustments so the new breast looks even more like the natural, remaining breast. It is very common in plastic surgery to have to complete a job in stages. You may have a very talented surgeon, but in order to get the outcome you want it may require a couple of tries. During the second surgery, some women have the natural breast reshaped to fit the new one. Often this entails a breast reduction for very large-breasted women. Again, the silver lining of your breast cancer may be your opportunity to finally achieve the breast size you have always wanted.

LUMPECTOMY RECONSTRUCTIONS

It is also possible to have reconstruction after a lumpectomy. Having a significant piece of the breast removed can make it very tricky to give a full smooth appearance through clothing. A small prosthesis can fill in the area, but the location of the missing tissue sometimes makes it hard to keep the prosthesis in place.

In this case, the free flap technique is generally used, where a piece of tissue from another part of the body is put into the space where the lump was removed. Small implants are not used in lumpectomy reconstruc-

Remember that a nipple will not be added until later.

Breast implants tend to work best for smaller-breasted women.

tions because the implants will get in the way of mammograms when trying to detect additional cancer.

Expectations

Probably one of the greatest factors in feeling satisfied with your reconstruction is how well you are prepared for the outcome. If you start with a realistic expectation of what reconstruction can accomplish, you are much more likely to be happy with the outcome. First of all you need to know that no form of reconstruction will produce breast sensation. You might have a little sexual sensation left in the area, but much more than that is highly unlikely. Some women don't realize that the reconstruction will not fix the nerve damage that was done by the mastectomy and think their newly created breast will feel just like the one they lost. They are then disappointed to find out that their new breast has no feeling in it. Also, if they had flap surgery, they probably sustained nerve damage in the skin around the donor tissue site, leaving that area with some permanent numbness.

How your breasts look after the surgery may not be at all how you imagined they would. I strongly recommend that you ask your surgeon to show you some pictures of reconstructed breasts with both good outcomes and some less desirable outcomes. Remember that each breast job is unique and no surgeon can promise a precise result. The outcome of your reconstruction will be determined by how the surgery progresses as the surgeon works with your particular body. Knowing ahead of time that you will be without a nipple for a while is also a help.

Timing of Reconstruction

Even though many surgeons are doing immediate reconstructions at the same time as they perform the mastectomy, you do not have to have it done then. Finding a lump, having it biopsied, learning you have cancer and you need a mastectomy is a huge upset to your life. It is an incredibly stressful time when you have to make a lot of big decisions with huge implications for your future. We are told to try to avoid big decisions during stressful times, yet breast cancer forces us to do just that. Picking a surgeon, a type of surgery, and an approach for treating your cancer are just a few of the big decisions that will be forced on you at this time. This is also a vulnerable time when you can be easily talked into something because you feel overwhelmed and just want someone else to decide for you, or because someone is offering you something that seems to be a solution to minimizing your loss. Denial and attempting to hang on to what you are losing is a natural reaction and the first stage of the grief process. Being in the early stage of grief can greatly influence those first decisions and lead to later regrets.

It is my strong bias that women should give themselves time to heal from their mastectomy before having reconstruction done. The shock of having cancer and undergoing a mastectomy are hard enough without having to make decisions about whether or not to have reconstruction. There are a lot of pros and cons to consider about the reconstruction options and, in my opinion, you will come out feeling the best about your choice if you have had enough time and a clear head with which to weigh the anticipated benefits against the risks.

Many women are sure that they will eventually be having reconstruction but, by the time they have reached the point where they are ready to proceed, they conclude that they are doing very nicely without any additional surgery. They have come to accept their body, and find that wearing a prosthesis works just fine, so reconstruction seems unnecessary. On the other hand, some women have the time after surgery to experience being without a breast and they become even more certain that reconstruction is the best choice for them.

The other reason I recommend waiting to have reconstruction until you are healthy is that I believe your body deserves its best shot at attacking the cancer and healing. Survival should be our first concern. Major surgery is very hard on the body, especially the immune system, which is the part you need most for fighting cancer. Mastectomy reconstruction with an immediate tissue transfer puts your body through two major surgeries at the same time. A mastectomy with immediate reconstruction using an implant is a major surgery and adds a foreign object into your already over-stressed immune system. I think the more you can fo-

"In some ways reconstruction was worse than the disease. It was incredibly painful. Even so, it was the only choice for me and I would never advise anyone against it."

cus your attention on fighting cancer and building up your body's natural way of battling it, the better chance you have of recovery.

Reshaping a body that is more desirable to live in should come later when your body has returned to a healthy, strong state. There are many surgeons and oncologists who share my belief. Just because we have advanced medically to the point where immediate reconstruction is possible doesn't mean it is the wisest approach.

CHAPTER THIRTEEN

GETTING IN OVER OUR HEADS (AND GETTING HELP)

It is not uncommon for women to develop problems that they may need psychiatric help with following a mastectomy. Don't let the word psychiatric frighten you. Having a psychiatric condition does not automatically mean you are crazy or psychotic. Mental illness, nervous disorder, or psychiatric condition are three terms that mean the same thing. And many mental illnesses are short lived and very treatable. However, like most other medical diagnoses, if left untreated mental illness can have many serious negative consequences. I cannot emphasize enough how important it is to look after the mental and emotional aspects of yourself as you heal from a mastectomy.

As I explained in Chapter 4, the mind, emotions, and body work together to create a complete state of wellness. A mastectomy brings with it trauma, loss, and change, both physically and emotionally, all of which put tremendous strain on our nervous system. A certain amount of anxiety and depression is a natural part of a normal grieving process. Time alone does not heal grief, however. We have to work through the feelings that go along with our losses after a mastectomy. Talking to supportive friends and family and attending support groups are all very helpful in dealing with the emotional component of having breast cancer and losing a breast. Many women seek out a therapist in addition to or instead of attending a support group.

It is not a sign of
weakness to need
some help with your
emotional recovery
after a mastectomy.

Finding a Good Therapist

Finding a good therapist is a two-step process. First, you need to obtain a list of names of therapists. Your oncologist, surgeon, primary care physician, nursing staff from the clinic, prosthesis fitter, American or Canadian Cancer Society, church pastor, and local community health center are all possible resources for names. Your insurance company may designate therapists who are covered under your particular medical plan. Your employer may have an employee assistance program that will help you find a competent professional. Let the person you are requesting names from know what you want counseling for, so they can match your needs with the competency level and specialty of the therapist.

The second step is to select the right person for you from the list of names you have been given. Psychiatric nurses, clinical social workers, psychologists, and psychiatrists are all trained to conduct individual, couple, family, and group therapy and should all have the same basic knowledge about psychotherapy. Each type of therapist has knowledge that goes beyond therapy and is unique to their discipline. A nurse or social worker with less than a master's degree has very limited knowledge and skill in providing therapy. Psychiatric nurses are registered nurses first, then have additional training as therapists. In some areas psychiatric nurses may also prescribe medications and monitor patients on those medications. Social workers learn about social services, along with how to conduct therapy. Psychologists are usually trained to do psychological testing as well as therapy. Psychiatrists are medical doctors first, and then learn how to prescribe psychiatric medications along with how to conduct therapy. Psychiatry has changed a great deal over the years, in that psychiatrists primarily used to conduct therapy with some medication prescribing, but because there have been so many advances with psychiatric medications, most psychiatrists now tend to spend the majority of their time prescribing medication and do much less actual therapy. There are some psychiatrists who do not advocate the use of medications or only prescribe them infrequently, but they are in the minority.

Most people receive counseling from a psychiatric nurse, social worker, or psychologist because of the lower cost and greater availability of appointment times with these therapists. A psychiatrist's fee is usually two to two and a half times that of the fee for the other disciplines, and the waiting period is usually much longer to see a psychiatrist because of the demand for medication management. I would recommend that you choose a therapist with a minimum of a master's degree.

In Canada and in the U.S., most medical plans pay for services provided by a psychiatrist but will not always pay for other types of therapists. Make sure you check your mental health benefits to see what limits it may put on the frequency of sessions and what type of therapist is considered an eligible provider.

It is imperative that you and your therapist are well matched. You should quickly feel a comfortable connection with the person. Your therapist is someone you will be going to for support and direction and someone you will be vulnerable with. If the therapist does not demonstrate warmth, caring, and respect, he or she won't be able to provide an environment that fosters trust and openness. Be wary of the therapist with an air of having all the answers. A good therapist usually does not give you all the answers to your problems; instead she listens to you and helps you define and solve your own problems. Your therapist should provide you with information, feedback, and direction in a way that fits with your personality, belief system, strengths, and goals.

The therapist you choose should have experience working with grief issues and, ideally, with women who have gone through mastectomies. It may be difficult to find someone who specializes in working with post-mastectomy clients, but a therapist with grief counseling experience should be easy to find. The gender of the therapist only matters to the degree that it matters to you. There are many excellent male therapists who have worked very effectively with women who have had a mastectomy. Ask yourself if you typically find it easier to talk to a man or a woman. Sometimes postmastectomy women desire an outside male perspective. Some women start with a therapist of one gender, then move to a new therapist of the other gender because of the issues they are working on.

Your assessment of the therapist can start on the phone and should be concluded by the end of your first session. If you do not feel a connec-

A good therapist will not have an air of having all the answers.

Support groups can
be a wonderful
source of support
and encouragement.

tion by the end of your first session, I recommend you try a different person. Ask the therapist about her credentials, experience, and general approach to therapy and listen closely to your overall reaction to the therapist as she responds to your questions. There is a difference between being nervous and fearful about the unfamiliar process of therapy even though you are in the presence of a comfortable person, and being tense and uncomfortable because you are having a negative reaction to the person. It does not mean that person is a bad therapist; it just means that the match is not right for you. If you find yourself thinking that a therapist is "probably just fine," this may be a clue that you are settling for less than you deserve. You are far too important to stay with someone who doesn't meet your needs. Remembering that you have a choice in the therapist you choose is critical, and will remind you that you are not powerless or helpless during this very vulnerable time.

Your therapist should also have a good sense of boundaries. She should be clear about the financial agreement, missed appointments, availability of her time outside your therapy session, and the expectations that you can have of her and that she has of you. Your therapist should only disclose personal information about herself in order to help you. Remember, this is your time.

Support Groups

Support groups are probably the most common form of emotional care after a mastectomy. Support groups are an extremely valuable way to make sense out of what you are going through, and a good place to find people who have a deep understanding and empathy for your situation. Support groups offer hope, encouragement, and a chance to give back, which can make people feel worthwhile. Postmastectomy groups are usually offered by women's clinics; churches; community health centers; organizations whose purpose is to serve the needs of mastectomy and cancer patients, such as the American or Canadian Cancer Society; and organizations that serve the needs of women and families, such as Lutheran Social Services and Jewish Family and Children's Services.

There are two basic types of support groups. One is a short-term educational support group and the other is a group in which you can talk about your situation and receive support as you go through the process of recovering after a mastectomy. Often women start with a short-term support group that is sponsored through a formal organization, then several of the women from the group leave to form their own informal support group that lasts for many years. I have already discussed the benefits and selection of a suitable support group in Chapter 4.

In the earlier part of your recovery it can be very helpful to attend a formally organized support group because they offer a lot of information as well as the opportunity to share your feelings and experiences. Formalized groups will have a group leader who has some training in leading a group as well as in the issues involved in recovery from a mastectomy. Rules and structure are very important in running an effective group, especially when dealing with differing personalities and backgrounds. Informal groups usually don't need a leader because the connections have already taken place, and the group members have selected one another because of an established sense of compatibility. The same resources listed above for finding a therapist can also be used to locate a suitable support group.

A common reason I hear women give for not wanting to take part in a support group is because the sad stories overwhelm them and make them more depressed. This can become a problem because people do not know how to avoid taking on other people's feelings. Many women are chronic caretakers who are deeply affected by other people's feelings and think it is their job to make everyone happy. For a woman assuming this role, walking into a group of women who are all experiencing a lot of pain will certainly make her feel as if she wants to run away. But in this case a support group may be very helpful.

If this describes you, you can use a support group to learn how to separate yourself from other people's pain and practice receiving help. If you listen compassionately and let others listen to you as you share your painful struggle, you may be able to reverse a long-standing relationship problem at the same time you are grieving your lost breast.

"I didn't like the support groups. I didn't want to let cancer and my mastectomy rule my life and it seemed like that was what was happening in the group."

It is imperative that
you find a support
group that makes
you feel at home and
like you belong.

Where Do You Go for Support If You Never Had Breast Cancer But Have Lost A Breast?

One of the most compelling reasons I had for writing this book was that I wanted to help other women in my situation. I have never had breast cancer but needed support and direction after my implants ruptured and I had to learn how to adjust to no longer having breasts. I was told by my surgeon after my bilateral surgery that I had not made a bad choice and had not been too hasty about having the surgery because they had found abnormal cells in my breast tissue. Eighty-five percent of women who get breast cancer do not have a family history of breast cancer, so could not have prevented it as I could. I have never doubted my decision, and am incredibly grateful that I have not had breast cancer. All the same, I found that I felt very much alone. I did not feel comfortable going to one of the many well-established support groups that exist for women who have lost a breast as a result of breast cancer. Even though I have a great deal in common with breast cancer survivors, the fact remains that I have not had breast cancer.

This sense of not belonging has been reinforced as I collected data to write this book. It is not that I have been treated poorly by women who have had breast cancer; rather, it is as if they don't know how to react to me. When I say that I had a bilateral mastectomy fifteen years ago, other women frequently say, "Oh, you are a long-time survivor. Good for you." When I then explain that I did not have breast cancer, the other person will say in a surprised tone, "Oh." This is often followed by an uncomfortable lag in the conversation until I shift the focus.

I have never taken offense to this type of reaction because I know it is difficult to understand my different situation, and not an intentional rejection. Nevertheless, such responses are a constant reminder that I do not belong to the network of breast cancer women. I find people want to put me in the category of those who have joined the cause of fighting breast cancer but who have not experienced cancer. In some ways that is an accurate description, but it does not tell the whole story.

Every Mother's Day I walk in the Susan G. Komen Race for the Cure. Breast cancer survivors are given a pink ribbon to wear, along with a pink visor. In October, which is Breast Cancer Awareness Month, J.C. Penney's a very strong supporter of the battle against breast cancer, hands out the same pink ribbons. I have often wondered whether I should be wearing one or if they were really only intended for women who have had breast cancer. (I have since learned that the pink ribbon is simply a symbol to raise breast cancer awareness and can be worn by anyone.)

If you had a preventive bilateral mastectomy or lost a breast because of an accident, I recommend you not attend a support group for women who have lost a breast from breast cancer. There are not enough of us who have lost a breast for other reasons for there to be support groups available for our needs. Many generous group leaders would allow you to join a breast cancer grief group to help you to adjust to your mastectomy, but I can see many possible problems for you in such a situation. It is a natural, normal part of the grieving process after breast cancer to ask, "Why me?" which also means, "Why not someone else?" Women with breast cancer need a safe place to express this anger. If you are in the group, it could prevent women from expressing their anger, or conversely, you may inadvertently become a handy dumping ground for their anger. Such a situation is also likely to cause you to minimize your loss. Attending a breast cancer survivor's group may lead you to focus on your gratitude that you don't have cancer, so that you take on the role of a caretaker in the group, instead of feeling support and validation for your own loss.

Accepting that you are different and not comparing your pain with women who have breast cancer is the key to successfully working through your grief. Instead of going to a breast cancer support group, I recommend that you seek out an individual therapist. The therapist will see you as an individual rather than define your situation in the context of a group. Individual therapy will provide you with someone to listen closely to what you are going through, to validate your feelings of loss, and to help you to reclaim your life. Individual therapy should also prevent you from caretaking others, instead directing you to focus on yourself and your recovery.

There are many ways that you can relate to women who have had breast cancer and you may develop wonderful, mutually supportive relationships with them, but that is best done outside a group setting. As I

"I have done some counseling for friends of friends. I find it quite difficult because it brings it all back."

have mentioned earlier, I have two friends who have recently had breast cancer. We have been able to support each other and have become even closer because of our shared loss of a breast.

Psychiatric Conditions After a Mastectomy

Depression is very
common and to
some degree, even
normal after breast
cancer and a
mastectomy.

Sometimes our stress level before, during, and after our surgery is so great it pushes us beyond the level of depression and anxiety that can be managed through such supportive measures as a support group. A support group and/or therapy is likely to be all that you will need to get through the process of recovering from your mastectomy. However, you should inform yourself about depression and anxiety, as well as medications, so you can take a more active role in the decision-making process if you require additional treatment. The two psychiatric conditions I commonly see after a mastectomy are depression and anxiety disorders. The DSM-IV is currently recognized as the most up-to-date resource for descriptions of these disorders.[21]

DEPRESSION

A certain degree of depression is a normal part of the grief that follows a significant loss such as a mastectomy. We usually think of it as "feeling down" or having a "blue mood." A sense of despair can be expected, and even some fleeting thoughts about wishing you were dead are common and normal. You don't really want to be dead. After all, you have been fighting desperately to save your life. But your misery might lead you to think of wanting an end to your pain and fear. Almost as soon as we consider death, our minds shift to more constructive solutions or comforting thoughts which lessen the emotional and physical pain.

Prolonged periods of stress, such as that brought on by cancer and a mastectomy, can precipitate a depression that goes beyond the normal ups and downs of our daily moods. It can be hard for you to know the difference between down moods and a more serious depression and to tell at what point you need further treatment. I will describe the symptoms and treatment for serious depression, but you are not expected to make the determination yourself. If you are struggling and are in a support group or seeing an individual therapist, you should rely on your group leader or therapist to help you assess your depression level and direct you to the right kind of intervention. You may want to ask to see your group leader alone before or after the group meets, to discuss your depression level. Any one of your physicians can also help you discover whether intervention is needed for your symptoms. Persistent suicidal thinking that includes forming a plan of action should never be left untreated. You must tell a professional if you are having such thoughts so they can help you determine what you need beyond therapy.

There are several classifications of depression, but only two forms that are likely to be experienced after your mastectomy. One is commonly called a clinical depression or, to be more exact, a major depressive episode. The second form of depression is called dysthymic depression or dysthymia.

The majority of mental health professionals believe that clinical depression is the result of a chemical imbalance in the nervous system. We have come to believe that the chemical neurotransmitters that activate the nervous system are not working properly, specifically that the nervous system is not producing enough of the right neurotransmitters and the nervous pathways are having difficulty utilizing the neurotransmitters that are present.

Some people have a genetically based predisposition to clinical depression. They have other blood relatives through the generations who have also experienced depression. Pregnancy and menopause can set off a depression because of the dramatic shift in hormone levels, and any major demand on the immune system can also destabilize the nervous system. And, of course, cancer makes the immune system work long and hard as it tries to combat the cancer. The grief from a mastectomy creates a great deal of stress on the immune system, and when you add cancer or health problems from ruptured implants, and a family history of depression, you are very likely to develop a temporary clinical depression that will require more than counseling to treat.

Dysthymia disorder or dysthymic depression is very similar to a major depressive episode except that it is more of a chronic or ongoing mood disorder. Major depressive episodes can come on very quickly and with treatment be resolved in a short period of time. Dysthymia is a de-

Dysthymia is a depressed mood that has lasted for at least two years.

Clinical depression is
also known as a
major depressive
episode.

pressed mood that has been present for at least two years. The symptoms are usually less intense than with clinical depression but are chronically present. Dysthymia is considered less a physiologically based depression and more a result of one's circumstances, upbringing, and world view or attitudes.

Dysthymia consists of a whole set of beliefs that reinforce the feeling that the person is stuck in her misery. It is more of a breakdown in the thinking process than a breakdown of the nervous system. However, our thoughts directly affect our nervous system, so the symptoms of dysthymia can look as though they stem from a faulty nervous system. But the real problem is the affected person's thoughts. Her past experiences may have shaped her thinking so that her thoughts leave her feeling helpless, worthless, and trapped.

A woman without adequate coping skills and resources available to her after a mastectomy could respond with a low-grade level of depressed mood and despair that hangs on for several years after the mastectomy. Unless she seeks counseling she is likely to continue feeling stuck as a helpless victim, and never find a way to move forward to adjust to and accept the loss of her breast. Some women are depressed even before undergoing their mastectomies, and the stress and emotional pain from the mastectomy make the already existing dysthymic depression worse.

Symptoms of Major Depressive Episode
A clinical depression changes a person's chemical balance. This imbalance leads to a disturbance in the basic rhythms of the body. Clinical depression is a combination of symptoms. If you have only one or two of the following symptoms, you probably don't have a clinical depression. The severity and frequency of the symptoms also need to be taken into consideration when diagnosing clinical depression.

In order to be diagnosed with a clinical depression, you will have at least five of the following symptoms present during a two-week period and these will be a change from your previous functioning. The five symptoms must include depressed mood or loss of interest or pleasure.

1. Depressed mood most of the day, nearly every day, feeling sad or empty or looking sad and tearful to others.

2. Significant loss of interest or pleasure in all, or almost all, activities most of the day, nearly every day.

3. Change in appetite. The thought of food can be either nauseating or uninteresting. There may be weight loss without dieting or weight gain from nervous compulsive eating, with no real pleasure from the eating.

4. Not able to sleep or sleeping too much but still not feeling rested.

5. Psychomotor agitation or retardation, which means that you are restless and fidgety, or that your movement and speech are in slow motion.

6. Fatigue or loss of energy nearly every day. This is more than being tired from putting in a hard day. It feels as if your muscles are full of lead and everything is a physical effort. It feels as if you could fall asleep standing up even though you have not done anything to make you tired.

7. Feelings of worthlessness or excessive or inappropriate guilt nearly every day.

8. Poor concentration, an inability to think clearly, poor short term-memory, indecisiveness. It feels as if your mind has gone to mush and your head is fuzzy.

9. Recurrent thoughts of death (not just fear of dying), suicidal thoughts with or without a specific plan or suicide attempt. Difficulty shaking these thoughts and shifting over to more positive, constructive thoughts.

10. Loss of sex drive. You have a flat disinterest in sex. Your body does not have its usual craving for sex.

11. Feeling like crying all the time but too emotionally blunted to be able to cry, or crying a lot but not feeling better afterwards. You just feel drained in comparison to other times when you feel relief after having a good hard cry.

Our body and mind normally function with several automatic, natural rhythms. We should feel tired, go to sleep, sleep well, and feel rested in the morning, ready and enthusiastic about our day's activities. Our body should tell us that we need food and it should taste good to us. We should feel filled up or satiated after eating instead of having a nervous

The combination of depression and the after effects of a mastectomy can be devastating.

"My support group
was great. Still, the
average age was 50
and I was 27 and I felt
terribly young and
out of place."

hunger even though we just recently ate. Our body should tell us that we want to have sex. Our mind should think clearly, with good concentration, memory, and decisiveness. When we are depressed, our nervous system is not functioning well enough to allow the body and mind to operate these basic rhythms. Clinical depression is more than just feeling a little down. It is a temporary breakdown in the nervous system that throws off your natural, built-in cycles which allow you to get the most out of life.

Even though someone can be diagnosed with a major depressive episode after two weeks of symptoms it is rarely done that soon. Lack of appetite, fatigue, no sex drive, restless sleep, and crying spells are all common reactions to major surgery such as a mastectomy because of the trauma to the body. Your surgical area will be nearly healed in a couple of weeks but you will still have some fatigue. The immediate psychological shock from the changes that come with your mastectomy and cancer will cause a lot of intense emotions and mood swings. However, as time passes you may sense that your symptoms are staying the same or getting worse and are starting to interfere with your overall ability to cope. You should then consult your doctor or seek a therapist. You may come to this realization a month after your surgery or nine months later. There is no predicting when the need to seek help may arise for you. The important thing is to listen to yourself and not ignore the suspicion that you could really use some help.

Symptoms of Dysthymic Disorder

When I am assessing for dysthymia I look for a picture that includes a fairly long period of time which the person describes as a series of disappointments, during which they have felt depressed much of the time. I look for examples in their thought process that reflect helplessness and despair about being able to make their lives better. Women suffering from dysthymia will often say such things as, "Life just doesn't work out and I feel worn out from it," or "Nothing I try seems to work and I can't see it ever getting better."

The postmastectomy woman who is also suffering from a dysthymic depression will have a very difficult time believing she can be attractive and accepted after the loss of a breast. Feeling overwhelmed and terribly burdened by the changes that come from a mastectomy, such as clothing alterations and using prostheses, is more common and pervasive for the woman with a dysthymic depression than for a woman without depression. Giving up on a sex life is more likely for a woman in the grip of a dysthymic depression.

In order to be diagnosed with dysthymic disorder you would have had a depressed mood for most of the day, for more days than not, for at least two years with at least two of the following symptoms and you would not have been without the symptoms for longer than two months at a time.

1. Poor appetite or overeating.
2. Trouble sleeping or excessive sleeping.
3. Low energy or fatigue.
4. Low self-esteem.
5. Poor concentration or difficulty making decisions.
6. Feelings of hopelessness.

As you can see, the symptoms are a lot like those of a major depressive episode but their severity and length of time over which they occur differs. The dividing line between clinical and dysthymic depression is not clear cut. There is a great deal of overlap between the two types of depression and in fact someone can have both types at the same time. A dysthymic depression can eventually lead to a major depressive episode.

TREATING DEPRESSION

It is important to make a distinction between the two types of depression because the treatment is different for each type. Generally speaking, the treatment for clinical depression is psychotherapy and medication, whereas the treatment for dysthymia is psychotherapy (counseling). Since a clinical depression is a breakdown of the nervous system it is necessary to assist the nervous system in getting back on track. Dysthymia is a problem at the learning level, so we need to rework the thought process and related behavior patterns. Psychotherapy is by far the most important form of treatment for dysthymia, but sometimes putting someone with dysthymia on an antidepressant can also be helpful.

> Don't hesitate to ask your doctor or therapist questions about depression and medication.

If you are prescribed
an antidepressant,
you should be
monitored regularly
by your doctor or
therapist, especially
at first.

It has been observed that the body will heal itself of a major depressive episode in approximately nine to twelve months provided the stressor that triggered the depression has decreased during this time. A major depressive episode will probably take a much longer period of time to resolve itself if the depressed person has a strong family history of depression and has already experienced several episodes of depression. If your life remains stressful because you are undergoing cancer treatment or because of other stressful circumstances, or you do not want to wait nine to twelve months to see if your body will heal itself, then medication can be a valid option.

MEDICATIONS FOR DEPRESSION

Medications used for depression are called antidepressants. Antidepressants have been around for many years but have undergone a lot of changes recently. Before antidepressants, the only forms of treatment for severe depression were psychotherapy and shock treatment. The old antidepressants, called tricyclic antidepressants (TCAs), were very effective but they had frequent, very annoying side effects. The newer antidepressants, called selective serotonin reuptake inhibitors (SSRIs) are just as effective as the TCAs but typically have less serious and annoying side effects. The TCAs are still used because they are so effective and not everyone who uses them is bothered by their side effects. The other big advantage of TCAs is that they are usually very inexpensive.

We think TCAs work by stimulating the nervous system to produce more neurotransmitters on the premise that when we are depressed we do not have enough available neurotransmitters to allow the nervous system to work at its full capacity. We believe SSRIs work by helping the nervous system to better use the existing neurotransmitters. Some SSRIs also stimulate more production of neurotransmitters but most SSRIs work on the level of absorption.

The nervous system is made up of many long nerves that work through a chain reaction that starts in the brain and travels throughout the entire body. There are gaps between each nerve. Nerve impulses get from one nerve to the next by a chemical reaction that occurs in the spaces between nerves. This is the function of the neurotransmitters.

Normally when neurotransmitters, such as serotonin, are not used in the nervous system, they get absorbed into the rest of the body. The SS-RIs prevent the neurotransmitters from being absorbed so the nervous system has a better chance to use them to create the desired chemical reactions.

When our nervous system is not functioning properly it affects our ability to maintain a stable mood and we end up with a flat, depressed mood and a negative, despairing outlook. Problems with our nervous system also interrupt our natural body rhythms, cycles of sleep, appetite, energy level, and sex drive.

The names of the tricyclic antidepressants (TCAs) are as follows:

Generic Name	Brand Name
Amitriptyline	Elavil, Endep
Clomipramine	Anafranil
Doxepin	Sinequan
Imipramine	Janimine, Tofranil
Trimipramine	Surmontil
Desipramine	Norpramin
Nortriptyline	Aventyl, Pamelor
Protriptyline	Vivactil
Amoxapine	Ascendin
Maprotiline	Ludiomil

The names of the selective serotonin reuptake inhibitors (SSRIs) are as follows:

Generic Name	Brand Name
Fluoxetine	Prozac
Fluvoxamine	Luvox
Paroxetine	Paxil
Sertraline	Zoloft

There are four additional antidepressants which are technically not SSRIs but were discovered after the TCAs and work much like the SS-RIs. They do not produce many of the common TCAs side effects. These drugs are referred to as the Atypicals and are as follows:

Generic Name	Brand Name
Bupropion	Wellbutrin
Nefazodone	Serzone
Trazodone	Desyrel
Venlafaxine	Effexor

Side Effects

Side effects are undesirable reactions to medication. Because our bodies are unique, side effects will vary from person to person regarding if and when they occur and to what degree.

The best way to start on a medication is to take it as prescribed, and give it a fair chance to work, observing any warnings of what to avoid, such as not mixing it with alcohol. If you begin to have an undesirable reaction after taking the medication for a while check the list of side effects to see if it is listed. Most drug stores provide a list of possible side effects with each prescription. If you did not get a list with your prescription or if you threw it away, call your pharmacist and ask about its side effects. Your pharmacist is the most knowledgeable source about how the drug is supposed to work and may be able to tell you if you could be experiencing a side effect from the drug or from an interaction between that drug and some other drug you are taking.

If problems persist, you will need to go back to your doctor to have the medication changed.

The common side effects that are associated with the TCAs are as follows:

- Sedation
- Weight gain
- Low blood pressure or a drop in blood pressure when you stand up suddenly
- Lactation (secreting breast milk from remaining breast)
- Blurred vision
- Dry mouth
- Memory loss
- Dizziness
- Tachycardia (racing of the heart)

- Increased sweating
- Anxiety
- Constipation
- Diarrhea
- Nausea

The most commonly seen side effects from this list are dry mouth, constipation, drowsiness, weight gain, increased sweating, blurred vision, and a drop in blood pressure when suddenly changing positions, which can lead to temporary lightheadedness. For many people, the side effects are very mild and the positive effects of the medication greatly outweigh the negative reactions.

The possible side effects of the SSRIs and Atypical antidepressants are:

- Diarrhea
- Nausea and related weight loss
- Anxiety
- Sweating
- Insomnia
- Shakes or tremors
- Drowsiness
- Decrease in sex drive or inability to achieve an orgasm
- Constipation

The most commonly seen side effects are nausea, insomnia, tremors, and sexual dysfunction. Some of these side effects may seem the same as the symptoms you have from your depression. You are not expected to sort out what is part of your depression and what is a side effect from the medication. That is the job of your therapist and the doctor who has prescribed the medication. Your job is to be thorough in observing and reporting symptoms to the professionals who are working with you.

Wellbutrin (bupropion) has the fewest side effects, and is frequently used with elderly people because this population is much more prone to drug reactions than younger people. Wellbutrin cannot be taken by someone who has a seizure disorder because it can set off their seizures. A benefit of Wellbutrin is that it has proven to decrease the urge to smoke and so can help someone trying to give up cigarettes. The biggest drawback to Wellbutrin is that it has to be taken three times a day, whereas the SSRIs and Atypicals are usually taken once in the morning or once at bedtime.

One unique possible side effect which occurs with Desyrel (trazodone) is a persistent, painful erection in men. This is a very serious condition.

How To Take Antidepressants
Antidepressants are slow-acting drugs. They have to build up in the bloodstream to a therapeutic level before they begin to work. This usually takes about three to four weeks. This gradual process has its good and bad side. The good side is that people cannot become addicted to these drugs. One reason that people become addicted to drugs is because they cause an immediate desirable change in mood. There is no immediate high from antidepressants. Gradually, over several weeks, you will start to notice that you are feeling a little better. You have more energy and you are starting to sleep better. Your overall mood is improved and life looks more hopeful. The bad side of the gradual effect of antidepressants is that three to four weeks can seem like an eternity when you are feeling miserable. However, most people feel better simply because the problem has been identified and a solution has been started.

It is imperative that you be monitored closely by the doctor or nurse who prescribed the medication.

It is very important that you not miss any doses of your antidepressant and that you keep taking it even after you start to feel better. Taking an antidepressant is a lot like taking an antibiotic, only on a greater scale. After twenty-four hours on an antibiotic you may feel dramatically better but you will still have to take the full course of medication to treat the infection so it does not return. The nervous system takes a long time to restore itself. It takes about nine to twelve months to treat a major depressive episode. You will feel better in about three to four weeks, but it will take a lot longer for your nervous system to get back on track and function at full capacity again. If you stop the medication after taking it for six months or less you have a 50% chance of a relapse. Research

Do not stop taking antidepressants abruptly.

shows that if we treat a depression as soon as possible and for a long enough time we greatly reduce the chance of the person having an immediate relapse or a recurrence of depression in the future.

Your doctor will probably take you off your antidepressant after about nine to twelve months. Your body should have returned to functioning on its own but if the symptoms of depression start to return you will be put back on your medication for a while longer. You should discontinue your antidepressant under the supervision of the person who prescribed it because you may experience withdrawal symptoms with some of the antidepressants if you stop taking them abruptly. You will probably be tapered off the medication gradually. Coming off the medication abruptly is hard on the nervous system and can destabilize it and set off a shift in your mood again. Gradually decreasing the dose allows you to see if your symptoms are going to return without having to start over, requiring another three to four weeks to reach a therapeutic level in your body again. It is rare that someone has to be on an antidepressant for the rest of her life. Some people do have chronic depression and, for them, lifetime medication is appropriate, but they are the exception to the rule.

The nervous system responds to the presence of antidepressants by decreasing the number of receptor sites for serotonin, which is called the "down-regulation of serotonin receptors." Sometimes the dose of your medication has to be increased because the body needs more due to the decrease in available receptor sites. Once you decrease the dose or discontinue the medication, the body responds by creating more receptor sites. Many people with chronic depression have certain times of the year when they are naturally less depressed, such as when the days are longer. During these times they either go off the medication or have the dose reduced to help keep as many receptor sites as possible available.

You need to be very careful about adding alcohol to antidepressants. The combination of antidepressants and alcohol will make you intoxicated faster, and combining them in high doses can cause a toxicity that can produce an overdose.

Antidepressants may be taken at the same time you are receiving chemotherapy. You will need to check with your doctor about being on an antidepressant while undergoing radiation treatments, though, because

Educate yourself on depression and antidepressants if you have some concerns, but make sure that you know there are conflicting opinions and try and get a balanced perspective.

some antidepressants can make you more sensitive to sunlight and cause burns more easily.

Myths About Antidepressants.
The media has had a field day putting out all kinds of stories about what antidepressants can do to you. Prozac has been most under attack because it is the SSRI that has been around the longest, so it has been prescribed more often and many people recognize the name. Most of what is being reported about Prozac comes from individual stories and is missing the background facts necessary to understand what really took place. Prozac has been called the miracle drug and also a dangerous drug. No drug is a miracle drug. They all have a positive contribution, but they also come with side effects and limitations. Antidepressants cannot solve your problems. Just taking a drug will not magically give you answers or take away your pain. Our fast-paced, goal-oriented culture has made us look to medication as the quick cure-all, but therapy is where you will be able to sort out your situation and make changes. Real, permanent change will come from your own efforts.

The new antidepressants cannot make you into a whole new personality type, as has been suggested in some magazine articles and books, nor would we want them to. Antidepressants help with chemical imbalances in the brain. If you have felt very flat and emotionless, then it can feel to you and to others as if you are a new person when your imbalance is corrected. This will be even more true if you have been depressed for a very long time, even dating back to childhood.

Some of the antidepressants are helpful with obsessive compulsive traits, so that when people are started on a drug such as Paxil or Zoloft, not only do they become less depressed but also less worried about details. The medication just helps to get the person back to her natural, healthy self. I should also mention that Paxil and Zoloft will not completely change obsessive compulsive personality traits, but will only modify them so they are less frequent and intense.

Another fear floating around is that Prozac can make you go into wild killing rages. If a person is homicidal in addition to being depressed, treating the depression may give the person the energy to possibly act out their rage. But Prozac would not cause the rage or the acting out. Nor will it make you suicidal.

Some people are very suicidal, but do not have the energy or motivation to carry out the act. Mental health professionals know that someone who is severely depressed and very suicidal is at risk of committing suicide when the medication has given her more energy but has not yet treated the rest of the negative thinking. No one should be put on an antidepressant without a thorough assessment of their suicide risk and close supervision for the first few months after they start the medication. A patient should never be started on an antidepressant without a follow-up appointment in two or three weeks, or sooner if they are at a higher suicide risk. A high suicide risk patient should be receiving intensive psychotherapy or be hospitalized. Psychotherapy is a very important part of dealing with repressed anger or suicidal thinking and it should not be overlooked as a necessary part of treatment for depression.

Sleep disorders can lead to depression and vice versa.

For those postmastectomy women who are considering taking an antidepressant or other medication and who are also in a recovery program for substance abuse, you should make that decision with your doctor or therapist. There are many well-informed and open-minded people in recovery programs, but there are also many people who are ill informed about medication. Such people think that antidepressants are addictive simply because they treat mood disorders. They may suggest that to take an antidepressant is "copping" out and actually running away from dealing with life, because they think antidepressants blunt your emotions so the emotional pain that leads to substance abuse is never dealt with. They may consider it a "slip" to take any psychiatric medication.

As I stated before, antidepressants are not addictive. Antidepressants do not blunt or suppress your emotions. They restore your nervous system so that you react normally to your emotions. If you are experiencing a major depressive episode, the antidepressant will get you back to where you can do your emotional healing and problem-solving through therapy.

Sleep Disorders

The sleep problems that commonly accompany depression can have a devastating effect on our physical and emotional recovery. Normally we

Staying up for 36
hours has been
shown to be an
effective treatment
for short-term sleep
disorders.

feel tired, lie down, fall asleep, and proceed through the various stages of sleep which allow for a good balance between dream activity for our mental health, and deep muscle relaxation for body restoration. We should be able to remain asleep consistently through the night so we can get the full benefit of each stage of sleep and feel rested and able to function the next day.

There are three basic types of sleep. The first is the superficial light sleep phase; followed by the rapid eye movement (REM) phase, in which we actively dream; and the third, the deep relaxation phase. Once we pass through the superficial level we rotate through periods of REM sleep and deep relaxation sleep. REM sleep is important for good mental health. It is widely believed that we work through a lot of our emotional issues while we are asleep. During REM sleep your body is very active, whereas during deep relaxation sleep the body processes slow down. Pulse rate, body temperature, and breathing rate all decrease in deep relaxation sleep. Our muscles become so relaxed that we actually become slightly paralyzed. Our muscles feel like dead weights and there is no movement in them. It is the combination of these three stages that make for a good night's sleep and allows you to wake up feeling rested and prepared to meet the day.

Some people have problems falling asleep. They find themselves restless and unable to shut their minds down enough to fall asleep. They may feel sleepy when they go to bed but once their head hits the pillow they are wide awake with their mind going full speed. They may obsess about an actual problem but most of the time they report that their mind just goes from one insignificant thought to the next. They start making lists in their head of things to do and walking through possible situations or rehashing old situations. None of the thinking is necessary or productive, yet they cannot seem to get their minds to turn off.

Other people fall asleep without any trouble but find that they wake up after a few hours and cannot get back to sleep. Their minds kick into gear and will not let go. Many wake up around 4:00 or 5:00 A.M. and are unable to fall back to sleep or, if they do fall back to sleep, it happens about fifteen minutes before they have to get up for the day.

If we cannot get a good night's sleep we become sleep deprived, which leads to symptoms that interfere with our normal daily functioning. Poor concentration, poor short-term memory, irritability, fatigue, indecisiveness, muscle aches and pain, and headaches can all result from insufficient sleep. Often when we become fatigued due to a lack of sleep we end up feeling and acting like a child who badly needs a nap, becoming irritable, negative, and unreasonable. Sleep deprivation can also bring on physical pain or intensify existing pain because the muscles don't get to relax if the deepest stage of sleep is not reached.

Worry before and after surgery, drainage tubes, physical pain, and the lack of exercise can all contribute to poor sleep for women who have undergone a mastectomy. Each stage of adjustment after being diagnosed with cancer and losing a breast brings on a new set of worries and fears that can prevent us from being relaxed enough to fall asleep, and/or emotional distress that can come out in very restless dreaming which can interfere with reaching the deepest stage of sleep. Sleep disorders following surgery should be temporary but sleeping patterns can become permanent so it is important not to wait a long time to treat a problem.

Many of the symptoms of sleep deprivation are the same as those of depression. That is because sleep deprivation weakens the nervous system and plays an important role in creating many depressive symptoms. Once proper sleep is restored, a lot of the symptoms of depression start to go away. If we start out with a sleep disturbance and it goes unchecked, it can lead to a full-blown depression.

Sleep Disorder Questionnaire and Suggested Treatments
There are a number of things you can do to treat your sleeplessness. First you should make an assessment of your sleeping habits and see where you may be able to make some changes. Ask yourself the following questions:

1. Do you have a regular sleep schedule? Your body works best when it can settle into a regular schedule. We have a natural inner clock, or circadian rhythm, that should regulate our sleep patterns if we sleep on a consistent schedule. You should go to bed at a set time that will allow you to get about eight hours of sleep every night.

2. Do you avoid substances that can interfere with sleep? Alcohol can

Regulating your sleeping habits can help to cure sleep disorders.

Ongoing anxiety can
interfere seriously
with the
postmastectomy
woman's quality
of life.

make you sleepy, but will prevent you from reaching the deep relaxation stage of sleep by causing too much REM sleep, which will leave you feeling as if you were running a race all night. Nicotine and caffeine are stimulants that will prevent you from falling asleep. They contribute to racing thoughts and keyed-up feelings.

3. Are you giving yourself enough wind-down time before you try to sleep? Being very active right up until the time you go to sleep will keep your mind too busy and can cause racing thoughts. Light reading, light TV, relaxation exercises, a warm bath, and relaxing music are just a few things people find helpful to quiet the mind before sleep.

4. Do you have a good sleeping environment? It is amazing how important simple things, such as the temperature of your bedroom, background noise, or light, are in getting a good night's sleep. I tend to sleep poorly when I am slightly chilled. My husband sleeps restlessly if he is too warm, which makes for lots of room to practice negotiating compromise in our marriage! When I forget to put a towel under the blinds when the window is open in the summer and the blinds keep banging, it drives me crazy and I cannot get to sleep, but that noise totally escapes my husband. Look carefully around your bedroom to see whether you can change anything to help you sleep.

5. Are you saving your sleep mostly for night or are you taking long naps that interfere with your sleep at night? Oversleeping by staying in bed too long or taking lengthy naps will both cause a poor night's sleep. It can become a vicious cycle when you nap to make up for lost sleep from the night before, but then cannot sleep well again that night. If you feel sleepy during the day and you take a very short nap, between ten and twenty minutes, you will feel alert and rested when you get up and be able to get through the remainder of your day. On the other hand, if you take a long nap, you are likely to wake up feeling groggy, sluggish, and irritable. You may feel that way the rest of the day or it may take a fairly long time to recover and feel alert again. The short nap allows you to make a quick recovery utilizing the first two stages of sleep, whereas a longer nap puts you into deep sleep that will take longer to wake up from and will interrupt your night sleep cycle. If you want to nap, but don't want to sleep for too long, set an alarm, sleep sitting up, or have someone

wake you. One of my clients said she used to sleep with her arms under her head and her head on the library table when studying at school. That way her arms would go numb and this would wake her up in about fifteen minutes.

6. Are you getting enough physical exercise? Physical exercise drains the body of the extra energy which can cause restlessness at night. Don't exercise too close to bedtime because it is likely to energize you and prevent you from falling asleep. Exercising earlier in the day will help reduce sluggishness and make your body more ready for relaxation at bedtime.

Besides working to build good sleep patterns by paying attention to the factors mentioned above, there are two other ways to treat sleep disturbance. One is to use sleep deprivation to regain your body's normal cycle and the other is to use medication.

Often you can fix a temporary sleep disturbance by depriving yourself of sleep for a thirty-six-hour period. If you are having trouble getting to sleep or constantly waking up during the night, if you force yourself to stay awake for thirty-six hours the body will reclaim its natural sleep rhythm. You can repeat this process every six days if necessary. Obviously, this is not a healthy or practical approach for someone who is having a frequent ongoing problem with sleep. But if you are experiencing one of those rare times when you are having trouble sleeping for a few nights, and your daily demands can allow you to go without sleep for thirty-six hours, you may want to try this. This approach has been shown to be effective 50% of the time.

MEDICATIONS FOR SLEEP DISORDERS

There are a few over-the-counter medications available to treat sleep disorders, but they are not terribly effective because they only make you drowsy instead of assisting you to reach the deeper stage of sleep. Some may actually interfere with the deeper stages of sleep. I do not recommend them.

Melatonin is another common over-the-counter sleeping medication in the U.S. This is a natural hormone made in the pineal gland that acts as a catalyst for serotonin, which affects sleep. Melatonin was first found to be helpful for people suffering from jet lag. It is supposed to help you get back on your inner clock, which is called your circadian rhythm. People are using melatonin for all types of sleep problems and are reporting good results. You will find this in the vitamin section of your pharmacy in the U.S. but it is not legal in Canada, although some health food stores are reported to sell it. Research has shown melatonin to be effective with jet lag and several other studies are in progress, which may shed light on how melatonin acts in a clinical setting with other types of sleep disturbances.[22] There are no research results yet that explain how melatonin works to treat sleep disorders.

There are two types of prescription drugs I consider relatively safe for treating sleep disturbances. Antidepressants and benzodiazephines, which are also called anti-anxiety agents or tranquilizers, can be used to treat sleep disorders. Antidepressants are the safest of the two but under proper supervision, and in the right situation, such as the night before surgery, benzodiazephines can be a viable option.

Benzodiazephines help with anxiety and racing thoughts and will make you drowsy. Most are short-acting so they will help you to fall asleep, but they do not help you to stay asleep through the night. One type, Dalmane, can be very detrimental to older people, causing confusion and falls, and should be avoided. These drugs can also be addictive and should only be used on a very short-term basis. If they are used over a long term, they will cause increased tolerance and you will require more and more to get the desired effect. Your body becomes dependent on the medication to be able to sleep so when you stop taking them you will once again have trouble sleeping. If you take benzodiazephines for any length of time you will also become physically dependent, and when you stop taking them you could have withdrawal symptoms. Mixing alcohol with this type of medication is very dangerous and can lead to overdose. There are some benzodiazephines that last longer in the system and can make you sleep longer, but these carry an even greater risk of addiction. Valium and Librium are examples of the longer-acting type.

Hypnotics and barbiturates are two other classes of drugs that may be prescribed for sleep problems. These drug types are highly addictive, will cause physical withdrawal, result in a bad hangover the morning after, and take away your natural ability to sleep. I strongly recommend that you refuse to take either of these types of drugs to help you sleep.

A number of antidepressants have the side effect of making you quite drowsy. This side effect can come in handy for addressing sleep problems. As with benzodiazephines, antidepressants will help you fall asleep but will also help you remain asleep. Antidepressants work on sleep problems in two ways. They make you drowsy enough to get you to sleep initially and the rest of their chemical reaction works with the nervous system to keep you asleep by prompting all of the stages of sleep.

One antidepressant that is widely used for treating sleep disorders is trazodone. Trazodone was the first new antidepressant to be discovered after the TCAs. To be effective for depression it is necessary to take 200 to 400 mg of trazodone per day. Most people cannot stand up, let alone walk, on that amount because of the extreme drowsiness it causes, so it is seldom used to treat depression. Then Prozac came along and replaced trazodone, without the sedating effect. However, for several years now trazodone has been used for sleep disturbance. The usual dose is 50 – 100 mg taken immediately before going to bed. It helps people fall asleep, stay asleep, and not feel drugged or hung over in the morning.

Trazodone has been widely used with older people because it has few and mild side effects. Some of the SSRIs used to treat depression, such as Prozac and Zoloft, may cause insomnia, so frequently a small dose of trazodone is added to help with sleep. The other antidepressants will take up to a month to start to correct a sleep problem resulting from depression, whereas the trazodone will work on the sleep problem the first night it is taken.

This drug should not be taken by people with serious heart conditions because it can cause heart arrhythmias. People with mild heart conditions seem to tolerate it in small doses. Dosages do vary and are tapered back as people age, depending on physical health.

Trazodone can safely be taken every night for years or it can be taken for only a few nights. You will not risk addiction, physical withdrawal, or an interruption of your normal ability to sleep by taking it. You do not have to go to a psychiatrist to get this medication. Most family practice doctors are very knowledgeable about how to use trazodone for sleep disorders and regularly prescribe it for that purpose. Trazodone has also proven effective for treating chronic pain because it allows the body to reach a state of deep relaxation. If you have chronic pain from complications after having ruptured implants or other health conditions, trazodone may help with your pain and your sleep problem.

Small doses of some of the more sedating TCAs can also be used in the same way as trazodone but they will cause dry mouth and constipation. However, in lower doses, the side effects are not as noticeable. The TCAs can also cause heart problems, but again, in small doses they are safe for most people.

By now you realize the seriousness of a sleep disturbance and I strongly encourage you to ask for help earlier rather than later. If you are experiencing a lot of fear and worry before surgery it may help to take a medication such as trazodone for a few nights. Treating a sleep disorder is not like treating depression, where you are committing to using a drug for nearly a year. You can use medication off and on as your sleep is affected during the long months of recovery. However, you should challenge yourself to do the things that you can do on your own, such as developing better sleeping habits, before or in addition to turning to medication.

ANXIETY

As with depression, there are several conditions that fall under the category of anxiety disorders. Phobias, agoraphobia, post-traumatic stress disorder, and obsessive compulsive disorder are all anxiety disorders. But the two conditions I have most commonly seen after a mastectomy are generalized anxiety disorder and panic disorder.

Let's face it, after cancer and a mastectomy we have a lot to be scared and anxious about. When you first go to the doctor to check out the lump you found, worrying about what the lump will turn out to be, going through a biopsy, waiting for the pathology report, going through general anesthetic and having your mastectomy, looking at your chest after surgery, worrying if the cancer can be completely eradicated or if you will die from it, facing how to dress after a mastectomy, reconsidering your sexuality and sex life—all these produce anxiety. Our fears will range from being insignificant and immediate to huge and prolonged.

Getting in Over
Our Heads
241

Losing a breast alone is enough of a change and loss to give us tremendous anxiety and set off panic attacks. Adding cancer to the picture can make us very fearful about our bodies and about life itself. Our foundation has been badly shaken, which often means we don't feel able to manage or control our lives. This is a very frightening proposition. Some women get through the surgery very well but many months later, especially after all the cancer treatments are over, begin to obsess about their health and become very anxious and panicky. The slightest unexpected sensation is interpreted as a new sign of cancer.

As you progress through your recovery you will begin to return to your normal life. As you resume normal activities you will be able to observe how much your anxiety and feelings of panic are interfering with normal functioning. If you seem to be limited more by anxiety than you had been in the past even when under stress, you are likely experiencing an anxiety disorder.

Your first step should be to consult with your doctor or find a therapist who can help you sort out what is a normal reaction to your circumstances and what is an actual anxiety disorder that needs treatment. Knowing the symptoms and forms of treatment will help you to ask the right questions about what you are experiencing sooner, and help you to make sense out of what your doctor or therapist recommends. Knowledge allows you to be an active participant in your recovery.

You may be wondering which category you fall into because you experience both depression and anxiety. I have written about them separately to build a clear picture of what depression is and what anxiety and panic attacks consist of, but they often co-exist.

Generalized Anxiety Disorder
To meet the criteria for generalized anxiety disorder you would experience the following:
1. Excessive anxiety and worry that occurs more days than not, over at least a six-month period, about a number of events or activities.

2. You find it difficult to control worry.

3. The anxiety and worry are associated with three or more of the following symptoms:

- Restlessness or feeling keyed-up or being on edge
- Being easily fatigued
- Difficulty concentrating or finding that your mind goes blank
- Irritability
- Muscle tension
- Sleep disturbance
- The worry, anxiety, and physical symptoms cause significant distress or impairment in your social, occupational, or other important areas of your life.

Panic Disorder

To meet the criteria for panic disorder you would experience the following:

1. Recurrent unexpected panic attacks

2. At least one of the attacks has been followed by one month or more of one or more of the following:

- Persistent concern about having additional attacks
- Worry about the implications of the attack or its consequences (e.g., losing control, having a heart attack, "going crazy")
- A significant change in behavior related to the attacks

A panic attack is not a disorder; it is something that happens as part of several different types of anxiety disorders. During a panic attack, you experience a discrete period of intense fear or discomfort, in which four or more of the following symptoms develop abruptly and reach a peak within ten minutes:

- Palpitations, pounding heart, or accelerated heart rate
- Sweating
- Trembling or shaking
- Sensations of shortness of breath or smothering
- Feeling of choking
- Chest pain or discomfort

- Nausea or abdominal distress
- Feeling dizzy, unsteady, lightheaded, or faint
- Derealization (feelings of unreality) or depersonalization (being detached from oneself)
- Fear of losing control or going crazy
- Fear of dying
- Paresthesias (numbness or tingling sensations)
- Chills or hot flashes

TREATING ANXIETY

The treatment for generalized anxiety disorder and panic attacks is very similar to the treatment for depression. A combination of psychotherapy and medication usually works best. Because anxiety and panic attacks are treated much the same I will address their treatment together. Sometimes psychotherapy is enough and sometimes medication alone is used, but the most complete and effective way to deal with generalized anxiety disorder and panic attacks is by undergoing some counseling and often by adding some medication. I do not recommend treating these conditions only with medication because I believe therapy should be considered the primary form of treatment and medication a possible adjunct to the therapy.

Cognitive and behavioral therapy are the most effective forms of psychotherapy for anxiety disorders. Changing how you think and interrupting behaviors that reinforce the anxiety and panic are crucial for controlling the anxiety. Analyzing your past or dwelling on the symptoms will only make the anxiety worse by feeding the mental obsession that accompanies anxiety. Breaking anxiety requires being able to move away from looking at the symptoms and refocusing on solutions. Anxiety and panic are fed by catastrophic thinking, which entails obsessing about the ways that a situation can go bad.

Learning to identify your negative, fear-based thoughts and to reframe situations into manageable ones should be the aim of your therapy. Behavioral changes may include distracting yourself with an activity when the worrisome mental obsessing starts up, in order to break the

Cognitive and behavioral therapy will help you to change how you think and interrupt behaviors that reinforce feelings of panic and anxiety.

negative thought process. Desensitizing yourself by gradually exposing yourself to and building up a tolerance for whatever it is that makes you extremely anxious is another behavioral approach.

Often, when a major part of our life is rearranged or tampered with, we feel a loss of control. Feeling as though we are losing or might lose control of our lives can produce a great deal of anxiety. The more we try to deny or suppress our feelings and face our losses like troopers, the more we put ourselves at risk of developing anxiety and panic. Your psychotherapy should help you to identify your real fears so they can be dealt with directly and rationally. If pushed aside, your fears may pop out at any time, which can leave you very confused about the real source of your anxiety.

When we are going through surgery and recovery we are often too close to the situation to have much perspective. So much happens so fast when we have a mastectomy that we cannot always process it all as it occurs, which is one of the reasons that an anxiety disorder can sneak up on us. Supportive psychotherapy, either in the form of individual sessions or in a support group, can help us take time out to realize what we are thinking and feeling. This will allow us to accept reassurance and discover new ways of coping.

If your anxiety is very persistent and causing a lot of disruption to your daily functioning, and you are already taking part in some form of therapy, it may be time to ask if your symptoms could be helped with medication. The psychiatric profession is still learning about anxiety disorders and their treatment. We know that, just as with depression, there may be a physiological base to anxiety. There is a definite interplay between our thought processes and our neurological functioning, which is why medication may be used as part of the solution for anxiety and panic disorders.

MEDICATIONS FOR ANXIETY

The two types of drugs most often used for anxiety disorders are antidepressants and antianxiety agents. Antidepressants are often used to treat anxiety disorders, especially if the anxiety has persisted for a long time. The SSRIs are being used with good results. Paxil, Luvox, Zoloft, Serzone, and Effexor are all showing good results. Trazodone and Wellbutrin arc not effective for panic attacks. Prozac is also not usually helpful with anxiety. SSRIs do not carry the risk of addiction that benzodiazephines do. Frequently an antidepressant is used as the main drug, with benzodiazephine prescribed in conjunction, to be used on occasion for a severe panic attack.

Benzodiazephines are antianxiety medications. There are quite a lot of benzodiazephines. I have limited this list to a few of the most commonly used benzodiazephines with the least risk of addiction.

The names of these benzodiazephines are as follows:

Generic Name	*Brand Name*
Alprazolam	Xanax
Clonazepam	Klonopin
Clorazepate	Tranxene
Oxazepam	Serax
Buspirone	BuSpar

The drugs from this list that work best for panic attacks are Xanax and Klonopin, but the entire list is effective for treating anxiety. BuSpar is becoming a very popular drug because it is believed to not cause addiction. BuSpar can be used for a longer period of time without the risk of physical dependency and potential withdrawal complications.

As I mentioned before in the sleep disorder section, benzodiazephines should only be used for a short period of time. By a short period of time, I mean one to two weeks.

Some people can take the medication for one or two days at a time and not need it again for many days or several weeks. This is true for anxiety as well as for panic attacks, but is much more the case with panic attacks. Anyone taking these drugs, except for BuSpar, will have physical withdrawal symptoms if they are taken daily for an extended period of time.

Side Effects

With the exception of BuSpar, the side effects seen with benzodiazephines are:

• Hypotension—drop in blood pressure that could cause fainting

Grief and mood
altering substances
are not a good mix.

- Dizziness, lightheadedness
- Tachycardia (racing of the heart)
- Dry mouth and throat
- Disturbed sexual function
- Blurred vision
- Nasal stuffiness
- Weakness, fatigue
- Clumsiness, in lack of coordination
- Drowsiness
- Depression
- Makes alcohol more potent, takes less alcohol to become intoxicated

The side effects you may see with BuSpar are dizziness and light-headedness, nausea, weakness and fatigue, headaches, drowsiness, and agitation or restlessness. Some of the side effects from these drugs are similar to the anxiety symptoms that you are trying to treat. It is important that you accurately report the effects of the medication to your doctor and therapist so they can make the necessary changes.

As I said before, the benzodiazephines can be very helpful and relatively safe when used under close supervision and in very specific circumstances for a short period of time.

Substance Abuse

Grief and mood-altering substances are not a good mix. The use of mood-altering substances, such as alcohol and marijuana, delay the grieving process because the drugs or alcohol will temporarily numb the emotions. Like any grief, the grief over the loss of your breast and all the associated fears and feelings that go along with your mastectomy and breast cancer experience are best handled at the time that the feelings begin to surface. Repressing emotions, whether with your conscious mind or with the help of mood-altering substances, takes a lot of energy and is experienced as stress on the body. Stress taxes the already overstressed immune system.

If you are receiving chemotherapy you need your liver to be as strong as possible, and alcohol will compete with the chemotherapy chemicals that need to be detoxified by the liver. If you are trying to beat cancer,

adding alcohol is not a smart move. In addition, alcohol is a depressant.
Many people consider it a stimulant because they say they get high on it.
It makes you feel high because it lowers your inhibitions after the first
few drinks. After this, the alcohol starts to have more of a depressive action.

It has been well documented for many years that using marijuana
(pot) on a regular basis leads to apathy and lack of motivation. The last
thing a woman who is trying to feel positive about her life after a mastectomy needs is a drug that makes her apathetic and takes away her motivation.

If you are having trouble staying away from alcohol, pot, or any other
mood altering substance I strongly encourage you to seek help. Twelve-
step groups such as Alcoholics Anonymous or Narcotics Anonymous
are excellent for substance abuse recovery. Depending on how serious
your problem is, you may need a formal detoxification or treatment program first, which you can follow up with an ongoing twelve-step group, a
Women for Sobriety group, or another self-help group.

Besides alcohol and illegal drugs, caffeine can cause problems for
many people. It is a stimulant which makes your nervous system work
harder. Too much caffeine causes anxiety and restlessness and is hard on
your already overworked immune system. Caffeine is found in colas,
coffee, teas, and chocolate. If you have been a regular caffeine consumer
you will experience some withdrawal when you first stop using it. I
stopped consuming caffeine in 1981 when I had my bilateral mastectomy because at the time it was thought that caffeine could cause breast
cancer, although further research has disproved that theory. I was a
three-cup-a-day coffee drinker. For about a week I felt drowsy in the
mornings and I had a couple of headaches. If you consume a lot of
caffeine, you will likely experience withdrawal for up to two weeks, with
headaches, shaky feelings, restlessness, and trouble getting going in the
mornings. I have remained off coffee because I feel better without it, but
I must confess I am not willing to give up chocolate just to avoid caffeine.

Nicotine and the other substances found in cigarettes are believed to
be carcinogenic, which means they cause cancer. Nicotine is also a stimulant, so it overloads your nervous system. Nicotine withdrawal takes at

least two weeks, with some minor symptoms continuing for another four to six weeks. One of the reasons some people have more trouble than others giving up smoking and caffeine is that they are self-medicating a depression. They may be using a stimulant to try to fight a low level of depression. This is definitely not the right way to go about treating depression because you are getting only temporary symptom relief rather than actually treating the underlying depression. Many good programs are available to help you "kick the habit." The American Cancer Society and the American Lung Association and the Canadian Cancer Society are excellent resources to help you stop smoking. They provide suggestions on how to go about quitting, and lists of support groups. Many people find a group of friends who also want to quit and form their own informal support group.

CHAPTER FOURTEEN

MOVING ON:
THE LIGHTER SIDE

One of the surest signs of a healthy recovery is the return of your sense of humor. Undergoing breast cancer and a mastectomy is a deadly serious matter. Most of us find little to laugh about in the early stages as our shock and fear tend to make us focus on ourselves and our self-preservation. But with time our sense of perspective returns and we find ourselves able to laugh once again. Eventually, we are even able to laugh about our illness and the changes that surgery has wrought. It is well known that laughter is a great healer. It is also an essential part of life. Once I was able to find the humor in the little mishaps I encountered after my last surgery I knew that I was truly on the mend.

The first person to show me that there is a lighter side to having a mastectomy was the woman who visited me from the Cancer Society's Reach For Recovery Program. As she explained how she used her two external prostheses following her double mastectomy she told me about the time she had forgotten to put them in her bra before heading off to her volunteer job. She related her surprise at looking down at herself to discover that she had left her breasts at home. She was a very attractive and bright young woman and her honesty and openness about the mistake made a bigger impression on me than anything else she said in her visit. I could see that she was doing more than just coping, she was also laughing and smiling again.

I have since made several such blunders of my own. I have found the health club a likely place to run into breast mishaps. Going to the health club is like traveling in that you generally have to remember several

Prostheses seem to
lend themselves to
ridiculous situations.

different outfits for different purposes, such as swimwear, workout clothes, and work clothes. If you also use different sets of prostheses for different activities, it all becomes a lot to remember. One morning I did not have my usual eight o'clock client so I decided to go to the health club on the way to work. I stretched, used the treadmill, and finished up with a few minutes in the hot tub. Everything felt great until I realized that, to my surprise and horror, I had forgotten to pack my silicone prostheses and now my fiber-filled ones were soaking wet and would take at least twelve hours to dry. I only had a short time before I had to meet my first client and I was too far from home to go get my silicone breast forms.

Initially, I felt panicked and wanted to burst into tears. So I had a matter-of-fact talk with myself and decided that falling apart was not the solution. I needed a plan, so I hunted through my gym bag for something to fill out my bra. Normally, I keep an extra pair of gym socks in it, but wouldn't you know it, not that day! The only option was my sweaty gym socks. I rolled them up and put one in each cup. Now, socks do not make very attractive breasts, but I had on a loose sweater and hoped that my lumpy chest was not too obvious. Leaving my private curtained dressing room to use the mirrors in the open part of the change room to adjust my "socks" was embarrassing but I got through it. The fact that I was in a hurry helped me to cope and I made it to work feeling a bit insecure but basically all right. When my husband called later that day to ask how my day was going we had a good laugh about me and my smelly gym sock breasts.

Another time Jim and I were relaxing in the sauna after our workouts and I noticed that my breasts felt funny. I tried to adjust them and discovered that I had put them into my swimsuit on the wrong sides. My fiber-filled forms are a butterfly shape with fuller padding in the center and a more tapered thickness on the outer sides that match the left and right sides of my body. In other words, they are not interchangeable! I felt like a little kid who has gotten her shoes on the wrong feet. Jim assured me that it did not look too obvious that my breasts were on backwards and we had a bit of a private giggle about it as we continued on to the hot tub.

The last "breast incident" at the health club was a different matter altogether. When I first began going back to the gym after my mastectomy I used my fiber-filled breast forms inside a sports bra while exercising. I eventually became tired of that and began wearing a sports bra with no prostheses and an oversized sweatshirt. When I wear my T-shirt without my prostheses it is obvious that I either never grew breasts or had them removed, but I decided that I was more comfortable exercising without my breast forms, which I would save for swimming and the hot tub. Jim was unaware of my new resolve and we had been walking along on our treadmills, side by side, for several minutes when a worried look came over his face. He leaned over and asked me if I had gotten my bra on backwards. I was wearing a large sweatshirt with no prostheses and the extra material around the chest area had pushed back as I walked, creating a bulge in the area of my wing bones. Jim's eyesight is not very good and at first glance it looked to him as if I was wearing my prostheses on my back.

When I finished laughing uncontrollably and was able to speak again, I explained that it was just my sweatshirt puckering and that I was not wearing my breast forms. Jim was quite relieved for me, not because he cared whether or not I wore my prostheses to the club, but because he cared very much about how I felt and was worried that I would be upset if I had made another mistake with my prostheses. The poor guy had been through me putting my breasts on the wrong side, so he reasoned why couldn't I also put them on back to front? I will probably make a lot of gaffes with my prostheses over the course of my life, but I am reasonably sure that I will never wear my breasts in the back.

One of my clients told me an endearing story about her grandma, who had been a breast cancer survivor. Her grandma took a lot of pride in her appearance as she lived her busy, public life. But her family saw another side of her. Connie remembers that her grandmother was forever taking her fake breast out and putting it back because she found it hot and uncomfortable. When she was at home with her family she would just take her prosthesis out and lay it on the closest table top. Then when she was in a hurry to go somewhere she would inevitably end up running

If you can laugh
again, you know you
have come out the
other side.

around the house saying, "Where is my boob? I can't find my boob. Has anyone seen it?" And everyone in the family would have to help her look for it so she could be on her way. It was obvious to me that being allowed to see this part of her grandma's life allowed for a special connection between Connie and her grandma.

Her story reminded me of the poet and writer Michael Ondaatje writing about his grandmother. He writes in *Running in the Family:*

> Lalla's great claim to fame was that she was the first woman in Ceylon to have a mastectomy. It turned out to be unnecessary but she always claimed to support modern science, throwing herself into new causes. (Even in death her generosity exceeded the physically possible for she had donated her body to six hospitals.) The false breast would never be still for long. She was an energetic person. It would crawl over to join its twin on the right hand side or sometimes appear on her back, "for dancing" she smirked. She would yell at the grandchildren in the middle of a formal dinner to fetch her tit as she had forgotten to put it on. She kept losing the contraption to servants who were mystified by it as well as to the dog, Chindit, who would be found gnawing at the foam as if it were tender chicken. She went through four breasts in her lifetime. One she left on a branch of a tree in Hakgalle Gardens to dry out after a rainstorm, one flew off when she was riding behind Vere on his motorbike, and the third she was very mysterious about, almost embarrassed though Lalla was never embarrassed. Most believed it had been forgotten after a romantic assignation in Trincomalee with a man who may or may not have been in the Cabinet.

The story of Lalla reminds me that losing a breast does not mean the end of laughter and lightness. It is instead a part of our unique history. I have a group of friends and each year the four of us go up to stay at a remote cabin for a long weekend. Three of us have had mastectomies and we are all in our forties. Out of eight breasts we have only three left. And all four of us have become much closer as we have taken turns helping each other through surgery and treatment. We have reassured Suzie that she does not have to get breast cancer to be fully included in our foursome, and for her part she says that she is so small-breasted that she fits in without having to have a mastectomy. Over our weekend together we do a lot of sharing and laughing about our changed bodies and lives. And we remember that laughter is truly a sign of returning life.

My most memorable incident in the life of my own postmastectomy body took place about two years after my surgery. We were on a family vacation in Carlsbad, California. We were at a beach basking in the sun and sand. I was wearing a one-piece swimsuit and using my fiber-filled prostheses, in which by this time I was very comfortable. We were diving into waves and riding their crests to shore. A particularly big wave washed over me and I stood up to find that I had lost both of my prostheses! The wave had been so powerful that it had grabbed my foam breasts and thrown them aside. I was now standing in the shallow water, breastless, and my renegade prostheses were bobbing along somewhere in the crowded water.

A little desperate, I called Jim and Carly over to tell them that my boobs had been lost. Jim stood in front of me while Carly ran to get my T-shirt, which was sitting on the beach. Clothed, I could focus a bit more on the missing breast forms. I turned and looked to see one floating just behind me. The other was washing up on the beach about thirty yards from where I stood, next to some children playing in the sand. How I prayed they wouldn't pick it up! Jim couldn't see well enough without his glasses to go and get it so Carly ran off to rescue it. I saw a young couple point to it as they walked past. When Carly breathlessly returned with the form in hand, she told us that she had rehearsed what she was going to say if anyone had questioned her or given her a funny look. "What's your problem? Haven't you seen one of these before?"

We carried on and had a great time. I was just careful to keep my T-shirt tied around my waist to catch my breasts if they tried to escape again. Walking back to the hotel, I had to shake my head in total disbelief. I had lost both my breasts in front of hundreds of people. And it had barely phased me. Now that's recovery! Looking back later, after the laughter had passed, it dawned on me that snaps on the side of my swimsuit prostheses pockets would have kept my forms in their place and another innovation was born.

I have written a great deal about the grief and pain that accompany a mastectomy. I hope that you will also take away with you a sense of the hidden rewards that also accompany your recovery. Learning to love yourself and redefine your worth, to put your relationships on a new footing, and to develop a sense of your own heroism are just a few of the hidden benefits of your surgery. And coming to laugh and take joy in life again is a process that will make living in your postmastectomy body not just tolerable, but a cause for celebration.

GLOSSARY

anesthesiologist—A doctor who specializes solely in administering anesthetics.

anesthetic—A medication that depresses the nervous system, resulting in loss of pain and/or sensation. General anesthetic includes the loss of consciousness.

anesthetize—To produce the loss of sensation.

areola—The circular area that surrounds the nipple. It is pigmented (has a darker skin tone) and contains glands that produce tiny bumps.

arthritis—Inflammation of a joint.

atypical antidepressants—A class of antidepressants used to treat such conditions as depression, anxiety disorders, sleep disorders, and nicotine cravings.

atypical connective tissue disease—One of the categories used in a class action suit against manufacturers of silicone implants. It describes symptoms reported by some women after having silicone implants.

atypical rheumatic syndrome—One of the categories used in a class action suit against manufacturers of silicone implants. It describes symptoms reported by some women after having silicone implants.

autoimmune disease—A condition where the body's immune system responds as if it has an allergy to its own tissue.

axilla—Armpit.

axillary—Referring to the area of the armpit.

barbiturate—A highly addictive class of medication used to induce sleep.

basilic vein—A vein that runs from the armpit down the arm and into the hand that can become shortened during a lymph node dissection.

benzodiazephines—A potentially addictive class of antianxiety medication used to treat such conditions as anxiety and sleep disorders (e.g. Xanax, Serax, Klonopin, Valium, Librium).

bilateral mastectomy—Removal of both breasts (a double mastectomy).

bioenergetics analysis—A psychological theory that states that a person's psychological experiences shape the development of their body and should be treated by working directly with the body.

breast enhancer—A small breast prosthesis that is used to smooth out, fill in, and equalize breast size after a lumpectomy or mastectomy.

breast equalizer—Breast enhancer.

breast form—Breast prosthesis.

breast reconstruction—A type of plastic surgery that creates a breast after some or all of a breast has been removed.

cancer—A general word that describes over 100 diseases in which there is abnormal and uncontrollable growth of cells that consume all the nutrition, glucose, and oxygen needed to sustain a functioning body.

cancer stages—A method of describing how far the cancer has spread that is used to determine the appropriate treatment. See also TNM.

capsular contracture—Scar tissue that may develop around a breast implant as the body tries to wall off the foreign object, which makes the implant hard and can cause pain.

carcinogenic—Anything that causes cancer.

carcinoma—Cancer arising in the epithelial tissue (skin, glands, and lining of the internal organs). Most cancers are of this type.

charley horse—A common term for a severe muscle spasm usually experienced in the foot or calf.

chemotherapy—The use of a drug to treat a disease. Usually thought of as referring to a cancer treatment.

circadian rhythms—Natural biological rhythms with a cycle of about twenty-four hours.

complex decongestive physical therapy (CDPT)—A massage method used to treat lymphedema.

connective tissue diseases—Diseases in the tissue that provides a solid structure that holds the entire body together, such as ligaments and tendons, and includes rheumatoid arthritis, lupus, fibromyalgia.

contralateral mastectomy—Removal of the unaffected breast (contra means opposite or other) for cosmetic reasons or as an attempt to prevent breast cancer in the healthy breast.

depressant—A chemical that depresses the action of the nervous system, such as alcohol.

drainage tube—A tube with a suction bulb that is inserted into a surgical area to facilitate healing by draining off builtup fluid.

duct—A tubular structure in the body that allows gland secretions and fluids to flow. Milk travels to the nipple through ducts.

ductal cancer in situ—Ductal cancer cells that have not grown outside their site of origin.

ductal carcinoma—Ductal cancer.

estrogen receptor assay—A test used to determine whether a tumor is nourished by estrogen.

estrogen receptor positive—Result of estrogen receptor assay that shows that the tumor is nourished by estrogen.

explant surgery—Surgical removal of a breast implant.

fascia—A sheet of fibrous tissue that envelops the body under the skin and encloses and separates muscles and groups of muscles.

fatty tissue (adipose tissue)—A type of connective tissue that consists primarily of fat cells.

FDA (Federal Food & Drug Administration)—U.S. governmental organization that is responsible for approving the use of drugs and medical devices.

fibrocystic disease (lumpy breasts)—A meaningless catch-all term for differences in the density of breast tissue that were considered to increase a woman's risk factor for breast cancer.

fibromyalgia syndrome—A chronic condition that primarily consists of sleep disturbances, fatigue, and pain in the muscles and the fibrous tissue that connects the muscles to the bones.

fibrous tissue—Tissue of white fibers found between connective tissue, (i.e.tendons, ligaments).

fitter—A professional who is trained to fit women with postmastectomy clothes and prostheses.

free TRAM flap—A breast reconstruction method of removing a flap of the abdominal muscle, skin, and fat and reattaching it to the chest to create a breast.

gamma interferon—A naturally occurring protein in the body that strengthens the effectiveness of the immune system.

gene—A functional unit of heredity which is capable of reproducing itself exactly at each cell division and directing the formation of an enzyme or other protein.

glandular tissue—Refers to glands which are tissue, that secrete or excrete, such as lymph nodes, thyroid gland.

gluteal free flap—A breast reconstruction method of removing a flap of the buttocks muscle, skin, and fat and reattaching it to the chest to create a breast.

hormone therapy—A form of cancer treatment used when a breast cancer patient is estrogen receptor positive.

hypnotic—A potentially addictive class of medication used to induce sleep.

image imprinting—A method that uses mental imagery to treat phantom breast pain.

immune system—A complete system of the body that protects against foreign invaders, such as infections or toxins.

implant—An artificial product that is put inside the body. A breast implant is a fluid-filled sac shaped like a breast, which is placed behind the chest muscle to form a breast.

infiltrating cancer—Cancer that has grown into surrounding tissue and possibly other locations in the body, from its initial location in the breast ducts or lobules. Also referred to as invasive cancer.

In situ—In its original place. Refers to tumors that have not grown beyond their site of origin and invaded neighboring tissue.

intraductal cancer—Cancer that is present in the breast ducts. Can be benign or malignant.

invasive cancer—Infiltrating cancer.

irritable bowel syndrome—An irritative and inflammatory disorder of the intestine that causes cramplike pain in the lower abdomen, nausea, bloating and gas, headache, rectal pain, backache, loss of appetite, and alternating diarrhea and constipation.

latissimus dorsi muscle transfer—A breast reconstruction method that transfers the latissimus dorsi (back) muscle, skin fat, and blood vessels that nourish the tissue through a tunnel from the back to the chest to create a breast.

living will—A legal document that states your wishes for the way you want to be medically cared for if you are unable to breathe or circulate your blood without the use of machines.

lobular cancer—Cancer that starts in the breast lobules.

lobules—The part of a breast that can make milk.

lumpectomy—Surgical procedure that removes a breast lump (tumor) and some surrounding tissue. Sometimes called partial mastectomy.

lupus—An inflammatory connective tissue disease.

lymphatic system—A complex system in the body that consists of lymph nodes, lymph vessels, lymph fluid, bone marrow, spleen, and thymus, which produces, stores, and circulates cells that fight infection (lymphocytes).

lymphedema—Swelling in an extremity from the build-up of lymph fluid due to fewer available functioning lymph nodes, which can occur after the removal of lymph nodes.

lymphatic system—A complex system in the body that consists of lymph nodes, lymph vessels, lymph fluid, bone marrow, spleen, and thymus which produces, stores and circulates cells that fight infection (lymphocytes).

mastectomy—Surgical procedure that removes all or part of the breast.

melatonin—A natural hormone produced in the pineal gland that acts as a catalyst for serotonin, which assists the body to maintain a normal sleep cycle. Manufactured in a pill form as a sleep aid.

metastasis—Spread of cancer cells to other organs in the body through the lymphatic system or bloodstream.

modified radical mastectomy—Surgical removal of breast, skin, nipple, areola, and some of the axillary lymph nodes.

MRI (magnetic resonance imaging)—A method of looking inside the body similar to an X-ray, but more effective.

multiple sclerosis (MS)—A disease of the central nervous system that causes patches of sclerosis (plaques) in the brain and spinal cord.

mutation—A change in the chemistry of a gene that leads to the production of an abnormal type of cell.

myofascial—Of or relating to the fascia surrounding and separating muscle tissue.

neurotransmitter—A specific chemical agent in the body that assists with the completion of necessary chemical reactions in the nervous system.

nipple—The tip of the breast that projects from the middle of the areola. It contains the opening of milk ducts from the breast.

noninvasive breast cancer—Breast cancer that has not grown outside of the duct or lobule.

Paget's disease—Breast cancer that begins in the milk ducts and involves the skin of the nipple and areola, causing a crusting, scaly, red, inflamed lesion on the nipple.

partial mastectomy—Removal of the breast tumor and some surrounding breast tissue. Also known as lumpectomy.

pectoralis muscles—The large muscles that attach to the front of the chest wall and upper arms which lie under the breast.

phantom pain—Pain experienced in a missing body part and usually referring to a limb after an amputation, but also present after the loss of a breast.

phantom sensation—The sensation that a missing body part is still attached to the body.

prosthesis—A fabricated substitute for a missing body part. A breast prosthesis is an object that is shaped like a breast and filled with different substances, intended to feel like a real breast.

psychiatrist—A medical doctor with a specialty in psychiatry.

psychologist—A psychotherapist with education in psychological testing.

psychotherapist—A person trained to provide individual, couple, group, and family counselling.

quadrantectomy—A type of partial mastectomy in which a quarter of the breast is removed.

radiation treatment—A treatment for cancer that uses radiation to kill cancer cells. Also called irradiation or radiation therapy.

radical mastectomy—Involved removing the whole breast as well as the pectoralis major and minor muscles, and all of the lymph nodes up to the collarbone. No longer performed except in very rare cases.

rapid eye movement (REM)—A physiologically active stage of sleep during which a person dreams. Too much of this stage of sleep is associated with depression and sleep disorders.

rheumatism—Pain and stiffness associated with arthritis and related disorders of the joints, muscles, and bones.

rheumatologist—A physician who specializes in the study, diagnosis, and treatment of rheumatic conditions.

ruptured breast implant—A tear or leak in the sac or shell of a breast implant, which allows either silicone or saline to enter the body.

saline—Sterile salt water used to make a type of a breast implant.

selective serotonin reuptake inhibitors (SSRIs)—A newer class of antidepressants used to treat such conditions as depression, anxiety disorders, sleep disorders, and chronic pain (i.e. Prozac, Paxil, Zoloft, Luvox).

sensate focus—A progressive touching exercise developed by Masters and Johnson that is used in counseling couples to help build sexual sensation and nonverbal communication, and reduce sexual performance anxiety.

serotonin—A neurotransmitter, a chemical produced in nerve cells (neurons), that affects a person's mood and sleep.

silicone—A type of gel that is used to make a breast implant or prosthesis. Also made in a solid form that is used for the breast implant shell.

somatic—Relating to the body.

spastic colon—One aspect of irritable bowel syndrome, that causes cramplike pain in the lower abdomen.

stem cell—Specialized part of bone marrow that fights disease.

stem cell transplant—A cancer treatment in which the patient's stem cells are removed before high doses of chemotherapy are administered and then returned to the body.

stimulant—A chemical that stimulates the action of the nervous system, such as nicotine and caffeine.

stockinette—An elastic, tube-shaped machine-knitted cloth used in making undergarments and bandages.

systemic—Relating to the body as a whole. A systemic treatment means that intervention is administered internally and affects all the systems of the body as it works on all the cells in the body. Chemotherapy is a systemic treatment.

tender points—Diagnostic points on the body that are very painful when pressure is applied, which indicate the presence of fibromyalgia.

TNM (tumor, nodes, metastases)—A four-stage system used to describe the progression of cancer.

TRAM flap (abdominal)—A breast reconstruction method that transfers the transverse rectus abdominis muscle, fat, skin, and blood vessels through a tunnel from the abdomen up to the chest to create a breast.

transcutaneous electrical nerve stimulation (TENS)—A tiny machine that sends low-level stimulation to a part of the nerves, interfering with the pain messages to the brain.

tricyclic antidepressants (TCAs)—The original class of antidepressants used to treat such conditions as depression, sleep disorders, anxiety disorders, and chronic pain (i.e. Imipramine, Doxepin, Amitriptyline).

tumor—A non-inflammatory growth arising from existing tissue but in which the cells grow out of control. Also known as a neoplasm.

RESOURCES

Cancer Resources

American Cancer Society—Provides a wide range of services to women with breast cancer and their significant others. To reach your local chapter call 1-800-227-2345.

Booklet—*Sexuality & Cancer: For the Woman Who Has Cancer, and Her Partner,* by Leslie R. Schover, Ph.D. 1994. Call number listed above to request a free copy.

Community Connections—Program that provides medication assistance for indigent cancer patients; mutual support groups; cancer education; and gift items such as wigs, head coverings, breast prostheses, and postmastectomy bras.

Kids Count Too—Support and education program on how to cope with a parent with cancer.

Looking Good Feeling Good—An education/support group that is led by a cosmetologist who provides direction to deal with some of the side effects of treatment.

Reach For Recovery—Visitation program for women with a personal concern about breast cancer that addresses emotional, physical, and cosmetic needs related to breast cancer and treatment. Provides a shopping list of places to purchase postmastectomy products.

Road to Recovery—Program that provides transportation to medical appointments for cancer treatment, as well as housekeeping and transportation reimbursement during cancer treatment.

Tapes—"A Significant Journey: Breast Cancer Survivors and the Men Who Love Them" is a videotape on sexuality after a mastectomy. "Finding Your Way" is a series of videotapes for families of cancer patients. Videotapes are free of charge. Send a request to: American Cancer Society, Attention: Library Videotapes Loan,

3316 W. 66th Street, Minneapolis, MN 55435, or call 1-800-582-5152.

"tlc"—Catalog of postmastectomy products. Call 1-800-850-9445. (U.S.)

Coping: Living With Cancer—A magazine for cancer survivors. Cost: $18 U.S. per year for 6 issues. To subscribe write to: Coping, P.O. Box 682268, Franklin, TN 37068-2268 or call (615) 791-3859.

The Cancer Information Service—A hotline to answer questions about any type of cancer, and provides statistics and directs to services. (Canada) 1-888-939-3333

Canadian Cancer Society—Provides transportation, support groups, Reach for Recovery volunteers, and educational information.

Foundation for Canadians Facing Cancer—National resource directory of products and services to assist with appearance for cancer survivors. 1 (800) 387-9954

JC Penny Catalog—Specialty catalog of Jodee postmastectomy products, including bras, prostheses, and lumpectomy accessories. Request a catalog by calling 1-800-932-4115. (U.S.)

National Alliance of Breast Cancer Organizations (NABCO)—NABCO is a breast cancer resource for patients and professionals. Its annual "Breast Cancer Resource List," provides names of services including over 300 support groups. It also publishes a newsletter. Materials are available in English and Spanish. NABCO's Hotline is (212) 719-0154.

National Cancer Institute—A resource center for information on cancer. (U.S.) Call 1-800-422-6237.

Nordstrom Department Store—Most Nordstrom stores provide a full line of prostheses and postmastectomy garments and also do bra and swimsuit alterations.

Sisters Network—A national African-American breast cancer survivor's support organization that offers emotional support through in-home sister-to-sister visits, resource networking, community education, and a national newsletter. Call Sisters Network national headquarters at (713) 781-0255 to get the number of your local chapter.

The Susan G. Komen Breast Cancer Foundation—A public charity foundation with a mission of eradicating breast cancer as a life-threatening
disease by advancing research, education, screening, and treatment.

National Komen Breast Cancer Helpline—Accommodates English and Spanish-speaking callers. Call 1-800-462-9273.

Race For The Cure—Largest 5k run-fitness walk in the United
States to help with the fight against breast cancer. Call 1 800-
462-9273.

Fibromyalgia Resources

Arthritis Foundation—call 1-800 283-7800. (U.S.)

Books

Fibromyalgia and Chronic Myofascial Pain Syndrome: A Survivor's
Manual. Mary Ellen Copeland and Devin Starlanyl. Oakland, CA: New
Harbinger Publishing, 1996.

The Fibromyalgia Survivor. Mark J. Pellegrino. Columbus, Ohio: Ana-
dem Publishing, 1995.

Canada: The Arthritis Society Canada, 1-800-321-1433,
http://www.arthritis.ca.

REFERENCES

1. American Cancer Society. *Breast Cancer Facts & Figures* 1997 pp 6–7.
2. Ibid.
3. Fisher B, Anderson S, Redmond CK, Wolmark N et al. Reanalysis results after 12 years of follow-up in a randomized clinical trial comparing total mastectomy with lumpectomy with or without irradiation in the treatment of breast cancer. *New England Journal of Medicine* 1995: 333: 1456–1461.
4. Love SM with Lindsey K. *Dr. Susan Love's Breast Book* 2nd ed. Reading MA: Addison Wesley, 1995.
5. Ibid.
6. Krydas, I, Fentiman IS, Habib F, Hyward JL. Sensory changes after treatment of operable breast cancer. *Breast Cancer Research & Treatment* 1986: 8(1): 55–59.
7. News Services. Stress over cancer may lower defenses. *Minneapolis Star Tribune:* 7 January 1998: p A14.
8. Dise-Lewis JE: Psychological adaptation to limb loss, in Atkins DJ, Meier RH III (eds): *Comprehensive Management of Upper Limb Amputee.* New York, Springer-Verlag NY Inc, 1989, pp 165–172.
9. Mitchell-Lipp M, Malone SJ. Group rehabilitation of vascular surgery patients. *Arch Phys Med Rehabil* 1976; 57: 180.
10. Immen, Wallace. Scientists trace phantom pain. *The Globe and Mail*
11. Brownlee S with Mitchell K. The route of phantom pain. *U.S. News & World Report* 2 October 1995 pp 76, 78.
12. Ibid.
13. Kwekkeboom K. Postmastectomy pain syndromes. *Cancer Nursing* 1996; 19(1): 37–43.
14. Fukushima R. Doctor draws on own illness in treating lymph disease. *St. Paul Pioneer Press,* 14 August 1997 p 12D.
15. Rosenberg SK, Modified lymphedema treatment: a part of the continuum of rehabilitative cancer care. Arch Phys Med. Rehab. 1996, August: Vol. 77.

References
268

16. Masters WH, Johnson VE, Kolodny RC. *Human Sexuality* (4th ed.) New York: Harper Collins: 1992: pp 256–258.

17. Guthrie RH. *The Truth About Breast Implants*. New York: John Wiley & Sons: 1993: p 90.

18. Gabriel SE, O'Fallon WM, Kurland LT, Besrd CM, Woods JE, Melton LJ III. Risk of connective tissue diseases and other disorders after breast implantation. *New England Journal of Medicine:* 1994: 300: 1697–1702.

19. Slovut G. Breast implant complications higher for cancer patients, Mayo study finds. *Minneapolis Star Tribune:* 6 March 1997: p A5.

20 Guthrie

21. American Psychiatric Association. Diagnostic and Statistical Manual of Mental Disorders. 4th Ed. Washington, DC. 1994.

22. Cowley G. Melatonin Mania. *Newsweek:* 6 November 1995: p 63.

INDEX

The book talks to people from a very real and upfront perspective. It addresses real issues from someone who has actually lived the experience. I would recommend this book to women who are looking at potential mastectomy and/or lumpectomy due to its frank and compassionate and truly educational content. The book is also a wonderful resource for those of us in the oncology healthcare provider roles who hope to more fully understand the experience so many of our patients endure.

—Mary Kay Johnston, RN, MS, OCN
Administrator/Nursing Manager

Rebecca Zuckweiler's extensive clinical experience combined with her personal journey through the life-changing experience of mastectomy, brings a rare and comprehensive outlook to the subject. She answers the questions I didn't even know how to ask. How I wish I had had this guide when I embarked on a similar journey.

—Chris Forth Lasley, Actress and Breast Cancer Survivor

I read with captivated interest *Living in the Postmastectomy Body* and Becky Zuckweiler's account of her and her family's reaction to her mastectomies, especially the words of her husband. Hers is a touching and deep story which chronicles not only the changes on the outside, but also the powerful changes on the inside as a woman confronts the reality of life after a mastectomy. It is an inspiring story with enough detail to satisfy anyone's medical curiosity and enough warmth and insight to help anyone facing a similar life challenge.

—Bruce L. Cunningham, MD
Professor of Surgery
Director, Division of Plastic and Reconstructive Surgery
University of Minnesota

the new soy cookbook

TEMPTING RECIPES FOR TOFU, TEMPEH, SOYBEANS & SOYMILK

by **Lorna Sass**

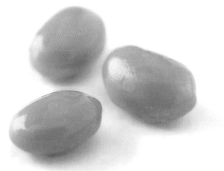

photographs by Jonelle Weaver

CHRONICLE BOOKS
SAN FRANCISCO

Library of Congress Cataloging-in-Publication Data:

Sass, Lorna J.
        The new soy cookbook : tempting recipes for
    tofu, tempeh, soybeans, and soymilk / by Lorna Sass ;
    photographs by Jonelle Weaver.
            p.   cm.
        Includes index.
        ISBN 0-8118-1682-6 (pb)
        1. Cookery (Soybeans) 2. Soyfoods.   I. Title.
    TX803.S6S27   1998   97-34151
    641.6'5655—dc21   CIP

Printed in Hong Kong.

Designed by Carole Goodman
Composition by Suzanne Scott
Food styling by Kimberly Huson
Food styling assistance by Alexandra Lieben-Dougherty
Prop styling by Christina Wressel
The photographer wishes to thank Heather Weston,
    David Land, Amy Osburne, and Jackie Adler.

Distributed in Canada by Raincoast Books
8680 Cambie Street
Vancouver, B.C. V6P 6M9

10 9 8 7 6 5 4 3 2 1

Chronicle Books
85 Second Street
San Francisco, CA 94105
Web Site: www.chronbooks.com

For Richard

Acknowledgments

This book embodies the inventiveness, hard work, and generous spirit of many kind people. I would like to express my gratitude to:

Bill LeBlond, for inviting me to further explore a subject so delicious and close to my heart;

Chronicle assistant editor Sarah Putman, who saw to every last detail and is the most efficient E-mail buddy an author could ever hope for;

William Shurtleff and Aikiko Aoyagi, for their masterful and comprehensive tomes, *The Book of Tofu*, *The Book of Tempeh*, and *The Book of Miso*. Writing on these subjects, I felt like I was standing on the shoulders of giants. Special thanks to Bill for sharing with me so wholeheartedly and articulately his rich knowledge of soyfoods;

My dear assistant and friend, Rosemary Serviss, for her cheerful and intelligent kitchen companionship and her uncompromising quest for great taste and health-promoting food;

My many devoted "elves," home cooks who volunteered to test and comment on the recipes, including Penelope Bareau, Judy Bloom, Heather and Gerhard Bock, Munro Bonnell, Evelyne Chemouny, Joyce Curwin, Cathy Roberts, Tristan Roberts, Barbara Spiegel, Cathy Walthers, and Alisa Zlotnikoff. Special thanks to "super elf" Joan Carlton, who tested every last one!;

Eden Foods, Inc., Gold Mine Natural Food Co., and Wildwood Foods for providing superb organic ingredients for recipe testing;

Elizabeth Schneider, Sarah Jane Freymann, Dorie Greenspan, Jean Richardson, and Michele Urvater for support and feedback of the most useful and collaborative sort;

Richard Isaacson, to whom this book is dedicated, for love, understanding, and patience when "tempeh fugit" were the operative words in my life.

contents

SOY ON THE SIDE 79

Vegetables and Grains

Salads, Slaws, and Dressings

Scones and A Few Desserts

introduction

Benjamin Franklin and I share a passion for soybeans.

During a visit to France in the late eighteenth century, Franklin was so excited when he learned about tofu—"a cheese made of soybeans in China"—that he arranged for soy seedlings from Le Jardin des Plantes in Paris to be shipped to eight Pennsylvania farmers. Thus the seeds were sown—literally and figuratively—for the American soybean industry.

Soy is now the nation's third largest crop. Each year over twenty million bushels of beans are processed into soyfoods, double the amount used for this purpose less than a decade ago. Who is drinking soymilk? Who is exploring the delights of tofu, miso, and tempeh? And why are they doing so now?

Although soyfoods have been a staple of the Asian diet for millennia, few Americans took much interest in cooking them until recently. However, word is now out that this "miracle bean" may help to prevent cancer, lower cholesterol, reduce heart disease, relieve menopausal symptoms, and prevent osteoporosis.

That's quite a roster for a humble legume, but soybeans are an extremely rich source of phytochemicals—those mysterious, non-nutritional compounds that appear to help the body defend itself against illness. In what is being hailed as the Second Golden Age of Nutrition, researchers are currently hard at work documenting phytochemicals' beneficial effects.

It's exciting to discover that the Japanese, who've been eating soy for eons, have no word in their language for hot flashes. However, as a cook I am fascinated by soy for other reasons: I am in awe of its infinite culinary potential. What starts out as a simple bean has been transformed by human ingenuity into myriad superb ingredients.

Over the past ten years, I've experimented with four traditional soyfoods—soybeans, tofu, tempeh, and soymilk—and two condiments, miso and shoyu (soy sauce). I've been intrigued and delighted with the results. Although I've consulted Asian cookbooks off and on during this time, I've made no concerted attempt to prepare these ingredients in traditional ways. Rather, I've allowed my own culinary muse to prevail. Consequently, the recipes reflect a delicious fusion of East and West simmered over time. Since many people turn to soyfoods as a cholesterol-free alternative to animal protein, this recipe collection contains no meat and very little dairy.

Discovering the exquisite complexity of long-brewed soy sauce and masterfully aged miso, experiencing the infinite varieties of braised tofu and marinated tempeh, savoring the extraordinary taste of fresh, green soybeans—these are only a few of the pleasures that await you in these pages.

THE SOY OF COOKING

Soyfoods are remarkably versatile and user-friendly ingredients. As you'll see in the recipes, the flavor of soy marries well with many foods common in the American kitchen—tomatoes, mustard, wine, and chiles, to name only a few.

But let's not get ahead of ourselves. Before you begin cooking, have a glance at the following pages for an introduction to the six soyfoods I've featured in this book. You'll find specifics on selection, storage, and recommended cooking techniques.

soybeans

High in protein and rich in nutrients, soybeans are often referred to as "the meat of the fields." When harvested young and immature, boiled and eaten straight from the pod, green soybeans are a delectable treat—richer and nuttier than any fresh bean I've tasted.

By all means, order them at a Japanese restaurant, or if you're lucky enough to find some in an Asian grocery, prepare these edible gems at your first opportunity. (Have a look at the simple recipe on page 20.) However, because fresh soybeans are seasonal and not commonly available, I've focused my soybean recipes on cooked, dried beans.

While there are hundreds of varieties of dried soybeans, I consider black soybeans in a class of their own. At their best, these elegant ebony beans have a taste reminiscent of chestnuts and a texture so creamy that they can be enjoyed with nothing more than a sprinkling of soy sauce to enhance their taste and a smattering of chopped scallions to add contrast and color.

selecting and storing: There are numerous varieties of black soybeans, but your health-food store is likely to have just one. (If not, you can easily order them by mail; see page 115.) While some have more intense flavor than others, all black soybeans tend to have better taste and texture than the average beige variety. Just make sure that your source has a good turnover so you won't be dealing with beans from the time of the Ming dynasty.

Recently harvested, high-quality beans should have shiny black skins that are smooth and intact. If they've been properly dried and stored, there should be few broken or skinless beans in the batch. Store the beans in a cool, dry place. Theoretically, they last indefinitely, but they'll taste best if eaten within six months.

cooking soybeans: Cooking soybeans from scratch can be a nuisance unless you own a pressure cooker, which does a terrific job of tenderizing the beans in about half an hour. If you don't mind simmering beans for three hours, you can cook them the standard way (instructions follow), but I don't encourage it. Simmered beans almost never attain the mellow, creamy texture of their pressure-cooked cousins.

To shorten cooking time, insure even cooking, and improve digestibility, soak the beans before cooking them. Alternatively, pan-roast them as directed at the end of the recipe. This latter technique accentuates their nuttiness and obviates the need to soak the beans.

Here's my basic recipe for pressure-cooking black soybeans. (You can follow the same instructions for cooking beige soybeans.) Since soybeans have delicate skins, soak and cook the beans with a bit of salt to keep their skins intact. If you wish, add a strip of dried kombu sea vegetable, a variety of kelp that is sold in Japanese groceries and in health-food stores. Japanese cooks believe it makes the beans more digestible. After the beans are done, if you like the taste of the cooking liquid, reserve it for use as soup stock or to thin soy-based spreads and purées.

be forewarned: Although they start out jet black, cooked soybeans fade to a color somewhere between mahogany and chestnut brown.

basic black soybeans

1½ cups black soybeans, preferably organic,
   picked over and rinsed.

Water

1 teaspoon salt

1 large clove garlic, peeled and thinly sliced

1 onion, peeled and quartered

2-inch strip kombu sea vegetable, rinsed (optional)

1 tablespoon vegetable oil (see note)

Place the beans in a large bowl with 4 cups of water and ½ teaspoon of the salt. Cover and refrigerate for 8 to 12 hours. Drain and rinse the beans. Discard any loose skins. (Alternatively, see the directions for pan-roasting, following.)

Place the beans in a 6-quart pressure cooker with ample water to cover and add the remaining ½ teaspoon salt. (Take care not to exceed the maximum fill-line of the cooker.) Over medium-high heat, bring to a boil uncovered. Reduce the heat to simmer and skim off any whitish gray foam on top. Bring to a boil again, reduce the heat to a simmer, and skim off most of the remaining foam. Rinse any beans that come out of the pot with the skimmer and return them to the pot. Add the garlic, onion, kombu (if using), and oil.

Lock the lid in place and over high heat, bring to high pressure. Reduce the heat just enough to maintain high pressure and cook for 20 minutes. Allow the pressure to come down naturally, 10 to 12 minutes. Remove the lid, tilting it away from you to allow any excess steam to escape.

If the beans are not tender, set (but do not lock) the lid in place and simmer them until done. Remove the onion and kombu and discard (or chop up and munch). Drain, reserving the cooking liquid if you wish, and refrigerate the beans and liquid separately for up to 3 days or freeze separately for up to 2 months.

Makes about **4½** cups cooked beans

Note: Don't be tempted to omit the oil; it is necessary to control foaming action under pressure.

pan-roasting dried soybeans: Instead of soaking the beans, set the rinsed soybeans in a large, nonstick skillet and turn the heat to high. When the water begins to sizzle, stir the soybeans until their surfaces are dry. Continue stirring as the skins shrivel, then smooth out again and split open to reveal the light interior of the bean, about 3 minutes. Turn off the heat and continue stirring for 1 minute. Transfer the beans to a bowl to cool slightly before cooking. Roasted soybeans tend to lose their skins when cooked, but are very delicious.

standard stove-top instructions: Drain off the soaking water and rinse the beans. Place them in a heavy saucepan and pour in enough water to reach 1 inch above the beans. Bring to a boil over high heat and skim off foam. Cover, reduce the heat to a gentle boil, and cook, occasionally skimming off foam, until the beans are tender, 2½ to 3 hours. Replenish water as needed to keep the beans covered.

cooking with soybeans: All of the recipes in this book that call for soybeans presume that they are already cooked. If you have neither the time nor inclination to cook them from scratch, you need not compromise on quality or flavor. Look for Eden Foods' organic black soybeans in fifteen-ounce cans. I have made it a point always to use 1½ cups beans (the approximate contents of a can) so that you can easily use home-cooked or canned interchangeably in the recipes.

Cooked soybeans freeze fairly well but, like most other beans, lose some flavor and texture. Beans that have been frozen are best suited for soups or stews. For salads, which require firm beans, rely on freshly cooked or canned.

Thanks to their creamy texture, soybeans do an impressive job of replacing chickpeas in a low-fat Black Soybean Hummus (page 21). Because they have such a delicate flavor, soybeans marry well with a wide variety of seasonings and benefit from a period of marinating or simmering, as you'll see in recipes such as Black Soybean Salsa (page 59) and Seasoned Black Soybeans (page 80).

soymilk

To make soymilk, soaked soybeans are ground, briefly simmered, and then pressed to release a nutrient-rich beige liquid. Shelf-stable, one-liter "bricks" of aseptic-packed soymilk are now widely available, but you may notice that they are never called milk. The label will read soy beverage or soybean drink, in accordance with United States Department of Agriculture (USDA) requirements. I hope the USDA will forgive me, but I shall conform to modern parlance and continue referring to this versatile dairy alternative as soymilk.

selecting and storing: My comparison tasting of a half-dozen brands quickly revealed that not all soymilks are created equal. Tastes ranged from light, fresh, and pleasantly sweet to musky, chalky, oily, and intensely "beany." Color ranged from creamy white to dark caramel, with lots of shades in between.

Since many people turn to soymilk as a cholesterol- and lactose-free alternative to dairy milk, it makes sense to opt for one fortified with calcium and vitamins. I also prefer full-fat soymilk for its creamy richness, but I avoid any brands that have added oil. I have used Edensoy Extra Original in testing the recipes for this book, since it fulfills these requirements, is widely available, and has the best nutrient profile among brands I compared. (For best results when preparing these recipes, choose among the aseptic-packed soymilks sold in health-food stores and supermarkets, the fresh soymilk available in Asian markets has less body.)

Aseptic-packed soymilk is shelf stable and will last until the expiration date marked on the container—usually a year or more from the date of purchase. Once opened, it must be refrigerated and should be used within five days.

cooking with soymilk: It's easy to cook with soymilk if you keep a few of its characteristics in mind. Since most aseptic-packed soymilk is sweetened (usually with some kind of malted cereal), it's a natural ingredient for desserts. Indeed, it can be used very successfully in fairly concentrated form, as I have done in the Pineapple-Coconut Rice Pudding (page 108). Keep in mind, however, that soymilk's beige color results in a darker pudding than you might normally expect if using dairy milk. For other recipes, such as Sage-Scented Cornmeal Scones (page 105) or Pumpkin Tart with Pecan Crust (page 113), color is not altered.

In savory dishes, a cup or two of soymilk in a soup to serve four adds good body and taste as long as the flavor of the other ingredients harmonizes with the soymilk's "beany" overtones and faint sweetness. Such is the case in the Red Lentil Soup with Indian Spices (page 37).

Soymilk will curdle when boiled, but the looks and taste of dishes that are chunky and have multiple ingredients do not suffer from this fact. If curdling is undesirable, as in the Creamy Dilled Spinach Soup (page 39), use soymilk only in recipes that contain little to no acid, add it at the very end, and do not let it come to a boil.

tofu

Tofu (aka bean curd) is made through a process that closely resembles cheese making. A coagulant such as magnesium chloride is added to soymilk, and the milk separates into curds and whey. Before the curds are drained, they retain a high water content and a custardlike texture. These curds, remarkably delicious when just made, are known as silken tofu. Curds drained more thoroughly and pressed into blocks are labeled soft, medium, firm, and extra-firm tofu, depending upon how much water has been released.

Most of the recipes in this book call for extra-firm or firm tofu, since these types hold their shape and contain the most protein. Silken soft tofu, with its high water content and smooth texture, is ideal for dressings and sauces.

selecting and storing: Vacuum packing makes it possible for us to refrigerate tofu—a fresh and perishable food—for weeks at a time. I recommend buying sealed one-pound plastic tubs of organic tofu, found in the refrigerator section of natural-food stores and many supermarkets. These are a more reliable choice than the small squares of tofu left soaking in water and open to the air and contamination. (Although nothing can beat a shelf-stable, ten-ounce box of aseptic-packed tofu for convenience, its taste and texture are not as appealing as fresh.)

If more than one brand of fresh tofu is available in your area, it pays to sample them side by side and see which you prefer. You will be surprised at the range of taste and texture, even among the blocks labeled extra-firm! If calcium is a concern, compare labels; calcium content varies according to the coagulant used. I used Nasoya—a reliably consistent brand that is readily available in my part of the world—to test the recipes in this book.

When purchasing tofu, always check the expiration date. Unless you plan to use the tofu immediately, reach toward the back of the refrigerator case for one with the latest date. If the expiration date approaches before you've had a chance to use it, pop the unopened tub into the freezer (see the section on freezing tofu that follows).

Once you have opened the container, store any leftover tofu in water to cover in a tightly sealed container. Change the water daily and the tofu will remain fresh for about five days. The aroma of fresh tofu is mildly beany and faintly sweet. Once the smell becomes slightly sour and the tofu darkens around the edges, toss it.

cooking with tofu: The Chinese say that tofu has "the taste of a hundred things" and with good reason. Tofu has a protean capacity for transformation, and the limits of tofu cookery are equal only to the limits of the cook's imagination. What other ingredient can you boil, fry, steam, broil, bake, freeze, marinate, or eat fresh—and achieve such diverse and satisfying results?

Here are some explanations for tofu-cooking techniques you'll encounter in the recipes:

draining tofu: Remove the tofu from the soaking water. It's not necessary to set the tofu in a strainer unless the recipe specifies doing so.

pressing tofu: Pressing tofu is the single most important step in producing a delicious final dish. Pressed tofu offers pleasing resistance to the tooth and, perhaps more importantly, the watery liquid released by pressing can be replaced with a flavor-packed marinade or sauce. For example, a one-pound block of extra-firm tofu releases three to four tablespoons of liquid during the first fifteen minutes of pressing. The pressed tofu will then, in a spongelike manner, absorb about that amount of marinade.

The most efficient way to press tofu is to purchase a Tofu Squeeze, an inexpensive and cleverly designed gadget that gently presses the water out of a 1-pound block (see Mail-Order Sources).

If you're not gadget oriented, loosely wrap the block of tofu in multiple layers of a clean kitchen towel. Set it on a plate and place a 1-pound bag of beans on top. Let rest for 15 minutes. Rewrap the tofu in a dry section of the towel, set the beans on top, and set aside for an additional 15 minutes (or overnight in the refrigerator).

cutting a block of tofu into cubes: Set the tofu on a cutting board with the longer side facing you. Use a large serrated knife to cut horizontal slices ½ inch thick. Cut vertical slices ½ inch thick. Give the board a quarter turn. Gently hold the block together and cut vertical slices ½ inch thick in the opposite direction to create cubes. (To dice tofu, use the same technique but make ¼-inch-thick slices.)

freezing tofu: Freezing tofu turns it a few shades darker, results in a distinctively chewy texture, and dramatically increases the tofu's capacity to absorb flavor.

To freeze, set the unopened tub of tofu in the freezer until it is rock hard, a minimum of 36 hours. (It can be frozen for up to three months.) For a quick defrost, puncture the plastic top with a paring knife in about 10 places, set the tub on a plate, and defrost in a microwave on high for 5 to 7 minutes.

Alternatively, defrost at room temperature; it should take about 3 hours. (You can speed up the process by setting the tub in a large bowl of hot water.) Drain and press as directed in the recipe. Slice with a serrated knife.

Freezing is not advised for silken tofu because it ruins the texture.

tempeh

Tempeh is a fermented soybean cake that originated many centuries ago in Indonesia, where it is still the country's most popular soyfood. In the tradition of the world's great blue-veined cheeses, tempeh is made by injecting hulled, cooked soybeans (or a combination of soybeans and grains or seeds) with mold. The mixture is sealed in flat, rectangular plastic bags and, as it ferments, the mold binds the soybeans together. The result is a firm, slab-shaped cake whose taste is often described as "yeasty" or "mushroomy." Fermentation breaks down the proteins and natural sugars in the beans, eliminating the digestive challenges other soyfoods may cause.

selecting and storing: Tempeh is stored in the refrigerator or freezer section of most natural-food stores. Depending upon the regional producer, you'll find either eight-ounce or sixteen-ounce organic cakes with clearly marked expiration dates, usually a number of months from the time of purchase.

Store tempeh in your refrigerator until the expiration date, or freeze it for up to three months (assuming it has not already been frozen). For a quick defrost, remove the plastic wrapping, set on a paper towel, and microwave on high for 45 to 60 seconds. Alternatively defrost either at room temperature (set the sealed tempeh in a bowl of hot water to speed this process) or overnight in the refrigerator.

Wrap any partially used cakes in a few layers of plastic wrap and refrigerate for up to five days after opening. If any gray or blackish spots are visible, simply cut them away. (These indicate that the mold is alive and well and are nothing to worry about.) Fresh tempeh should have a mild, slightly sweet aroma. If you detect the smell of ammonia or the tempeh feels slippery to the touch, throw it out.

cooking with tempeh: Despite its unusual looks, tempeh is an extraordinary food that has become a personal favorite. Like tofu, it has a spongelike capacity to absorb flavor. Perhaps even more appealing to the cook, however, is the fact that tempeh has a toothsome meatiness and a flavor profile more complex than most ingredients in the vegetarian kitchen.

Tempeh comes in many varieties, depending upon what other ingredients are mixed with the soybeans. Straight soy tempeh has the most assertive flavor and is well suited to hearty recipes like Country Tempeh Pâté (page 26) or Tempeh Simmered in Red Wine with Herbes de Provence (page 42). For general cooking, however, I prefer tempeh that includes one or more grains. Mixed-grain tempeh has a milder taste than straight soy tempeh and harmonizes more readily with subtle seasonings.

I used Lightlife tempeh for recipe testing, since it's the brand carried by my local natural-food store. Lightlife tempeh comes in rectangular slabs about three-quarters inch thick. If your brand of tempeh is thicker, halve it horizontally to expose more surface area.

Creating delicious tempeh-based dishes is guaranteed if you observe two basic rules.

1 Infuse the tempeh with lots of good flavor. This is easily done by cutting the cake to maximize exposed surfaces and then marinating or simmering the pieces in a tasty sauce.

2 Enhance the looks and texture by sautéing the tempeh until brown and slightly crusty. Since raw tempeh immediately guzzles up any oil in the skillet, it's most efficient to brush the surfaces lightly with oil before browning them.

Alternatively, to keep added fat to a minimum, brown the pieces after they have been cooked and saturated with liquid. In either case, use a high-quality nonstick skillet and cover the pan for part of the time. I have come to rely on my All-Clad 12-inch frying pan, which does the job remarkably well.

miso

Like tempeh, the pastelike condiment called miso is a fermented soyfood. The art of miso making, however, is much more varied and complex. Although details vary according to type, most miso is made by mixing cooked soybeans with koji, a grain inoculated with aspergillus mold, plus water and salt. As the mixture ferments, wild microorganisms from the environment and enzymes in the koji break down the soybeans and grains into amino and fatty acids and simple sugars.

Depending upon the type of grain used, the balance of koji to beans, the amount of added salt, and the conditions and duration of fermentation, a mind-boggling array of misos results. (To further obfuscate matters for the westerner, misos are frequently referred to by their Japanese names.)

Therefore, as with wine, becoming a true connoisseur of miso requires lifetime attention. But I can assure you that even the smallest effort will reap extraordinary rewards, as more and more American chefs are in the process of discovering.

For a wealth of information on the subject, I refer you to the encyclopedic *Book of Miso* by William Shurtleff and Akiko Aoyagi. In the meanwhile, here are a few simple guidelines, plus suggestions for purchasing the finest misos available.

types of miso: For ease of discussion, misos can be classified by color as "light" and "dark." In general (but not always!), light misos are fermented for only a few months. They are yellowish beige, smooth in texture, high in simple sugars, and relatively low in salt. Sweet white and shiro misos are two good examples of light misos. High-quality light misos have a mellow sweetness and a vibrant taste.

Dark misos, on the other hand, are fermented for two or three years and range in color from chestnut to chocolate brown. Often chunky, they have a higher proportion of soybeans and are considerably saltier than light misos. Barley (*mugi*) and soybean (*hatcho*) misos are two superb dark varieties. The best dark misos have a lively, complex character, an intriguing aroma, and a deep, rich taste.

As with other soyfoods, it's extremely informative to do a blind tasting of a variety of misos. In this category, more than any other, the disparities among brands are worth paying attention to: your choice will have a noteworthy effect on the taste of your dish.

selecting and storing: Look in the refrigerated section of your natural-food store, where you will find plastic tubs of the best-tasting misos. Shelf-stable misos have been pasteurized to halt fermentation, and as a result usually lack the vitality and complexity of those that contain living enzymes.

In the United States, we are extremely fortunate to have many superb organic misos from which to choose. For an experience of miso made completely by hand in the traditional way, look for varieties of rustic and full-flavored South River Miso, produced in Massachusetts and available in many natural-food stores and by mail order. You can also order by mail (from a California source) a wide range of superb unpasteurized misos made by small Japanese producers. High-quality misos produced on a larger scale by Miso Master of Rutherfordton, North Carolina, are probably the most widely available in health-food stores.

Although it may take a bit of effort to get your hands on the best misos available, they last upward of a year under refrigeration. I suggest that you begin with two—a light and a dark—and expand your collection slowly. To simplify matters, I have called for only two types of miso in the recipes: sweet white miso and barley miso. I tested with Miso Master's sweet white miso and Ohsawa Yamaki barley miso imported from Japan. If you're game to keep a third miso on hand, I recommend South River's full-bodied and unique regional creation, dandelion-leek miso.

cooking with miso: The subtle sweetness and simple, buttery freshness of light misos make them a good choice for dressings and sauces, as you'll see in the recipe for

Peanut Miso Dressing and Dipping Sauce (page 102). Dark misos have an intense earthy (almost beefy) flavor that works like a top-notch bouillon in soups, such as the Meal-in-a-Bowl Noodle Vegetable Hot Pot (page 63). For variety and increased complexity, it's intriguing to blend two or more types of miso, as I have suggested in many of the recipes.

Because the saltiness of miso varies by type and maker, it's impossible to suggest an amount that will work perfectly each time. In general, about one tablespoon of sweet miso and two teaspoons of dark blended into a cup of water will provide the right amount of flavor. Once you become familiar with the misos in your refrigerator, you'll know what proportion works best for you.

Miso is typically stirred in at the end of cooking, ideally after the heat is turned off, so that none of its lively flavor components are burned off by high temperatures. To avoid unpleasant clumps of miso in the final dish, be sure to blend the miso into hot water or broth before adding it.

Aside from offering complex flavor by the spoonful, miso does an extraordinary job of unifying diverse ingredients, creating a whole that is greater than the sum of its parts. For a good example of this characteristic at work, try the recipe for Shrimps, Mussels, and Tofu in Lemongrass-Miso Broth (page 65) and do the before-and-after taste test I suggest.

soy sauce

Surely the best-known soyfood in America, soy sauce is the least understood and appreciated. Most of the brands available in supermarkets are an abomination—an unfortunate combination of quick industrialized manufacturing and artificial coloring, sweeteners, and additives that bear no resemblance to the real thing.

With apologies to specialists in Chinese gastronomy, I must admit that having grown up (culinarily speaking) on traditionally brewed Japanese shoyu and tamari, I have little appreciation for the assertive, harsh saltiness of Chinese soy sauces. I was gratified to find my opinion shared in print by Ken Hom, who states in his book *Chinese Kitchen* that when compared to light Chinese varieties, "naturally brewed Japanese soy sauces . . . have a more complex flavor."

Traditional shoyu is made by inoculating toasted cracked wheat and steamed soybeans with the spores of an aspergillus mold. The resulting mixture, known as *koji*, is combined with a brine and fermented for a year or two in large wooden vats. Finally, the mixture is pressed through cotton sacks. The liquid extracted is a mixture of soy oil and shoyu. The oil rises to the surface and is removed, and the shoyu is pasteurized and bottled.

According to Jan and John Belleme, authors of *Cooking with Japanese Foods*, less than one percent of Japanese shoyu is produced in this time-honored way. Fortunately, this highly prized shoyu is available in America and at quite a reasonable price.

selecting and storing: In a tasting of numerous brands of organic shoyu brewed and aged traditionally, two stood out for their complex winy, fermented flavor: Eden Organic Shoyu and Ohsawa Nama Shoyu. With other brands, an initial jolt of saltiness detracted from the rich bouquet and balance of flavors. For those concerned about salt intake, Eden's reduced-sodium shoyu is also superb. Anyone allergic to wheat may opt for tamari (similar to shoyu, but wheat-free) as a substitute.

Store shoyu in the refrigerator. Screw the cap on tightly and it will last for a year or more, although the vitality will fade as time goes on.

cooking with soy sauce: I have used shoyu exclusively in all of the recipes in this book primarily because I prefer its flavor. In addition, it seemed a practical way to avoid confusion about the quantity to suggest, given the wide range of saltiness in the broad category of soy sauces.

A good way to think of shoyu is as "salt plus." Shoyu contains glutamic acid, a natural form of monosodium glutamate (MSG) that enhances flavor. At the same time, a well-made shoyu imparts a subtle sweetness (somewhat like dry sherry) and a delicate, fermented, winy flavor to a dish. It also deepens color, giving sauces and dressings an appealing earthy tone. (See, for example, Tempeh with Quick Homemade Tomato Sauce and Olives, page 52.)

Shoyu marries remarkably well with olive oil, and I love using it to make vinaigrettes and other dressings. Try the Lime-Shoyu Vinaigrette (page 101), and you will see how it brings considerable complexity to a simple dressing. Shoyu offers the same depth of flavor to marinades, as evidenced in the Down-Home "Barbecued" Tofu (page 72).

For a simple weeknight meal, I sometimes toss pasta with a splash-on sauce of nothing more than a good-quality olive oil and shoyu—the best! Use toasted Asian sesame oil instead of olive oil, and the personality of the sauce changes entirely, as you will see in the recipe for Double-Sesame Skillet Brown Rice (page 92).

When practical, it's ideal to add shoyu at the end of cooking— as you would a good balsamic vinegar—to maximize enjoyment of the flavor nuances of this superb condiment.

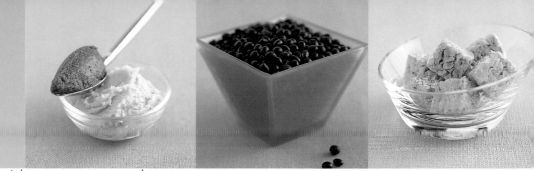

appetizers and soups

Appetizers provide a miniature window onto the vast world of soyfoods. Among them, we move from the simplest of soy recipes—boiled Fresh Green Soybeans—to the complex taste of Country Tempeh Pâté and Black Soybean Hummus.

In this chapter, you'll get a first glimpse of tofu's versatility. In Thai-Inspired Shrimp and Tofu Cocktail, the tofu absorbs the intense flavor of fish sauce to become a separate but equal partner with shrimp. Mesclun with Maple-Mustard Tofu Points reveals how the taste and texture of tofu can be transformed from mellow and soft to assertive and chewy.

Thanks to the skills of traditional miso masters who produce a product with such depth and character, the simple Impromptu Miso Soup offers many levels of flavor, providing soul-satisfying contentment and healing for all that ails us. Embellish the basic broth with vegetables and herbs for a Shiitake, Miso, and Barley Soup, and the results are fit for a royal feast.

And finally, you'll experience soymilk's remarkable ability to provide body and richness to Creamy Dilled Spinach Soup and Red Lentil Soup with Indian Spices. Just as a starter whets the appetite for a meal, the tantalizing and diverse recipes in this chapter will whet your appetite for soyfoods cookery.

fresh green soybeans

IF YOU'RE EVER LUCKY ENOUGH TO SPOT FRESH GREEN SOYBEANS FOR SALE IN AN ASIAN GROCERY OR FARMERS' MARKET, GRAB THEM FOR AN UNFORGETTABLE TASTE TREAT. YOU'LL RECOGNIZE THESE DIMINUTIVE SPECIMENS—ABOUT TWO INCHES LONG—BY THE DELICATE BROWN FUZZ COVERING THEIR GREEN PODS. (BACKYARD GARDENERS, TAKE NOTE: I'VE BEEN TOLD THAT THEY'RE EXTREMELY EASY TO GROW.) MORE READILY AVAILABLE, BUT SLIGHTLY SECOND-BEST, ARE THE FROZEN GREEN SOYBEANS FOUND IN MANY ASIAN GROCERIES. DEFROST THEM, THEN FOLLOW THE SAME DIRECTIONS FOR PREPARATION.

CALLED *EDAMAME* BY THE JAPANESE, SOYBEANS IN THE POD ARE TRADITIONALLY SERVED AS FINGER FOOD. BEFORE COOKING, THEY ARE OFTEN RUBBED IN SALT TO REMOVE THE FUZZ FROM THEIR PODS. ALTERNATIVELY, THEY ARE BOILED IN HEAVILY SALTED WATER TO FIX COLOR AND INTENSIFY FLAVOR. I DON'T BOTHER WITH EITHER APPROACH, FINDING THEIR LOOKS AND SUBTLE BUT EXTRAORDINARY FLAVOR NEED NO ENHANCEMENT.

SERVE *EDAMAME* IN A LARGE BOWL, INVITING EACH DINER TO SPLIT OPEN THE POD (EASILY DONE WITH A THUMBNAIL), REVEALING A FEW PRECIOUS GREEN BEANS THAT ARE SWEET, NUTTY, AND IRRESISTIBLY RICH. THEY TASTE BEST WHEN FRESHLY COOKED, ALTHOUGH THEY ARE STILL A TREAT AFTER A BRIEF SOJOURN IN THE REFRIGERATOR.

1 Bring a large pot of water to a boil. Add the beans and cook uncovered at a medium boil until the beans are creamy and tender but still firm, 5 to 10 minutes. (Timing and doneness vary according to batch and personal preference. Begin testing every minute after the first 5 minutes to avoid overcooking.)

2 When the beans are done, drain them and run under cold water to set the color and halt cooking. Drain well and transfer to a bowl. Serve at room temperature.

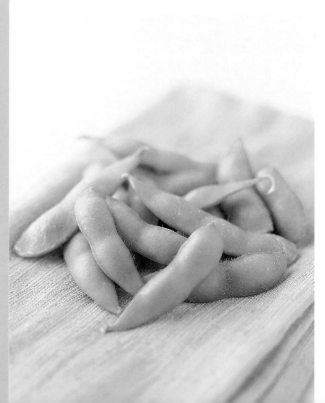

black soybean hummus

BLACK SOYBEANS ARE A TERRIFIC STAND-IN FOR CHICKPEAS IN THIS ROBUST HUMMUS. BECAUSE OF SOYBEANS' NUTTINESS AND CREAMY TEXTURE, NO OLIVE OIL AND VERY LITTLE TAHINI (SESAME-SEED PASTE) ARE REQUIRED TO GIVE THE DIP ITS TRADITIONALLY RICH FLAVOR. I LIKE TO GIVE THE HUMMUS SOME HEAT BY ADDING A BIT OF THE NORTH AFRICAN HOT PEPPER PASTE CALLED *HARISSA*. YOU'LL FIND *HARISSA* AND TAHINI AT MOST INTERNATIONAL GROCERIES; TAHINI IS ALSO AVAILABLE AT HEALTH-FOOD STORES.

SERVE THE HUMMUS IN A SMALL BOWL, GARNISHED WITH A SPRINKLING OF SWEET PAPRIKA AND A SCATTERING OF OIL-CURED OLIVES. SET A BASKET OF PITA TRIANGLES ON THE SIDE.

I OFTEN DOUBLE THE RECIPE SO I CAN MAKE A LUNCH OF HUMMUS AND THICK STRIPS OF ROASTED RED PEPPER STUFFED INTO A PITA POCKET.

1 CLOVE
garlic, peeled

1 ½ CUPS
cooked black soybeans (page 9) or 1 can (15 ounces) organic black soybeans, drained (reserve liquid)

2 TO 4 TABLESPOONS
freshly squeezed lemon juice

2 TO 3 TABLESPOONS
soybean cooking or canning liquid or water

1 ½ TABLESPOONS
tahini (sesame-seed paste)

½ TO ¾ TEASPOON
ground cumin

½ TO ¾ TEASPOON
salt

½ TO 1 TEASPOON
harissa or ⅛ to ¼ teaspoon ground cayenne pepper (optional)

Sweet paprika and oil-cured olives, for garnish

1 Mince the garlic in a food processor. Add the black soybeans and the minimum amounts of the remaining ingredients. Process to a fairly smooth paste, scraping down the sides of the work bowl as needed. Taste and blend in more of any ingredients required to give a smooth consistency and to suit your taste.

Makes about 1¼ cups

21

mesclun with maple-mustard tofu points

FOR THIS UNUSUAL SALAD, TASTY TRIANGLES OF PIQUANT, GOLDEN-CRUSTED TOFU ARE SET ATOP A BED OF MESCLUN THAT HAS BEEN LIGHTLY SPRINKLED WITH SEASONED RICE VINEGAR. (I LIKE MARUKAN-BRAND VINEGAR; IT'S READILY AVAILABLE IN ASIAN GROCERIES AND MANY SUPERMARKETS.) TO GIVE IT AN APPEALING CHEWINESS, THE TOFU IS FIRST FROZEN, THEN DEFROSTED AND PRESSED. THE SLICED TOFU IS DIPPED INTO A TANGY SAUCE AND QUICKLY BROILED. TO ACHIEVE THE BEST TEXTURE, MAKE THIS RECIPE WITH EXTRA-FIRM TOFU.

ALTHOUGH THIS SALAD MAKES A LOVELY STARTER, YOU CAN DOUBLE EACH PORTION TO CREATE A LIGHT LUNCHEON ENTRÉE FOR TWO. FOR A PLEASANT CHANGE, TRY A NEST OF THINLY SHREDDED RED AND GREEN CABBAGE INSTEAD OF THE MESCLUN.

2 TABLESPOONS
shoyu

2 TABLESPOONS
Dijon mustard

1 TABLESPOON
sweet white miso

1 TABLESPOON
maple syrup

1 TABLESPOON
water

1 TABLESPOON
toasted Asian sesame oil

A FEW DROPS
chili oil or hot pepper sesame oil
(optional)

1-POUND BLOCK
extra-firm tofu, frozen, defrosted,
and drained (page 13)

¼ POUND
mesclun or mixed salad greens

Seasoned rice vinegar

16 STRIPS
roasted red bell pepper, about
2 inches long and ½ inch wide

1 Line a broiling pan or baking sheet with aluminum foil. Set aside. Place the top oven rack 5 to 6 inches from the broiling element and turn on the broiler.

2 In a pie plate or shallow bowl, use a fork to mash and mix the shoyu, mustard, miso, maple syrup, water, sesame oil, and chili oil to taste (if using) until thoroughly blended. Set the shoyu mixture aside.

3 Set the block of defrosted tofu between 2 plates and, pressing the plates firmly together, tip them over the sink as the tofu releases excess water. Release the pressure slightly, then press the plates firmly together again 4 or 5 more times, or until no more water is expressed.

4 Set the block of tofu on a cutting board with the longer end facing you. With a serrated knife, cut the tofu crosswise into 8 slices, each about ½ inch thick. Cut each slice on the diagonal into 2 triangles. Dip the triangles into the shoyu mixture to coat all sides. Arrange the triangles on the prepared broiling pan as you go.

5 Broil until lightly browned and slightly crusty on the first side, 3 to 4 minutes. (If your broiler cooks unevenly, rotate the broiling pan halfway through.) Turn the triangles over with a spatula. If there's any remaining shoyu mixture, paint it on with a pastry brush. Broil until the second side is browned, about 3 minutes. (For a more barbecued taste, broil the triangles until they are slightly blackened around the edges, but take care not to burn them.) Remove the broiling pan from the oven and set aside to cool slightly. (Triangles may be served warm or at room temperature.)

6 Divide the mesclun among 4 luncheon-sized plates. Lightly drizzle the greens with the rice vinegar, about 1 teaspoon per portion. On top of the greens, arrange 4 tofu triangles per plate in a clover pattern, with the narrowest point of each triangle facing into the center. Place 4 red pepper strips on each serving, laying them between the triangles.

Serves **4**

thai-inspired shrimp and tofu cocktail

THIS UNUSUAL COCKTAIL IS BURSTING WITH EXOTIC FLAVORS AND INTERESTING TEXTURES, BEST EXPERIENCED WHEN FRESHLY MADE. AFTER THE TOFU IS BLANCHED, PRESSED, AND DICED, IT QUICKLY SOAKS UP THE FLAVOR OF A JAZZY SOUTHEAST ASIAN SAUCE THAT INCLUDES LEMONGRASS, CURRY PASTE, AND THAI FISH SAUCE, *NAM PLA*. YOU CAN ALSO USE THE VIETNAMESE FISH SAUCE, *NUOC MAM*. LOOK FOR BOTH TYPES IN ASIAN MARKETS.

IF YOU NEED TO PREPARE THIS DISH IN ADVANCE, HOLD BACK ON ADDING THE CUCUMBER UNTIL THE LAST MINUTE. FOR AN ELEGANT PRESENTATION, SERVE THE COCKTAIL IN SMALL GOBLETS OR GLASS BOWLS LINED WITH RADICCHIO. PERK UP ANY LEFTOVERS WITH AN EXTRA SPLASH OF LIME JUICE.

8 OUNCES
extra-firm or firm tofu

1 FOUR-INCH STALK
lemongrass (measure from fleshy bulb upward), bruised outer leaves removed, cut into 1-inch-long pieces (see note)

2 CLOVES
garlic, peeled

½ CUP
tightly packed cilantro leaves

½ TEASPOON
Thai red curry paste or ¼ teaspoon crushed red pepper flakes

3 TABLESPOONS
freshly squeezed lime juice

2 ½ TABLESPOONS
Thai fish sauce

2 TABLESPOONS
peanut or canola oil

8 OUNCES
raw shrimp, cooked, peeled, deveined, and cut into ½-inch chunks

½ CUP
finely diced red onion

½ CUP
peeled, seeded, and finely diced cucumber

Radicchio leaves, for garnish

Note: If fresh lemongrass is not available, Thai Kitchen's jarred lemongrass packed in water is a viable substitute.

1 Bring a small pot of water to a rapid boil. Set the block of tofu in the water, reduce the heat to low, and simmer for 5 minutes. Drain and, when cool enough to handle, press according to the directions on page 13. Set aside.

2 With the motor of the food processor running, pop the lemongrass through the feed tube. Process at full speed alternating with the pulsing action until the lemongrass is very finely chopped, about 2 minutes, stopping and scraping down the sides of the work bowl as needed. With the motor running, pop in the garlic cloves and chop finely. Add the cilantro, curry paste, lime juice, fish sauce, and oil and process until well blended.

3 Slice the tofu into ½-inch cubes. Cut each of the cubes in half to create triangles. In a medium-sized serving bowl, toss together the tofu, shrimp, red onion, and cucumber. Pour on the dressing while stirring. Gently toss until all of the ingredients are evenly coated with the dressing.

4 Line goblets or bowls with radicchio and fill with the mixture. Serve immediately.

Serves 4 or 5

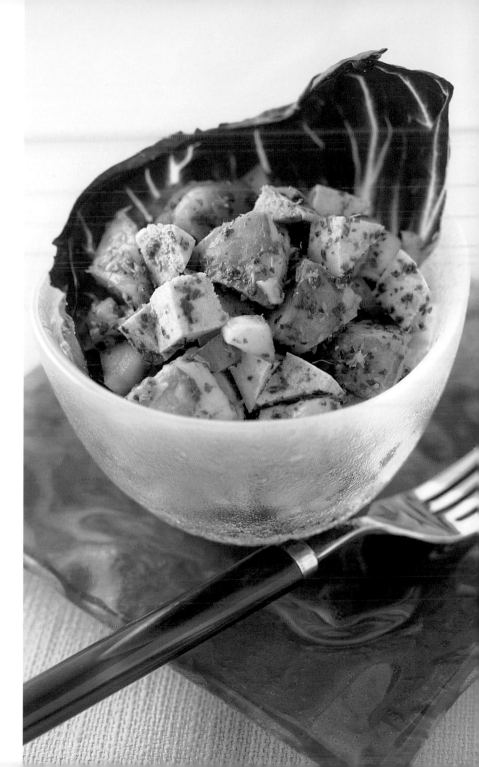

country tempeh pâté

INSPIRED BY THE CLASSIC PÂTÉS OF FRANCE, THIS
TEMPEH-BASED VERSION WINS RAVES FROM CONFIRMED MICHELIN-
TOTING CARNIVORES. IT'S AN IDEAL COMPANY DISH—FESTIVE,
WITH SOPHISTICATED FLAVOR AND A SUBLIMELY SMOOTH
TEXTURE THAT IS PUNCTUATED BY THE ACIDIC POP OF BRINED
GREEN PEPPERCORNS. FOR SOME LIVELY COLOR, I'VE ADDED
A CENTRAL AND A TOP LAYER OF ROASTED RED PEPPER, BUT IF
YOU PREFER A HOMESPUN LOOK, FEEL FREE TO OMIT THEM.
(DO, HOWEVER, INCLUDE HALF OF THE PEPPER IN THE PÂTÉ
MIXTURE ITSELF.)

FOR OPTIMUM TASTE, CHILL THE PÂTÉ OVERNIGHT
AND SERVE IT THE FOLLOWING DAY. AFTER THAT, THE SEASONINGS
AND BALANCE OF FLAVORS BEGIN TO FADE, ALTHOUGH THE LEFT-
OVERS ARE GOOD ON CRACKERS AND MAKE GREAT SANDWICHES.

TO PREPARE THIS PÂTÉ, YOU'LL NEED A SMALL
METAL BAKING PAN WITH A TWO-CUP CAPACITY. ALTHOUGH THE
PAN MAY STRIKE YOU AS TOO SMALL TO MAKE ENOUGH TO SERVE
EIGHT, TRUST ME, THIN SLICES OF THIS RICH APPETIZER WILL BE
JUST RIGHT.

I LIKE TO SERVE THE PÂTÉ WHOLE, UNMOLDED ON A
LAVISH BED OF GREENS AND GARNISHED WITH CORNICHONS AND
THIN SLICES OF SOURDOUGH BAGUETTE. YOU MAY PREFER TO SLICE
THE PÂTÉ AND PLATE INDIVIDUAL SERVINGS IN THE KITCHEN.

Olive oil for coating baking pan

8 OUNCES
tempeh, preferably soy,
cut into 1-inch squares

¾ CUP
Cognac, Armagnac, or other
good-quality brandy

1 TABLESPOON
olive oil

½ CUP
chopped shallots

2 LARGE CLOVES
garlic, peeled and minced

1 TEASPOON
herbes de Provence (see note)

½ CUP
diced celery

1 LARGE red bell pepper, roasted,
peeled, seeded, and halved

½ CUP
packed parsley leaves

½ CUP
walnuts, toasted

1 TABLESPOON
Dijon mustard

1 TEASPOON
salt

½ TEASPOON
freshly ground black pepper

1 TABLESPOON
green peppercorns in brine,
drained

Bed of greens, for garnish

2 TABLESPOONS
minced parsley, for garnish

1 Place a rack in the center of the oven. Preheat the oven to 350 degrees. Lightly coat a 5¾-by-3-by-2-inch loaf pan with oil and set aside.

2 In a small saucepan, combine the tempeh and brandy. Bring to a boil, reduce the heat to medium, cover, and simmer for 10 minutes. Uncover and continue simmering until all of the liquid is absorbed, 2 to 3 more minutes. Transfer to a food processor.

3 In a small skillet, heat the oil over medium-high heat. Sauté the shallots, garlic, herbes de Provence, and celery, stirring occasionally, until soft, about 5 minutes. Transfer to the food processor along with one half of the roasted red pepper and all of the remaining ingredients except the green peppercorns and the garnishes. Process until the mixture is completely blended and very smooth, stopping and scraping down the sides of the work bowl as needed. (This will take a bit of time. The mixture will be stiff at first.) Gently stir in the peppercorns by hand.

4 Press half the tempeh mixture into the prepared pan. Finely dice most of the remaining red pepper half (reserve some for garnish) and distribute it on top. Press the remaining tempeh mixture evenly over the red pepper. Cover tightly with aluminum foil and bake for 30 minutes. Remove the foil and bake until slightly brown around the edges, 15 to 20 minutes longer. Remove from the oven, cool to room temperature, then refrigerate for several hours or preferably overnight.

5 To serve, run a knife around the edges of the pan several times. Carefully invert the pâté onto a bed of greens. Gently press minced parsley into the top and sides. Cut the reserved red pepper into strips or decorative shapes and arrange on top, then serve. Refrigerate any leftovers for up to 3 days.

Serves **8**

Note: Herbes de Provence is an aromatic blend of herbs available in gourmet shops and many supermarkets.

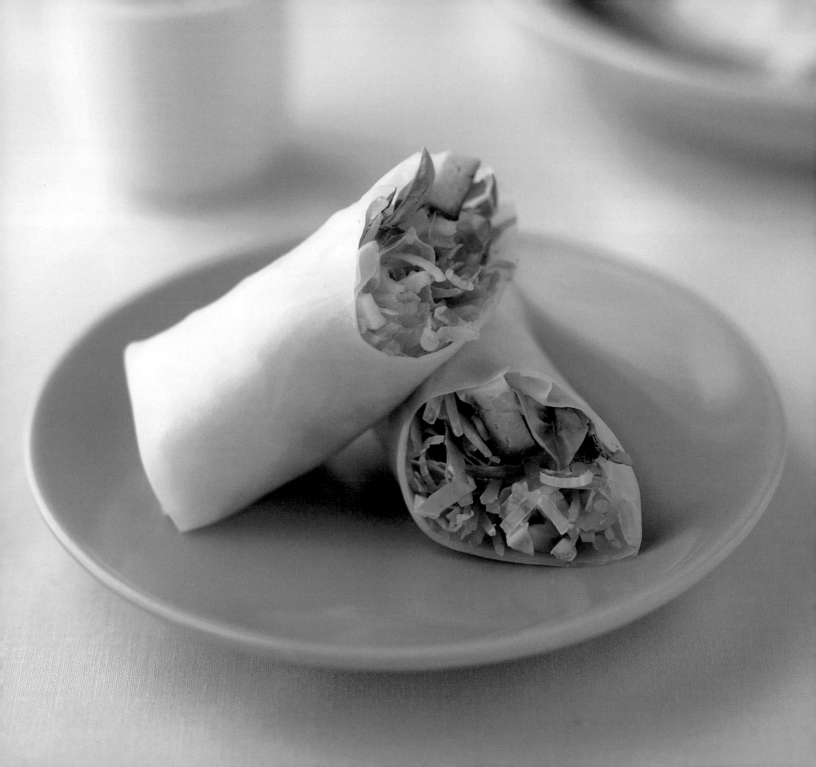

vegetable spring rolls with baked seasoned tofu and peanut miso dipping sauce

THESE COLORFUL SPRING ROLLS ARE FILLED WITH A MIXTURE OF BEAN THREAD NOODLES AND SHREDDED CABBAGE AND CARROT, AND DOTTED WITH TASTY MORSELS OF BAKED SEASONED TOFU. FRESH BASIL LEAVES CONTRIBUTE A SPRIGHTLY GREEN AND GIVE THE FILLING A REFRESHING LILT, BUT IT'S THE PEANUT MISO DIPPING SAUCE THAT USUALLY STEALS THE SHOW. SERVE THE SAUCE IN SMALL, INDIVIDUAL BOWLS SO THAT GUESTS CAN UNABASHEDLY DUNK AS THEY MAKE THEIR WAY THROUGH EACH ROLL.

YOU'LL BE ABLE TO BUY THE BEAN THREAD (MUNG BEAN) NOODLES AND RICE PAPER WRAPPERS IN MOST ASIAN GROCERIES, PARTICULARLY THOSE THAT SPECIALIZE IN THAI OR VIETNAMESE INGREDIENTS. (OR YOU CAN ORDER THEM BY MAIL; SEE PAGE 115.) THE WRAPPERS ARE FRAGILE AND BREAK OR TEAR EASILY, SO HAVE A FEW EXTRA ON HAND WHEN PREPARING THIS DISH.

1 OUNCE
bean thread noodles, cooked according to package directions and well drained

1 ½ CUPS
shredded napa or Chinese cabbage (rinse leaves and spin dry before shredding)

½ CUP
grated carrot

⅓ CUP
thinly sliced scallion greens

ABOUT 12
8-inch round rice papers (see introduction)

4 OUNCES
Baked Seasoned Tofu (page 90 or substitute store-bought), cut into ½-inch cubes (about 1 cup)

20 TO 24 large fresh basil leaves, rinsed and spun dry

Peanut Miso Dressing and Dipping Sauce (page 102)

1 Gently squeeze the cooked bean thread noodles to release excess moisture. Chop them coarsely. In a large bowl, toss together the noodles, cabbage, carrot, and scallion greens.

2 Fill a 10-inch pie plate with warm water. Submerge one of the rice papers in the water and soak just until pliable, 30 to 60 seconds. Transfer to a clean kitchen towel and blot gently to dry. Arrange about ¼ cup of the noodle mixture along the bottom third of the rice paper. Distribute 5 or 6 tofu cubes and 2 basil leaves on the noodles. Lift the bottom edge over the filling, fold the sides toward the center, and roll up as tightly as possible. Set on a plate, seam side down. Repeat with the remaining rice papers.

3 Serve the spring rolls immediately. Alternatively, refrigerate in a tightly sealed container for up to 2 days. (Return to room temperature before serving.) Divide the dipping sauce among several small bowls and serve alongside.

Makes **10** to **12** spring rolls

impromptu miso soup

MISO SOUP IS ONE OF THE WORLD'S MOST TONIC
POTIONS. THE GOOD NEWS IS THAT WITH HIGH-QUALITY MISO
ON HAND, YOU DON'T HAVE TO GO TO A JAPANESE RESTAURANT
TO ENJOY THIS RESTORATIVE SOUP. INDEED, MY VERSION IS
SO QUICK AND EASY TO MAKE THAT IT CAN EASILY BECOME A
REGULAR ON YOUR MENU—AS IT HAS ON MINE.

SO THAT I CAN PREPARE THIS SOUP AT A MOMENT'S
NOTICE, I HAVE NOT ATTEMPTED TO REPRODUCE A CLASSIC MISO
SOUP, WHICH REQUIRES THE INITIAL STEP OF PREPARING THE
STOCK CALLED *DASHI*. INSTEAD I CREATE AN INTERESTING BROTH
BY BLENDING TWO TYPES OF MISO AND ADDING A BRINY SEA
VEGETABLE CALLED *WAKAME*. EXPERIMENT BY SHIFTING THE
BALANCE OF LIGHT AND DARK MISOS UNTIL YOU ARRIVE AT THE
FORMULA THAT WORKS BEST FOR YOU. YOU CAN ALSO VARY THE
TASTE BY ADDING A TEASPOON OF GRATED FRESH GINGER OR
SHIITAKE MUSHROOM POWDER, OR A FEW CILANTRO LEAVES.

THIS RECIPE MAKES ENOUGH FOR TWO SMALL
RESTAURANT-SIZED PORTIONS OR ONE LARGE BOWLFUL. FEEL
FREE TO DOUBLE OR TRIPLE THE AMOUNTS.

2 ¼ CUPS
water

2 OUNCES
firm or extra-firm tofu, drained and
cut into ¼-inch dice (about ¼ cup)

1 TABLESPOON
sweet white miso

2 TEASPOONS
barley miso

1 TABLESPOON
instant *wakame* flakes (see note)
or ½ cup chopped fresh spinach or
bok choy leaves

1 scallion, very thinly sliced,
for garnish

1 Bring the water to a boil in a medium-sized saucepan.

2 Ladle out about ½ cup of the boiling water and pour it into a glass measuring cup. Add the tofu to the pan. Reduce the heat to medium, cover, and cook for 1 to 2 minutes.

3 While the tofu is cooking, blend the two misos into the hot water by mashing the paste against the sides of the cup with a fork and stirring vigorously.

4 Just before serving, add the *wakame* or fresh greens to the saucepan and simmer the soup uncovered until the *wakame* is reconstituted, about 30 seconds, or the fresh greens are tender, 1 to 2 minutes.

5 Turn off the heat and stir in the miso broth. Ladle into bowls, garnish with the scallion, and serve immediately.

Serves 1 or 2

Note: *Wakame* flakes reconstitute within about 30 seconds of being stirred into hot water. They are available in many natural-food stores and Asian groceries. Or you can purchase a package of whole *wakame* and snip the leaves into tiny bits. Discard any thick central ribs.

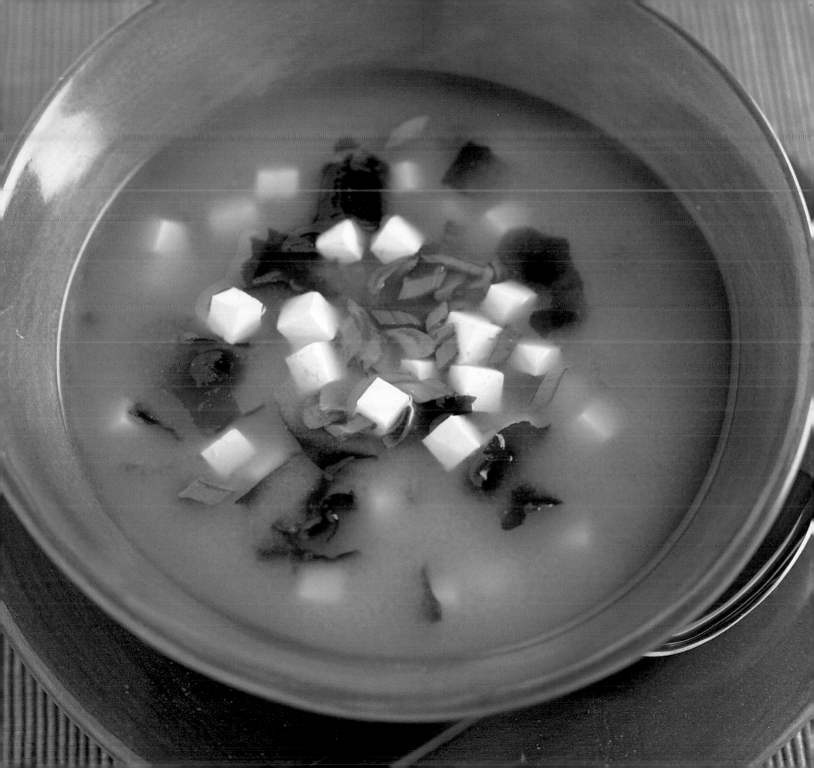

shiitake, miso, and barley soup

WITH ITS MEATY CHUNKS OF SHIITAKE AND THE CREAMY TEXTURE OF BARLEY, THIS ASIAN-INSPIRED VERSION OF A TRADITIONAL EASTERN EUROPEAN SOUP WILL WARM YOU ON SNOWY WINTER DAYS. ONCE COOKED, THE SOUP CONTINUES TO THICKEN AS IT SITS ON THE STOVE OR IN THE REFRIGERATOR. ENJOY IT AS IS OR THIN IT WITH EXTRA MISO BROTH.

1 OUNCE
dried shiitake mushrooms

1 TABLESPOON
olive oil

2 CUPS
thinly sliced leeks (white and light green parts), thoroughly rinsed

1 TEASPOON
minced garlic

½ TEASPOON
dried thyme or marjoram leaves

½ CUP
dry white wine or vermouth

6 CUPS
vegetable stock (see note)

3 LARGE carrots, trimmed, peeled, halved lengthwise, and cut into ½-inch-thick slices

½ CUP
pearl barley, rinsed

½ CUP
hot water

3 TO 4 TABLESPOONS
sweet white miso

salt, to taste

3 TABLESPOONS
minced parsley, for garnish

1 Break off the shiitake stems (or pry them out with a sharp paring knife). Discard the stems or reserve them for stock. Brush or chop the shiitake caps into tiny bits. Quickly rinse and drain. Set aside.

2 In a large, heavy soup pot, heat the oil over high heat. Sauté the leeks and garlic for 1 minute, stirring frequently. Add the thyme and wine and continue cooking over high heat until about half of the wine evaporates.

3 Add the vegetable stock, reserved shiitakes, carrots, and barley, and bring to a boil. Reduce the heat to low, cover, and cook at a gentle boil until the barley is tender, 30 to 45 minutes.

4 Pour the hot water into a large glass measuring cup and dissolve 3 tablespoons of the miso in it by mashing the paste against the sides of the cup and stirring vigorously with a whisk or fork. Turn off the heat and stir the miso broth into the soup. Taste and add the additional miso as needed for flavor, first dissolving the miso in a small amount of the soup's broth. Add salt, if needed. Ladle into bowls, garnish with the parsley, and serve immediately.

Serves 4 to 6

Note: Use your own favorite stock recipe or make stock with a high-quality instant vegetable stock powder, such as Vogue Vege Base (available in most natural-food stores).

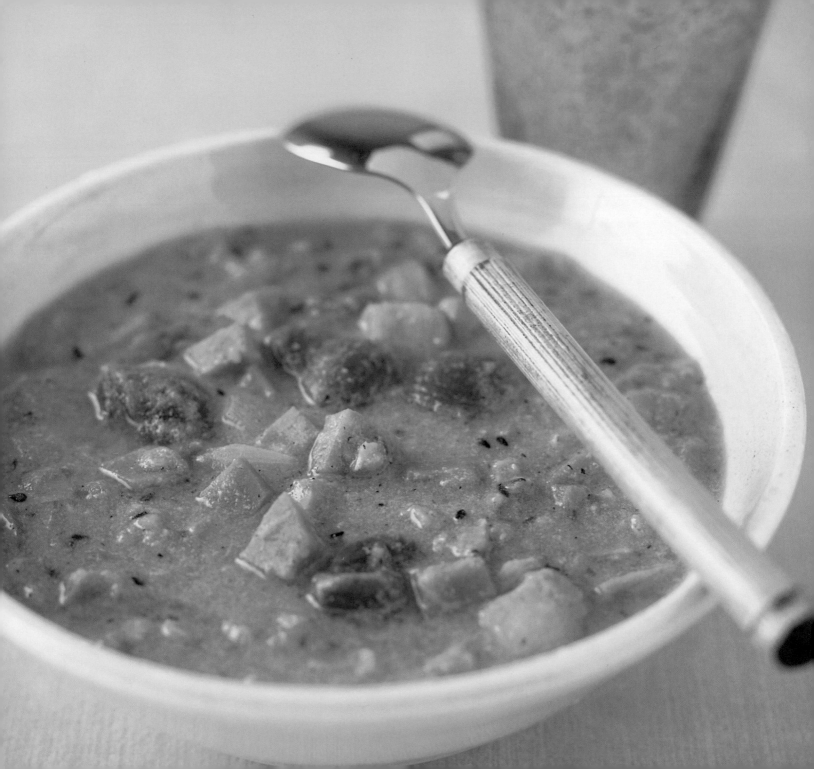

red lentil soup with indian spices

QUICK-COOKING RED LENTILS PRODUCE A LUSCIOUS SOUP WITH LONG-SIMMERED TASTE AND TEXTURE IN UNDER FORTY-FIVE MINUTES. AS THEY COOK, THE LENTILS DISSOLVE, THICKENING THE SOUP AND CREATING A COARSE PURÉE REMINISCENT OF DAL. BUT THIS SOUP IS MUCH MORE COLORFUL THAN ANY DAL I'VE EVER SEEN, WITH ITS DOTS OF BLACK MUSTARD SEED AND BRIGHT FLECKS OF TOMATO AND CARROT.

SOYMILK IS PART OF THE COOKING LIQUID, ENRICHING THE SOUP AND ROUNDING OUT THE LIVELY INDIAN FLAVORS. ALTHOUGH IT WILL CURDLE, THE FINAL LOOK, TASTE, AND TEXTURE OF THE SOUP ARE NOT ADVERSELY AFFECTED. FOR A CHANGE, I SOMETIMES USE AN IMMERSION BLENDER TO PURÉE ALL OR PART OF THE SOUP. THIS SOUP IS A MEAL IN ITSELF, EITHER ON ITS OWN OR LADLED OVER HOT BASMATI RICE.

2 TABLESPOONS
black mustard seeds

2 TEASPOONS
cumin seeds

2 TEASPOONS
fennel seeds

1 TABLESPOON
peanut oil or ghee (clarified butter)

2 CUPS
coarsely chopped onion

2 TABLESPOONS
finely minced fresh ginger

½ TO 1 TEASPOON
crushed red pepper flakes

2 CUPS
water

2 TO 2 ½ CUPS
soymilk

1 CAN (15 OUNCES)
diced tomatoes

1 ¼ CUPS
red lentils, picked over and rinsed

3 carrots, trimmed, peeled, and cut into ½-inch-thick slices

⅓ CUP
unsweetened grated dried coconut

1 TEASPOON
salt, or to taste

1 In a small bowl, combine the mustard seeds, cumin, and fennel seeds. Heat the oil in a large, heavy (preferably nonstick or enameled) soup pot over high heat. Add the seeds, cover, and sizzle until the mustard seeds begin to pop, 15 to 30 seconds. Immediately turn off the heat and let sit, covered, until the seeds stop popping, about 1 minute.

2 Stir in the onion, ginger, and red pepper flakes. Sauté over medium-high heat for 1 minute, stirring frequently and taking care to scrape up any seeds that have stuck to the bottom of the pot. Add the water, 2 cups of soymilk, and the tomatoes (with canning liquid), and bring to a gentle boil. Reduce the heat to medium-low (or the soymilk will froth and boil over) and stir in the red lentils, carrots, and coconut. Cover and cook at a gentle boil for 20 minutes, stirring from time to time.

3 Add the salt and continue cooking, covered, until the lentils have melted into a coarse purée, about 15 minutes more. If the soup is too thick, thin to the desired consistency with additional soymilk. Adjust seasonings before serving.

Serves **6**

creamy dilled spinach soup

IN THIS SIMPLE SOUP, DILL AND SPINACH MAKE
A SAVORY PAIR, AND THE SOYMILK ADDS BODY AND AN ELEGANT
SMOOTHNESS. PLAN TO MAKE THE RECIPE WHEN THE MARKET
OFFERS IRRESISTIBLE BUNCHES OF BABY SPINACH, WITH THEIR
TENDER LEAVES AND SLENDER STEMS. COOK THEM, ROOTS AND
ALL. (IF USING MATURE SPINACH, TRIM OFF THE ROOTS AND
COARSE STEMS.) ALWAYS RINSE THE SPINACH IN SEVERAL CHANGES
OF WATER TO AVOID ANY RESIDUAL GRIT, WHICH WOULD DEFI-
NITELY DETRACT FROM THE SOUP'S SMOOTH TEXTURE.

A SPRINKLING OF CAYENNE FOR GARNISH ADDS
A NICE JOLT OF HEAT AND COLOR. IF YOU PREFER, USE SWEET
PAPRIKA. THE SOUP TASTES GREAT EITHER HOT OR CHILLED.

1 TABLESPOON
olive oil

2 CUPS
thinly sliced leeks (white and light
green parts), thoroughly rinsed

3 CUPS
vegetable stock (see note)

1½ POUNDS
spinach, trimmed if needed and
coarsely chopped

1 CUP
loosely packed fresh dill
(stems removed)

¾ TEASPOON
salt, or to taste

1 CUP
soymilk

Ground cayenne pepper,
for garnish

1 Heat the oil in a large, heavy soup pot over medium-high heat. Sauté the leeks for 2 minutes, stirring frequently. Add the stock and bring it to a boil. Add the spinach, dill, and salt. Cover and cook until the spinach is very soft, about 4 minutes.

2 Transfer to a blender in two or three batches and process until very smooth. Return to the pot and bring to a gentle boil over medium heat. Reduce the heat to very low. Stir in the soymilk and additional salt, if needed. Heat thoroughly, but do not boil once the soymilk has been added. Serve in shallow soup bowls, garnished with a sprinkling of cayenne.

Serves **4** to **6**

Note: Use your own favorite stock recipe or make stock with a high-quality instant vegetable stock powder, such as Vogue Vege Base (available in most natural-food stores).

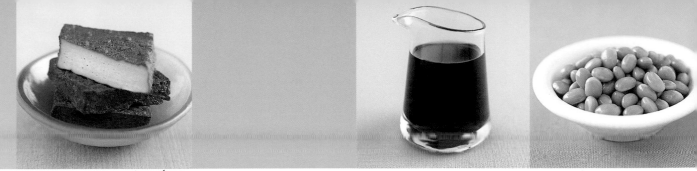

entrées

Soyfoods in the center of the plate provide genuine aesthetic pleasure and a real sense of satisfaction. To my mind, the most intriguing of all soyfoods is tempeh, an ingredient that is at home in a wide variety of culinary contexts. For a delightful French-inspired stew, opt for Tempeh Simmered in Red Wine with Herbes de Provence. A hearty Double-Soybean Chili, which includes crumbled tempeh and whole black soybeans, is infused with bold Southwest seasonings. To suit another mood, the more delicate Tempeh Braised in Coconut Milk with Lemongrass might be just the thing.

Among these entrées, you'll discover that glistening mahogany soybeans are not only beautiful to behold, but very receptive to marinades, making them lively components of a zesty salsa that accompanies strips of golden fried swordfish. Mellow and undemanding by nature, unseasoned black soybeans can be used to add hearty substance to main dishes, such as the Meal-in-a-Bowl Noodle Vegetable Hot Pot.

And finally, as you cook your way through this chapter, you'll witness the chameleon-like nature of tofu. Tossed in a curry paste with spinach and tomatoes, it's bright yellow. Braised in an assertive fermented bean sauce, it's robed in black. Floating placidly in a lemongrass miso broth, tofu is undisguised: a chewy, white morsel content to let the other ingredients steal the show.

tempeh simmered
in red wine with
herbes de provence

THE ASSERTIVE FLAVOR OF TEMPEH STANDS UP
BEAUTIFULLY TO THE INTENSITY OF RED WINE AND HERBS IN THIS
HEARTY STEW. IT'S A ROBUST COLD-WEATHER DISH WITH A
GENEROUS SUPPLY OF TASTY SAUCE. SERVE THE STEW IN SHALLOW
SOUP BOWLS OVER BROAD NOODLES OR ACCOMPANIED BY
CRISPLY ROASTED POTATOES.

12 OUNCES
tempeh, preferably soy

1½ TO 2 TABLESPOONS
olive oil

1½ CUPS
thinly sliced leeks (white and light
green parts), thoroughly rinsed, or
coarsely chopped onion

1 TABLESPOON
minced garlic

2 CUPS
good-quality dry red wine

1 CAN (15 OUNCES)
diced tomatoes

1 CUP
vegetable stock or water

2 LARGE carrots, trimmed, peeled,
and chopped

¼ POUND
pearl onions, trimmed and peeled,
or small white onions, halved

6 OUNCES
cremini or button mushrooms,
trimmed and halved

1 LARGE bay leaf

1½ TO 2 TEASPOONS
herbes de Provence (see note)

1 TEASPOON
coriander seeds, crushed

1 TEASPOON
fennel seeds, crushed

¾ TEASPOON
salt, or to taste

Freshly ground black pepper

2 TABLESPOONS
arrowroot, dissolved in
2 tablespoons water

3 TABLESPOONS
minced parsley, for garnish

1 Cut the tempeh in half crosswise. Cut each slab in half horizontally. Heat a large nonstick skillet over medium heat. Lightly brush both sides of each piece of tempeh with oil and set it in the skillet. Cover and cook until speckled with dark brown spots, about 2 minutes. Flip over, cover, and brown on the second side, 1 to 2 minutes.

2 Transfer the tempeh to a cutting board. When cool enough to handle, cut into 1-inch fingers. Then cut each "finger" into 1-inch squares. Set aside.

3 Heat 1 tablespoon of oil in a large, nonreactive saucepan over high heat. Sauté the leeks and garlic for 1 minute, stirring frequently. Stir in the wine, tomatoes (with canning liquid), stock, reserved tempeh, carrots, onions, mushrooms, bay leaf, 1½ teaspoons herbes de Provence, coriander, fennel, salt, and pepper to taste. Bring to a boil, then reduce the heat to medium, cover, and cook at a gentle boil for 30 minutes. Stir gently from time to time and add an additional ½ teaspoon of the herbs halfway through, if needed.

4 Stir the arrowroot mixture into the stew and continue to simmer gently, stirring occasionally, until the cooking liquid thickens slightly, about 3 minutes. Remove the bay leaf and adjust the seasonings. Garnish each serving with parsley.

Serves **4**

Note: Herbes de Provence is an aromatic blend of herbs available in gourmet shops and many supermarkets.

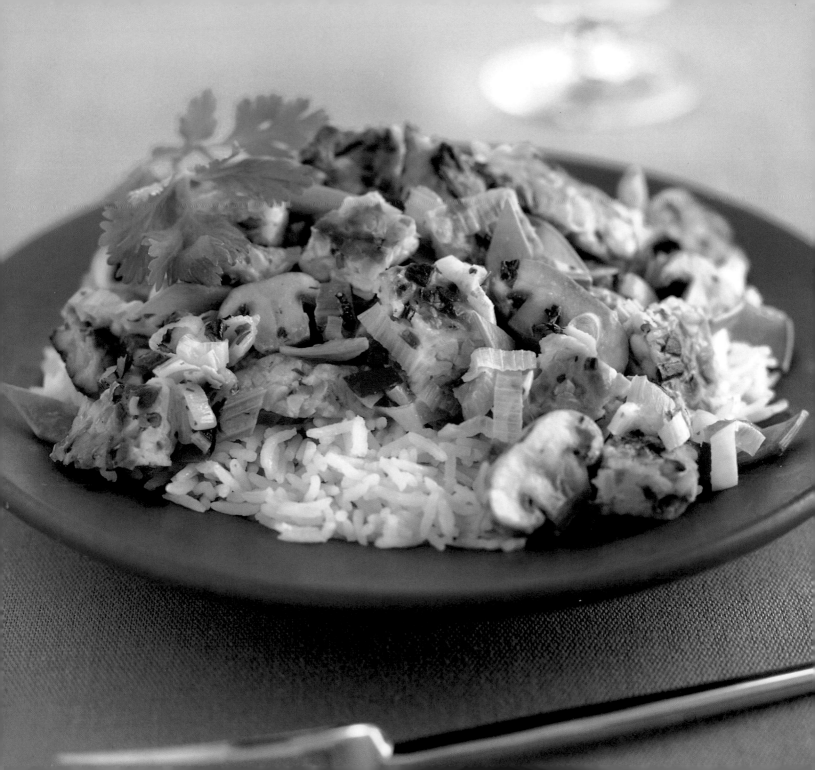

tempeh braised in coconut milk with lemongrass

SINCE INDONESIA IS TEMPEH'S LAND OF ORIGIN,
IT'S NO SURPRISE THAT IT TASTES SO GOOD WHEN PREPARED
WITH INGREDIENTS AND SEASONINGS COMMON TO THAT PART
OF THE WORLD, NAMELY COCONUT MILK AND LEMONGRASS.

THE REMAINING INGREDIENTS ARE MY OWN ADDI-
TIONS, RESULTING IN A LUSCIOUS STEW WITH LOTS OF RICH
SAUCE. BE SURE TO HAVE A LIME ON HAND: A LITTLE OF ITS
JUICE STIRRED IN AT THE VERY END MAKES ALL OF THE FLAVORS
POP. SERVE OVER STEAMED JASMINE OR BASMATI RICE OR
JAPANESE UDON, DELICIOUS WHEAT NOODLES.

8 OUNCES
tempeh, preferably mixed grain

1 ½ TO 2 TABLESPOONS
peanut oil

1 TABLESPOON
slivered garlic

1 ½ CUPS
thinly sliced leeks (white and light
green parts), thoroughly rinsed

1 CAN (14 OUNCES)
unsweetened coconut milk,
regular or low-fat

1 CUP
diced red bell pepper

1 CUP
diced celery

¼ POUND
cremini or button mushrooms,
trimmed and sliced

2 FOUR-INCH STALKS
lemongrass (measure from fleshy
bulb upward), bruised outer leaves
removed, sliced into 1-inch-long
pieces (see note)

½ TO ¾ TEASPOON
crushed red pepper flakes

1 ½ TABLESPOONS
barley miso dissolved in ¼ cup
hot water

4 OUNCES
snow peas, cut crosswise into
½-inch strips

Shoyu, to taste

½ CUP
loosely packed chopped cilantro

1 TO 2 TABLESPOONS
freshly squeezed lime juice

Sprigs of cilantro, for garnish

1 Cut the tempeh in half crosswise. Cut each slab in half horizontally. Heat a large nonstick skillet over medium heat. Lightly brush both sides of each piece of tempeh with oil and set it in the skillet. Cover and cook until speckled with dark brown spots, about 2 minutes. Flip over, cover, and brown on the second side, 1 to 2 minutes.

2 Transfer the tempeh to a cutting board. When cool enough to handle, cut into 1-inch "fingers." Holding the knife at a 45-degree angle, cut each finger on the bias into slices about ½ inch thick. Set aside.

3 Heat 1 tablespoon of oil in a large saucepan over medium heat. Lightly brown the garlic, add the leeks, and sauté for 1 minute, stirring frequently. Stir in the coconut milk, reserved tempeh, red pepper, celery, mushrooms, lemongrass, and crushed red pepper. Bring to a boil. Cover and cook at a gentle boil for 15 minutes.

4 Remove the pieces of lemongrass and stir in the dissolved miso and snow peas. If the mixture is not quite salty enough, add shoyu to taste. Just before serving, stir in the chopped cilantro and lime juice to taste. Garnish with cilantro sprigs.

Serves **3**

Note: If fresh lemongrass is not available, Thai Kitchen's jarred lemongrass packed in water is a viable substitute.

miso-mustard cabbage
with tempeh

THIS HEARTY DISH COMBINES MANY OF THE
ELEMENTS OF A RUSTIC PEASANT STEW—CABBAGE, MUSHROOMS,
CARROTS, AND LEEKS. BUT THE CREAMY MISO-MUSTARD SAUCE
RAISES THESE HUMBLE VEGETABLES FROM THEIR EARTHY ROOTS
AND GIVES THEM A REAL TOUCH OF CLASS.

THIS FILLING AND FLAVORFUL DISH STANDS QUITE
WELL ON ITS OWN. FOR BEST RESULTS, BE ACCURATE ON THE
MEASUREMENT OF CABBAGE TO KEEP THE FLAVORS IN BALANCE.

8 OUNCES
tempeh, preferably mixed grain

1 ½ TO 2 TABLESPOONS
olive oil

1 CUP
hot water

3 TABLESPOONS
sweet white miso

¼ CUP
Dijon mustard, plus 1 to 3 additional
tablespoons to add at the end

2 CUPS
thinly sliced leeks (white and light
green parts), thoroughly rinsed

2 LARGE CLOVES
garlic, peeled and minced

2 LARGE carrots, trimmed, peeled,
halved lengthwise, and cut into
½-inch-thick half-moons

½ POUND
cremini or button mushrooms,
trimmed and sliced

½ CUP
dry white wine or vermouth

1 SMALL green cabbage (about 1½
pounds), quartered, cored, and cut
crosswise into ½-inch slices

Salt and freshly ground black
pepper, to taste

1 Cut the tempeh in half crosswise. Cut each slab in half horizontally. Heat a large nonstick skillet over medium heat. Lightly brush both sides of each piece of tempeh with oil and set it in the skillet. Cover and cook until speckled with dark brown spots, about 2 minutes. Flip over, cover, and brown on the second side, 1 to 2 minutes.

2 Transfer the tempeh to a cutting board. When cool enough to handle, cut into 1-inch "fingers." Holding the knife at a 45-degree angle, cut each finger on the bias into slices about ½ inch thick. Set aside.

3 Prepare the sauce by pouring the hot water into a large glass measuring cup. Dissolve the miso in the water by mashing the paste against the sides of the cup and stirring vigorously with a whisk or fork. Blend in ¼ cup mustard.

4 Heat 1 tablespoon of oil in a large, nonreactive saucepan or enamel-lined Dutch oven over high heat. Sauté the leeks and garlic for 1 minute, stirring frequently. Add the miso-mustard sauce, reserved tempeh, carrots, and mushrooms. Stir gently. Bring to a boil, then cover and cook over medium heat for 15 minutes, stirring occasionally. Stir in the wine, then the cabbage. (It will seem like a lot, but will quickly wilt.) Cover and cook over medium heat, stirring occasionally, until the cabbage is tender but still a bit crunchy, 8 to 10 minutes. If the mixture becomes dry before the cabbage is cooked, stir in ¼ cup of hot water.

5 When the cabbage is done, add salt and pepper and additional mustard if needed to intensify the flavor of the sauce.

Serves **4**

quinoa salad with tempeh adobo nuggets and lime-shoyu vinaigrette

THIS BEAUTIFUL SALAD COMBINES A NUMBER OF NEW WORLD FOODS AND TEMPEH ADOBO WITH GREAT SUCCESS. QUINOA, CORN, AND JALAPEÑOS ARE A NATURAL SOUTH-OF-THE BORDER TRIO, AND THE HIGHLY SEASONED TEMPEH NUGGETS ADD POCKETS OF INTENSE FLAVOR. FOR A STRIKING PRESENTATION, MOUND THE SALAD ON A BED OF RADICCHIO.

1 ½ CUPS
quinoa (see note)

1 ½ CUPS
fresh or frozen (defrosted) corn kernels

Tempeh Adobo Nuggets
(see note, page 55)

1 CUP
finely diced red bell pepper

½ CUP
finely diced red onion

⅓ CUP
finely minced, tightly packed cilantro

1 TO 2 jalapeño chilies, seeded and finely diced

¼ TO ⅓ CUP
Lime-Shoyu Vinaigrette (page 101)

1 TO 2 TABLESPOONS
freshly squeezed lime juice (optional)

Radicchio leaves, for garnish

1 In a large saucepan, bring 3 quarts of water to a rolling boil. Meanwhile, swish the quinoa vigorously in a large bowl of warm water. Drain through a fine-mesh strainer. Repeat this process until the rinsing water remains just about clear. Drain.

2 Add the quinoa to the boiling water and cook over high heat until almost done, 11 to 12 minutes. Add the corn and cook until the quinoa is tender but still crunchy, about 1 minute more. Using a large, fine-mesh strainer, drain thoroughly, bouncing the strainer up and down to release excess water. Transfer to a large bowl and stir from time to time to accelerate cooling.

3 When the quinoa stops giving off steam, toss in the tempeh nuggets, red bell pepper, onion, cilantro, jalapeño(s), and enough vinaigrette to coat the ingredients lightly. Add the lime juice to taste, if desired. Serve warm or at room temperature on a bed of radicchio.

Serves **4**

Note: Quinoa is a protein-rich, quick-cooking grain from the Andes. It must be rinsed well to remove any residual saponin—a natural, bitter coating. Quinoa is available in natural-food stores and some supermarkets.

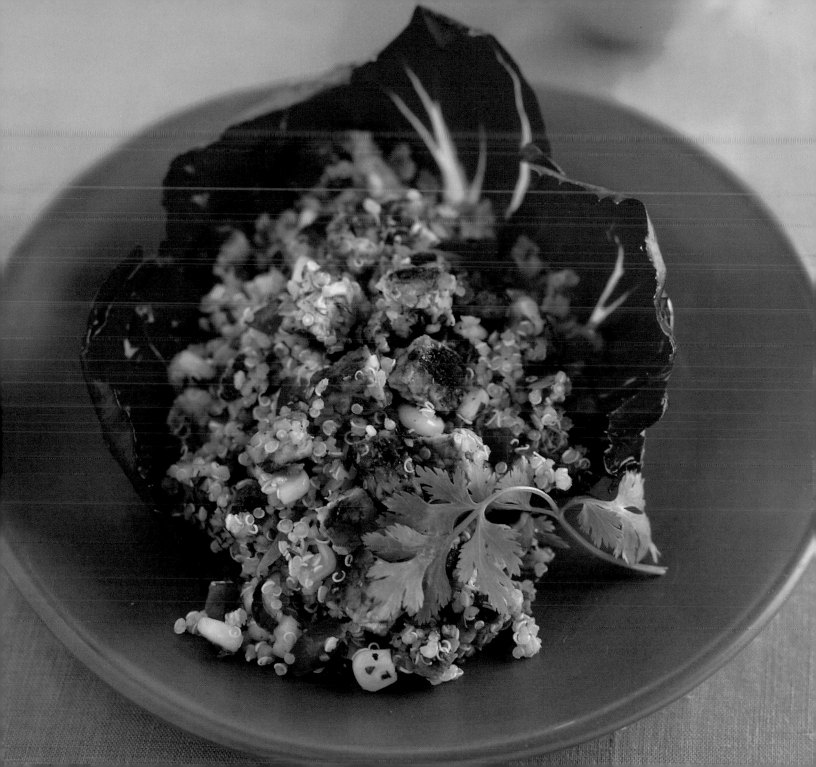

tempeh with quick homemade tomato sauce and olives

WHAT MAKES THIS STEW QUICK AND GOOD IS THE TEMPEH, WHICH CONTRIBUTES LONG-SIMMERED HEARTINESS IN RECORD TIME. THE SHOYU GIVES THE SAUCE AN EARTHY COLOR AND DEEP, RICH TASTE.

WHEN I SERVE THIS DISH ON ITS OWN, I LIKE TO CUT THE TEMPEH INTO "FINGERS" ABOUT ONE-THIRD INCH WIDE. IF I'M PLANNING TO LADLE THE STEW OVER SPAGHETTI, I PREFER TO HALVE THE TEMPEH HORIZONTALLY AND CUT IT INTO ONE-INCH SQUARES.

HOWEVER YOU PLAN TO SERVE IT, DON'T OMIT THE FINAL BROWNING OF THE TEMPEH, WHICH SEALS IN FLAVOR AND ENHANCES TEXTURE AND LOOKS.

2 TABLESPOONS
olive oil

2 LARGE CLOVES
garlic, peeled and thinly sliced

1 CUP
coarsely chopped onion

1 CUP
diced fennel or celery

2 ½ CUPS
water

1 CAN (6 OUNCES)
tomato paste

ABOUT 1 TABLESPOON
shoyu

1 TO 2 TABLESPOONS
drained capers (optional)

1 ½ TEASPOONS
fennel seeds

1 ½ TEASPOONS
dried leaf oregano

¾ TO 1 TEASPOON
crushed red pepper flakes

8 OUNCES
tempeh, preferably soy,
cut into fingers or squares
(see introduction)

⅓ TO ½ CUP
oil-cured black olives, pitted
and coarsely chopped

2 TABLESPOONS
finely chopped parsley, for
garnish

1 In a medium-sized saucepan, heat the oil over medium-high heat. Sauté the garlic, stirring frequently, until lightly browned, about 1 minute. Stir in the onion and fennel and sauté for 1 minute more, stirring frequently. Add the water and blend in the tomato paste and shoyu. Add the capers (if using), seasonings, tempeh, and olives, and bring to a boil. Cook uncovered over medium heat at a gentle boil, stirring occasionally, for 15 minutes. Reduce the heat to low and continue to simmer the sauce uncovered as you brown the tempeh.

2 With a slotted spoon, remove the tempeh from the sauce (let surplus sauce drip from the tempeh and brush away any bits of vegetable), and transfer it to a large nonstick skillet set over medium-high heat. Brown the tempeh on all sides, turning frequently with tongs or a spatula to avoid burning. (I have not found the need to use oil during this browning stage, but add a bit if you are experiencing sticking.)

3 Taste, and add more shoyu to the sauce, if necessary. If serving the tempeh as fingers, set them on a plate and spoon the sauce on top. Alternatively, ladle over spaghetti. Garnish each serving with parsley.

Serves **2** or **3**

tempeh adobo

TEMPEH HOLDS UP BEAUTIFULLY TO THE ASSERTIVE
SEASONINGS OF THE LATIN AMERICAN KITCHEN. ONCE MARI-
NATED AND COOKED, THESE FLAVORFUL ADOBO-RED SLABS MAY
BE SERVED ON THEIR OWN OR ON A BED OF FRIED PEPPERS
AND ONIONS. THEY MAKE A GREAT FILLING FOR TAMALES AND
ARE ALSO TASTY TUCKED INTO A KAISER ROLL WITH ROASTED
RED PEPPER OR SHREDDED LETTUCE AND TOMATO.

TRY DICING THE TEMPEH ADOBO INTO NUGGETS
(SEE VARIATION BELOW) AND TOSSING THE SPICY SNIPPETS WITH
QUINOA TO CREATE AN UNUSUAL PERUVIAN-INSPIRED MAIN-
DISH SALAD (PAGE 49).

8 OUNCES
tempeh, preferably mixed grain

3 TABLESPOONS
freshly squeezed lime juice

2 TABLESPOONS
olive oil

2 TABLESPOONS
shoyu

1 TABLESPOON
mild chili powder

1 TO 2 LARGE CLOVES
garlic, peeled and pushed
through a press

1 ½ TEASPOONS
dried leaf oregano

1 TEASPOON
ground cumin

1 TEASPOON
pureed chipotle in adobo or
⅛ to ¼ teaspoon ground chipotle
chili (see note) or ground cayenne
pepper

1 Cut the tempeh into 3 equal pieces crosswise. Cut each piece in half horizontally to create a total of 6 thin slabs.

2 Spoon the remaining ingredients into a 1-quart zipper-top storage bag or lidded container. Mix well. Add the tempeh, seal, and shake gently to coat the pieces. Marinate at room temperature for 1 hour or refrigerate overnight, shaking gently from time to time.

3 Gently transfer the tempeh to a large nonstick skillet. Set over high heat until the tempeh sizzles. Cover, reduce the heat to low, and cook for 3 minutes. Flip the tempeh over, cover, and cook an additional 3 minutes. Uncover and sauté over medium-high heat, flipping the tempeh as needed, until the slabs are browned and crusty on both sides.

Serves **2** or **3**

Tempeh Adobo Nuggets:
Cut the browned tempeh into ¼-inch dice. Eight ounces of tempeh yields about 2¼ cups nuggets.

Note: Chipotles in adobe is a thick paste of chipotles, vinegar, onions, garlic, and spices. Look for it in Hispanic groceries and gourmet shops. Chipotle chilies are dried jalapeños that impart a hot, smoky flavor. They may be purchased from gourmet shops either whole or ground To grind your own, stem and seed the chili, snip it into bits, and grind the bits to a powder in the spice grinder.

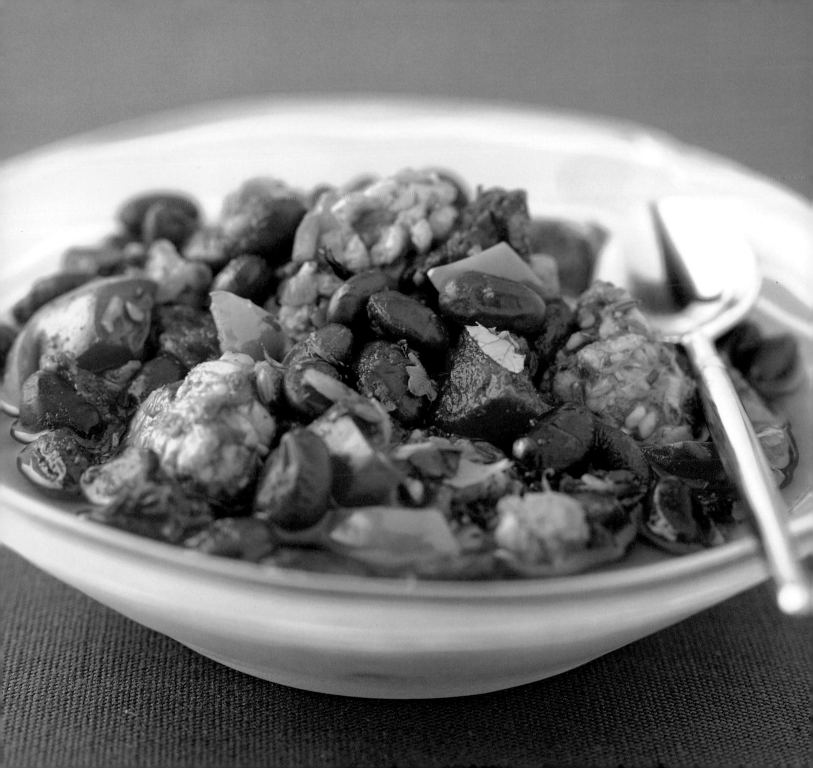

double-soybean chili

BLACK SOYBEANS AND CRUMBLED TEMPEH ARE THE TWO "SOYS" IN QUESTION. THESE PLUS A BOTTLE OF DARK BEER AND A GENEROUS ROUNDUP OF SOUTHWEST SEASONINGS ADD UP TO A HEARTY, COLORFUL, AND OUTRAGEOUSLY TASTY CHILI. USING SNIPPED DRIED ANCHO AND SMOKY CHIPOTLE CHILIES (AVAILABLE IN GOURMET SHOPS) IN ADDITION TO CHILI POWDER CREATES HAUNTING LAYERS OF FLAVOR. IF YOU CAN'T FIND THE DRIED CHILIES LOCALLY, IT'S WORTH ORDERING SOME BY MAIL (SEE PAGE 115). BE SURE TO WEAR RUBBER GLOVES WHEN HANDLING CHILIES.

THIS CHILI IS DELICIOUS ON ITS OWN OR LADLED ATOP POLENTA OR RICE. THERE'S ALREADY SO MUCH GOING ON THAT I WOULDN'T BOTHER WITH ANY OF THE USUAL FAT-LADEN TOPPINGS. BUT IT IS FUN TO SERVE THE CHILI WITH SOME WARM TORTILLAS FOR SOPPING UP THE LUSCIOUS SAUCE.

LIKE MOST STEWS, THIS ONE TASTES EVEN BETTER THE DAY AFTER IT'S MADE.

2 TABLESPOONS
olive oil

2 TEASPOONS
cumin seeds

3 CUPS
coarsely chopped onions

8 OUNCES
tempeh, preferably soy, crumbled into small bits or quartered and finely chopped in a food processor

1 LARGE green bell pepper, seeded and cut into 1-inch dice

1 LARGE red bell pepper, seeded and cut into 1-inch dice

1 TABLESPOON
minced garlic

1 TABLESPOON
chili powder

2 chipotle chilies, stemmed, seeded, and snipped into bits (see note)

1 ancho chili, stemmed, seeded, and snipped into bits (see note)

2 TEASPOONS
dried leaf oregano

1 BOTTLE (12 OUNCES)
dark beer

6 sun-dried tomato halves (dry pack, not marinated in oil), snipped into bits

1 ½ CUPS
cooked black soybeans (page 9)
or 1 can (15 ounces) organic black
soybeans, drained

1 CAN (15 OUNCES)
diced tomatoes or plum tomatoes,
coarsely chopped

1 TEASPOON
salt, or to taste

½ TO 1 CUP
coarsely chopped cilantro (use the
maximum if you are passionate
about this herb)

1 Heat the oil in a large saucepan over medium-high heat. Sizzle the cumin in the hot oil for 20 seconds. Add the onions and tempeh and sauté, stirring frequently, until the onions are golden brown, about 10 minutes. Add the bell peppers, garlic, chili powder, chili peppers, and oregano. Sauté for 1 minute more, stirring constantly.

2 Stir in the beer, dried tomatoes, soybeans, diced tomatoes (with canning liquid), and salt. Bring to a boil. Cover partially, reduce the heat to low, and simmer, stirring occasionally, until the flavors deepen and mingle, 20 to 30 minutes. Just before serving, stir in the cilantro and adjust the seasonings.

Serves **4** to **6**

Note: Chipotles are dried jalapeños that impart a hot, smoky flavor. Ancho chilies are dried poblanos and are relatively mild. Look for both in gourmet shops.

black soybean salsa with swordfish strips

ONCE BLACK SOYBEANS ARE MARINATED IN LIME-SHOYU VINAIGRETTE, THEY BECOME AN IDEAL COMPONENT FOR A ZESTY AND NUTRITIOUS SALSA (WHICH MAY BE PREPARED A DAY IN ADVANCE). THE COLORFUL TOMATO-RED MIXTURE IS SET IN THE CENTER OF THE PLATE WITH SPOKES OF SWORDFISH STRIPS RADIATING OUTWARD. IT'S A PRETTY AND FILLING DISH, WITH LOTS OF INTERESTING VISUAL AND TEXTURAL CONTRASTS.

1 ½ CUPS
cooked black soybeans (page 9) or 1 can (15 ounces) organic black soybeans, drained

⅓ CUP PLUS 2 TABLESPOONS
Lime-Shoyu Vinaigrette (page 101)

2 swordfish steaks (1½ pounds total), ¾ to 1 inch thick

Salt and freshly ground black pepper

1 LARGE CLOVE
garlic, peeled and finely minced

1 POUND
plum tomatoes, seeded and finely diced (about 3 cups)

½ CUP
finely diced red onion

1 TO 2 jalapeño chilies, seeded and diced

1 TO 2 TABLESPOONS
freshly squeezed lime juice

Sprigs of cilantro and lime wedges, for garnish

1 In a large bowl, mix the soy-beans and ⅓ cup of the vinai-grette. Cover and marinate in the refrigerator for at least 3 hours and preferably overnight. Stir occasionally.

2 Shortly before serving, cut each swordfish steak into 2 equal pieces. Brush both sides with the remaining 2 tablespoons vinai-grette, and dust lightly with salt and liberally with black pepper. Set aside.

3 Toss the remaining ingredients with the marinated black soy-beans and any unabsorbed mari-nade, adding salt and enough lime juice to give the mixture an assertive, puckery edge. Using a slotted spoon, spoon about ¾ cup of the salsa in the center of each of 4 large plates.

4 Heat a large nonstick skillet over high heat. Sauté the swordfish until both sides are deeply browned and the fish is no longer translucent in the center, 3 to 4 minutes per side. (If both sides are quite browned and the center is still raw, cover the skillet for the final minute or two of cooking, but take care not to overcook!)

5 Transfer the fish to a cutting board and cut on the bias into strips about ½ inch wide. Divide the strips among the 4 plates, setting them in spokes around the salsa. Garnish the salsa with sprigs of cilantro and place wedges of lime between the strips.

Serves **4**

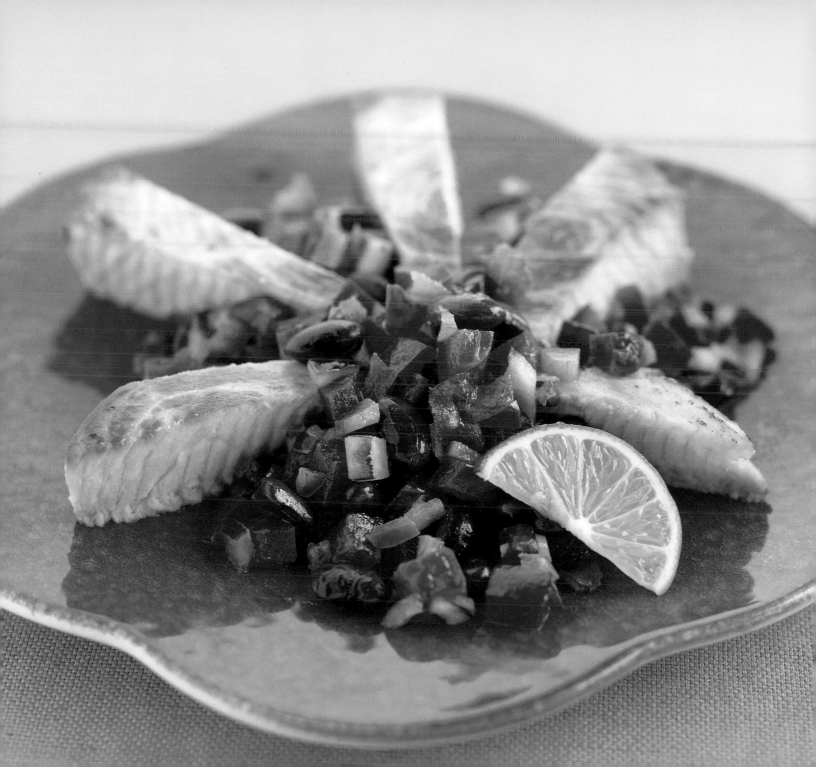

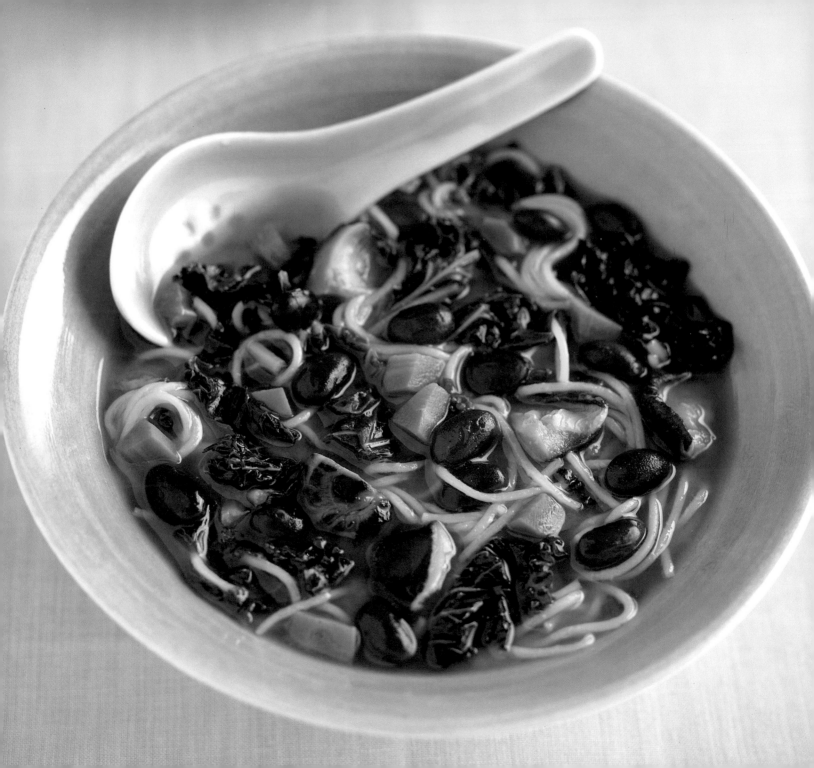

meal-in-a-bowl noodle vegetable hot pot

IF YOU LIKE THE IDEA OF DINNER IN A BOWL, THIS HEARTY HOT POT IS FOR YOU. THE MISO BROTH IS FULL OF GOOD THINGS: RICE VERMICELLI, BLACK SOYBEANS, KALE, AND DRIED SHIITAKE MUSHROOMS, TO NAME BUT A FEW.

THE RICE NOODLES ARE COOKED RIGHT IN THE HOT POT AND DRINK UP MUCH OF THE LIQUID, TRANSFORMING THE MIXTURE FROM A SOUP TO THE KIND OF SCRUMPTIOUS CASSEROLE YOU SEE PEOPLE ENTHUSIASTICALLY SLURPING UP IN ASIAN NOODLE SHOPS. AND YES, BE PREPARED, AS MY VERSION IS QUITE SLURPY, TOO.

6 CUPS
water (if available, use soybean cooking or canning liquid to replace some of the water)

1 carrot, peeled and finely diced

1 TABLESPOON PLUS 1 TEASPOON
finely minced fresh ginger

½ OUNCE
dried shiitake mushrooms

1 SMALL BUNCH
(about ¾ pound) kale

3 TO 4 OUNCES
rice vermicelli (see note)

1 ½ CUPS
cooked black soybeans (page 9) or 1 can (15 ounces) organic black soybeans, drained

¼ CUP
barley miso plus 2 tablespoons sweet white miso dissolved in 1 cup hot water

Chili oil or hot pepper sesame oil, to taste

1 In a large soup pot, bring the water, carrot, and 1 tablespoon of ginger to a boil. Meanwhile, break off the shiitake stems (or pry them out with a sharp paring knife). Discard the stems or reserve them for stock. Break or chop the shiitake caps into tiny bits. Quickly rinse and drain, and add them to the soup. Press the shiitake down into the water with the back of a large spoon. Cover and cook over medium heat while you prepare the kale, about 5 minutes.

2 Holding the kale in a bunch, chop off and discard the stems. Slice the kale as thinly as possible. (You should have about 5 cups very tightly packed. If you have more, put it aside for another use.) Rinse well and drain.

3 Return the soup to a rolling boil. Add the kale and push it under the water with the back of a large spoon. (It will seem like a lot, but will shrink dramatically.) Boil uncovered over medium-high heat until the kale is just short of tender, about 4 minutes. Add the rice vermicelli and soybeans. Press the vermicelli under the liquid and separate the strands. (The pot will seem very crowded at this point!) Continue cooking at a moderate boil, stirring occasionally and pressing the ingredients down into the water, until the vermicelli are tender, about 2 minutes.

4 Reduce the heat to low and stir in the dissolved miso, the remaining teaspoon of ginger, and chili oil to taste. Use a slotted spoon and a ladle to transfer portions to large, deep bowls. Serve the hot pot with chopsticks and soup spoons.

Serves **4**

Note: Angel-hair-thin rice vermicelli are also called rice sticks and *bifun*. You'll find them in Asian markets and some natural-food stores.

shrimps, mussels, and tofu in lemongrass miso broth

HERE IS AN ELEGANT SEAFOOD STEW IMBUED
WITH A PROFUSION OF ASIAN FLAVORS: LEMONGRASS, THAI RED
CURRY PASTE, CILANTRO, AND MISO. IN TRUTH, WHEN I FIRST
MADE THIS DISH AND TASTED IT BEFORE ADDING THE MISO, I
THOUGHT IT WASN'T GOING TO WORK. DESPITE THE FACT THAT
THESE INGREDIENTS ARE COMMONLY COMBINED IN THAI DISHES,
IN THIS STEW THE VARIOUS FLAVORS SEEMED TO BE FIGHTING
ONE ANOTHER.

THEN I STIRRED IN THE MISO AND VOILÀ: TRANS-
FORMATION. THE BROTH WAS SUDDENLY BALANCED, COMPLEX,
AND SOOTHING. THE CONTRAST WAS ASTONISHING. TRY
THE BEFORE-AND-AFTER EXPERIMENT YOURSELF, AND YOU WILL
UNDERSTAND THE HARMONIZING MIRACLE OF MISO BETTER
THAN I CAN EVER PUT INTO WORDS.

1 FOUR-INCH STALK
lemongrass (measure from fleshy
bulb upward), bruised outer leaves
removed, sliced into 1-inch-long
pieces (see note)

4 LARGE CLOVES
garlic, peeled

¼ POUND
shallots, peeled

¾ TEASPOON
Thai red curry paste or ½ teaspoon
crushed red pepper flakes

1 TABLESPOON
peanut oil

4 CUPS
water

8 OUNCES
extra-firm or firm tofu, drained and
cut into ½-inch cubes

½ CUP
diced red bell pepper

3 TO 4 TABLESPOONS
barley miso

1 ½ POUNDS
mussels, bearded if necessary

¾ POUND
medium shrimps, peeled and
deveined

½ CUP
tightly packed cilantro leaves

10 LARGE fresh basil leaves,
shredded

1 scallion, thinly sliced

1 TO 2 TABLESPOONS
freshly squeezed lime juice
(optional)

1 With the motor of the food processor running, pop the lemongrass through the feed tube. Process at full speed alternating with the pulsing action until the lemongrass is very finely chopped, about 2 minutes, stopping and scraping down the sides of the work bowl as needed. With the motor running, pop in the garlic cloves and chop finely. Toss in the shallots and curry paste and process until the mixture resembles a coarse paste, 30 to 60 seconds more.

2 Heat the oil in a 4-quart (or larger) nonstick saucepan over medium heat. (If you don't own a large nonstick saucepan, do this step in a nonstick skillet and transfer the mixture to a saucepan.) Sauté the lemongrass paste in the oil, stirring constantly, until the ingredients begin to brown and cling to the bottom of the pan, 3 to 5 minutes. Stir in the water, tofu, and red pepper. Bring to a boil, cover, and cook over medium heat for 5 minutes.

3 Ladle out about ½ cup of the broth into a glass measuring cup and blend 3 tablespoons of the miso into it. Set aside.

4 Return the soup liquid to a rapid boil and add the mussels. Cover and cook over high heat for 1 minute, then quickly toss in the shrimps. Cover and continue to cook just until the mussels open and the shrimps turn pink, 1 to 2 minutes. (Do not cook an instant longer than necessary or the seafood will become rubbery.)

5 Remove from the heat and stir in the miso solution, cilantro, basil, and scallion. Taste and, if needed, blend a bit more miso into ½ cup of the broth and add to the pot. If you'd like to add yet another marvelous flavor dimension, stir in lime juice to taste.

Serves **4**

Note: If fresh lemongrass is not available, Thai Kitchen's jarred lemongrass packed in water is a viable substitute.

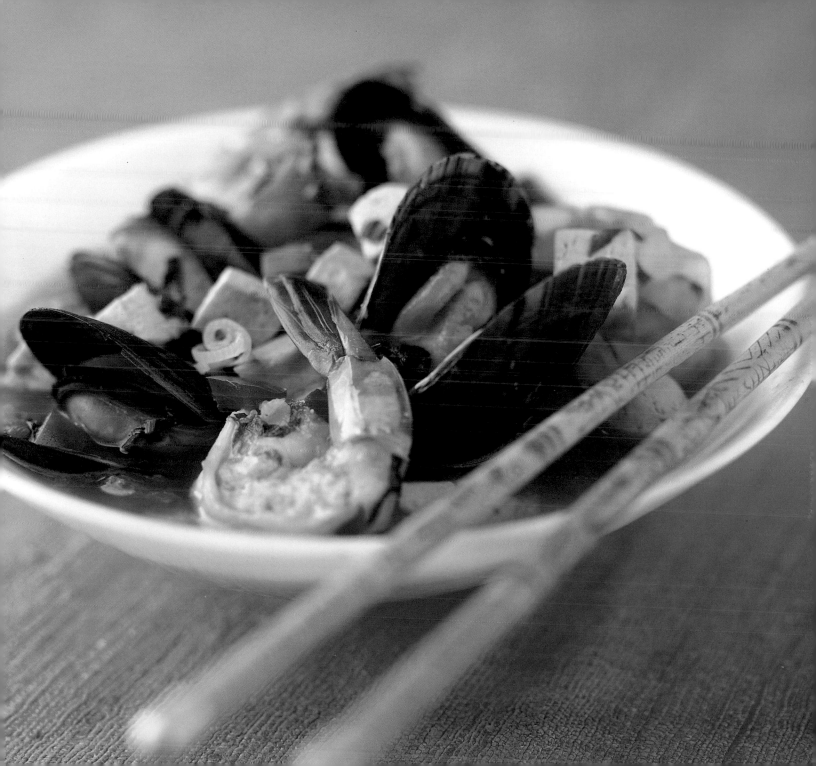

chunky codfish and clam chowder

THIS NEW TAKE ON A CLASSIC NEW ENGLAND FISH CHOWDER SUGGESTS THE RICHNESS AND GOOD FLAVOR OF THE ORIGINAL WITHOUT DEPENDING UPON BUTTER AND CREAM. I HAVE TWO SECRET WEAPONS. ONE IS COOKING THE POTATOES UNTIL THEY BECOME MELTINGLY SOFT, GIVING OFF THEIR STARCH TO ENRICH THE BROTH. THE OTHER IS ADDING SOYMILK AT THE VERY END TO ROUND OUT THE FLAVORS AND GIVE THE CHOWDER ITS CHARACTERISTIC CREAMINESS.

WITH SOME GOOD BREAD AND A GENEROUS PORTION OF MIXED GREEN SALAD OR A HEARTY SLAW—LIKE THE CAULIFLOWER SLAW ON PAGE 98—THIS CHOWDER MAKES A FINE MEAL.

1 TABLESPOON
olive oil

2 TEASPOONS
minced garlic

2 CUPS
thinly sliced leeks (white and light green parts), thoroughly rinsed

2 BOTTLES (8 OUNCES EACH)
clam juice

1 POUND
fingerling or Yukon Gold potatoes, peeled and cut into ¼-inch dice

½ CUP
diced red bell pepper

¾ TO 1 TEASPOON
dried thyme leaves or several sprigs of fresh thyme

½ TEASPOON
salt, or to taste

Freshly ground black pepper, to taste

½ CUP
water

8 littleneck clams

1½ POUNDS
cod or scrod fillets, cut into 1-inch chunks

1 CUP
soymilk, at room temperature

2 TO 3 TABLESPOONS
minced parsley, for garnish

1 Heat the oil in a large saucepan over medium high heat. Sauté the garlic, stirring frequently, until lightly browned, about 1 minute. Add the leeks and sauté for an additional minute. Add the clam juice, potatoes, red pepper, thyme, salt, and black pepper. Bring to a boil. Cover and cook over medium heat until the potatoes are very soft, 10 to 15 minutes.

2 Steam the clams while the potatoes are cooking: Bring the water to a rapid boil in a large saucepan. Add the clams, cover, and cook over high heat, shaking the pan vigorously once or twice, until the clams open, 2 to 8 minutes. (If some clams remain closed, remove those that have opened and continue cooking the others. Discard any clams that do not eventually open.) Set aside.

3 When the potatoes are done, stir the cod into the chowder. Cover and cook at a gentle boil until the fish turns pearly white and easily flakes, 2 to 4 minutes for the scrod or 5 to 8 minutes for the cod. Take care not to over-cook or the fish will become rubbery!

4 Divide the clams among 4 large, shallow soup bowls. Taking care that any sand or grit remains on the bottom of the pot, tip any remaining clam cooking liquid into the chowder. Stir the soymilk into the chowder, add more thyme, salt and pepper to taste, if needed, and heat briefly if necessary, but do not boil. Ladle the chowder over the clams and garnish each portion with the parsley.

Serves **4**

tofu and brussels sprouts with fermented black beans

CONNOISSEURS OF CHINESE FOOD ADORE THE
SALTY, INTENSE, AND VERY DISTINCTIVE TASTE OF FERMENTED
BLACK BEANS. UNBEKNOWNST TO MANY, THESE ARE ACTUALLY
BLACK SOYBEANS THAT HAVE BEEN INOCULATED WITH A MOLD,
THEN LEFT TO FERMENT IN A SALT-BRINE SOLUTION FOR ABOUT
SIX MONTHS. FERMENTED BLACK SOYBEANS ARE THOUGHT TO
BE THE EARLIEST CONDIMENT MADE OF SOY, PREDATING BOTH
SOY SAUCE AND MISO.

IN THIS DISH, I'VE COMBINED THE BLACK BEANS
WITH OTHER TRADITIONAL CHINESE SEASONINGS—GARLIC,
GINGER, AND ORANGE PEEL—TO CREATE A THICK PASTE. THIS
PASTE DARKENS THE TOFU AND COATS THE SURFACE WITH
FLAVOR, WHILE LEAVING THE INSIDE OF EACH CHUNK JUST AS
MILD MANNERED AS TOFU CAN BE. THE CONTRAST OF TASTE
AND COLOR IS QUITE APPEALING.

SLICED BRUSSELS SPROUTS WORK SURPRISINGLY
WELL IN THIS ASIAN CONTEXT. THERE IS LITTLE TO NO SAUCE,
SO I USUALLY SERVE THE MIXTURE ON ITS OWN RATHER THAN
OVER RICE. DO SERVE IT WITH CHOPSTICKS. I DON'T KNOW WHY,
BUT THE DISH TASTES BETTER THAT WAY.

2-INCH CHUNK
fresh ginger, trimmed and
quartered

4 LARGE CLOVES
garlic, peeled

2 ½ TABLESPOONS
fermented black beans (see note)

1 TABLESPOON
grated dried orange peel
(see note)

¼ TO ½ TEASPOON
crushed red pepper flakes

1 TABLESPOON
peanut oil

1 CUP
water

¼ CUP
dry sherry

ABOUT 1 ½ TABLESPOONS
shoyu

1-POUND BLOCK
extra-firm or firm tofu, drained,
pressed, and cut into ¾-inch
cubes

10 OUNCES
brussels sprouts, trimmed and cut
into ¼-inch-thick slices

2 LARGE carrots, peeled and thinly
sliced on the diagonal

1 With the food processor motor running, pop the ginger, garlic, and black beans through the feed tube. Process until finely chopped. Remove the cover, scrape down the sides of the work bowl, and add the orange peel and red pepper flakes. Pulse a few times to mix well.

2 Heat the oil in a large skillet or wok over medium-high heat. Add the black bean mixture and sauté, stirring constantly, for 10 seconds. Blend in the water, sherry, and shoyu, and bring to a boil. Add the tofu and stir gently to coat it with the sauce. Reduce the heat to medium, cover, and cook for 3 minutes, stirring occasionally.

3 Scatter the brussels sprouts and carrots on top of the tofu. Cover and cook over medium-high heat until the vegetables are crisp-tender, 3 to 5 minutes. If the mixture becomes dry before the vegetables are cooked, stir in a few additional tablespoons of water. Add shoyu to taste, if needed.

Serves 3

Notes: You'll find fermented black beans (also known as preserved beans and salted beans) in most Asian groceries, usually in small plastic bags. If you happen upon the Pearl River Bridge brand in a yellow box, these are considered best. Some fermented black beans are seasoned with ginger and orange peel, which is fine for this recipe. Once opened, refrigerate the beans in a tightly sealed jar and they will last indefinitely.

You may substitute 2 to 3 teaspoons of freshly grated orange zest for the dried orange peel; stir it in at the end.

down-home "barbecued" tofu

WE ALL NEED A ZESTY RECIPE TO PERK US UP ON A
WEARY WEEKDAY NIGHT, PREFERABLY ONE THAT REQUIRES LITTLE
PREPARATION, COOKS QUICKLY, AND DOESN'T NECESSITATE A
STOP AT THE SUPERMARKET ON THE WAY HOME. "BARBECUED" TOFU
FULFILLS ALL OF THESE PRACTICAL CRITERIA. THERE'S NOTHING
SUBTLE, ELEGANT, OR SOPHISTICATED ABOUT THESE TASTY
SQUARES, BUT THEY CAN BE THROWN TOGETHER AND BROILED
IN ABOUT TEN MINUTES, AND THEY ALWAYS TASTE GOOD.
EXTRA-FIRM TOFU WILL GIVE YOU THE BEST RESULTS.

LEFTOVERS MAKE GREAT SANDWICHES, GARNISHED
WITH THINLY SLICED TOMATO AND RED ONION. SINCE THE
FLAVORS MELLOW SLIGHTLY AFTER REFRIGERATION, YOU MIGHT
ALSO LIKE TO ADD A SMEAR OF MUSTARD.

1-POUND BLOCK
extra-firm tofu, drained

2 GENEROUS TABLESPOONS
Dijon mustard

2 GENEROUS TABLESPOONS
ketchup

1 ½ TO 2 TABLESPOONS
shoyu (depending upon desired saltiness)

1 LARGE CLOVE
garlic, peeled and pushed through a press

2 TEASPOONS
blackstrap molasses

2 TEASPOONS
toasted Asian sesame oil

1 TO 2 TEASPOONS
chipotle in adobo or ⅛ to ¼ teaspoon ground chipotle chili (see note) or cayenne pepper

Freshly ground black pepper, to taste

1 Wrap the tofu in several layers of a clean, absorbent kitchen towel and set a 1-pound bag of dried beans on top. Set the tofu aside until you are ready to slice it.

2 Line a broiling pan or baking sheet with aluminum foil. Set aside. Place the oven rack about 5 inches from the broiling element, and turn on the broiler.

3 In a pie plate or large, shallow bowl, prepare the barbecue sauce by blending together the remaining ingredients.

4 Unwrap the tofu and set the block on a cutting board with the longer side facing you. Cut the block crosswise into 9 slices, each slightly less than ½ inch thick. Dip the slices into the sauce to coat both sides heavily. Arrange the slices on the broiling pan as you work. (Reserve any remaining sauce.)

5 Broil the tofu until flecked with dark brown spots, 4 to 6 minutes. (If your broiler cooks unevenly, rotate the broiling pan halfway through.) Turn the tofu over with a spatula and slather any remaining sauce on the second side with a pastry brush or knife. Broil until deeply browned on the second side, 4 to 6 more minutes. Serve with the darker side up.

Serves **3** or **4**

Note: Chipotles in adobe is a thick paste of chipotles, vinegar, onions, garlic, and spices. Look for it in Hispanic groceries and gourmet shops. Chipotle chilies are dried jalapenos that impart a hot, smoky flavor. They may be purchased from gourmet shops either whole or ground. To grind your own, stem and seed the chili, snip it into bits, and grind the bits to a powder in a spice grinder.

fettuccine and broccoli
with miso pesto

1 LARGE BUNCH
(about 1½ pounds) broccoli

¾ POUND
fettuccine

⅓ TO ½ CUP
Miso Pesto (page 104)

Shoyu and freshly ground black
pepper, to taste (optional)

Grated Parmesan cheese,
for garnish (optional)

WHEN BASIL IS IN SEASON, I OFTEN WHIP UP A
BATCH OF MISO PESTO AND KEEP IT ON HAND IN THE REFRIGER-
ATOR. FOR A QUICK SUPPER, I NEVER TIRE OF THIS NO-FRILLS
APPROACH: COOK CHOPPED BROCCOLI ALONG WITH FETTUCCINE,
AND COAT THE MIXTURE WITH THE NUT-RICH PASTE. THE RESULT
IS A HARMONIOUS SYMPHONY OF COLOR, FLAVOR, AND TEXTURE.

1 Put a large pot of salted water over high heat and bring to a boil. Meanwhile, trim the broccoli into small florets, 1 to 1½ inches across the top. Trim and peel the stalks; cut any thick stalks in half lengthwise. Cut the stalks into ¼-inch thick slices. Rinse the broccoli and set aside.

2 Cook the fettuccine in the rapidly boiling water until 2 minutes short of al dente. (Check the package directions for timing.) Add the broccoli and press it down with the back of a large spoon to submerge it under the boiling water. Continue cooking at a rapid boil until the pasta is al dente. Pour the pasta and broccoli into a large colander, and bounce the colander up and down a few times to release excess water.

3 Transfer the noodles and broccoli to a bowl and rapidly toss with enough pesto to coat the ingredients thoroughly—about ⅓ cup usually does the trick. Add the shoyu and black pepper (if using). Serve hot or at room temperature, garnished with a sprinkling of Parmesan, if you wish.

Serves 4

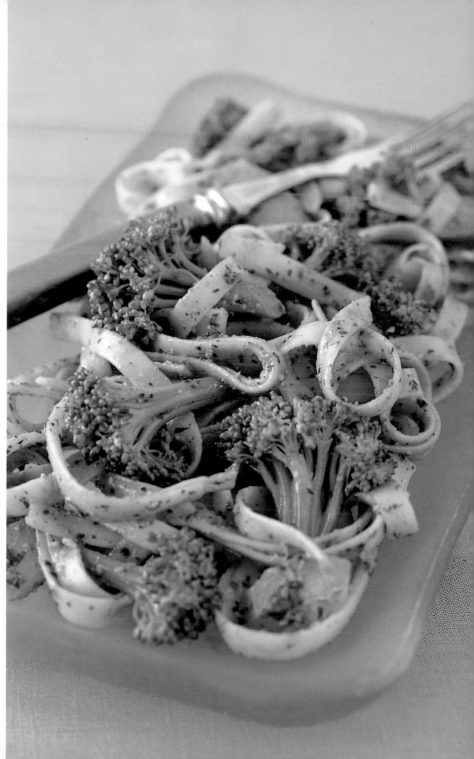

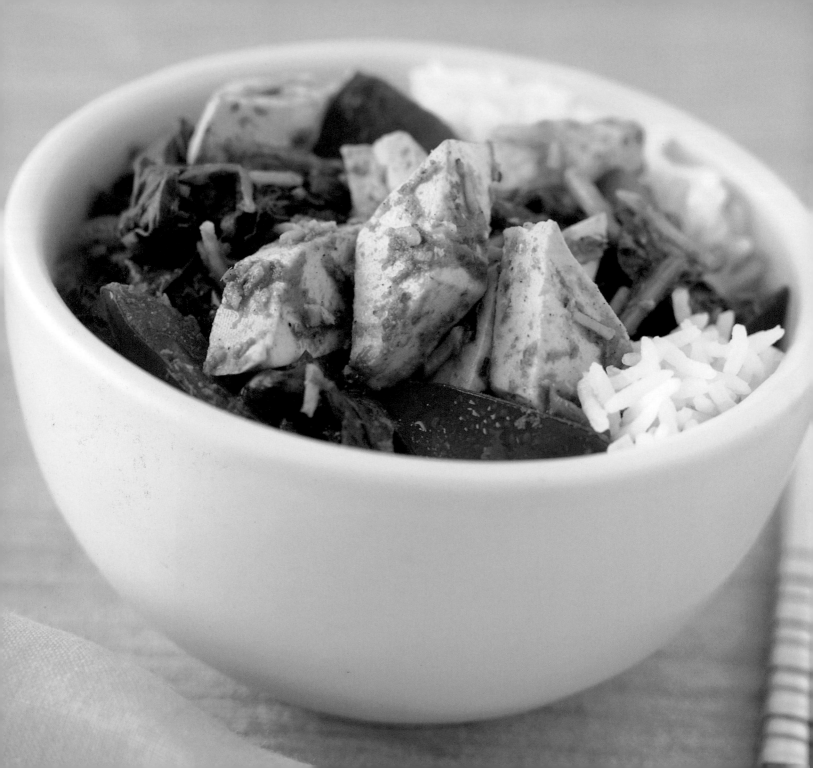

curried tofu with spinach and tomatoes

FOR A CASUAL SUPPER, I ALWAYS ENJOY THIS
COLORFUL MEDLEY WITH ITS CURRY-YELLOW TOFU, BRIGHT GREEN
SPLASHES OF SPINACH, AND CHEERY DOTS OF TOMATO. IT'S
RICHLY FLAVORED WITH PATAK'S PREPARED MILD CURRY PASTE,
A CONDIMENT I'VE COME TO RELY UPON FOR ITS INTENSELY
GOOD BALANCE OF SPICES. I PARTICULARLY LIKE MAKING THIS
CURRY WITH FROZEN TOFU, WHICH THIRSTILY DRINKS UP THE
SAUCE AND HAS A DELIGHTFULLY CHEWY TEXTURE. YOU'LL ALSO
HAVE GOOD RESULTS WITH PRESSED FRESH TOFU.

THE FRESH SPINACH WILL SEEM LIKE A HUGE QUAN-
TITY, BUT IT SHRINKS DRAMATICALLY WHEN COOKED. I ALWAYS
INCLUDE THE ROOTS AND STEMS IF THE SPINACH IS YOUNG AND
TENDER. DRAIN THE SPINACH WELL AFTER WASHING, LEAVING
JUST THE WATER CLINGING TO THE LEAVES.

SERVE THE CURRY IN SHALLOW BOWLS OVER
STEAMED BASMATI RICE, WITH YOUR FAVORITE SWEET MANGO
CHUTNEY ON THE SIDE.

1-POUND BLOCK
extra-firm or firm tofu, frozen, defrosted, and drained (page 13)

1 TABLESPOON
peanut oil or ghee (clarified butter)

1 CUP
coarsely chopped onions

1 CUP
water

¼ CUP
mild curry paste (see note)

3 TABLESPOONS
unsweetened grated dried coconut

3 LARGE plum tomatoes, cored and cut into eighths

¾ POUND
spinach, trimmed, coarsely chopped, and thoroughly washed

Salt, to taste

⅓ TO ½ CUP
chopped cilantro (optional)

1 Set the block of defrosted tofu between 2 plates and, pressing the plates firmly together, tip them over the sink as the tofu releases excess water. Release the pressure slightly, then press the plates firmly together again 4 or 5 more times, or until no more water is expressed. With a serrated knife, slice the tofu into 1-inch cubes. Set aside.

2 Heat the oil in a large, heavy saucepan or wok over medium-high heat. Sauté the onions, stirring frequently, until lightly browned, about 3 minutes. Add the water and blend in the curry paste and coconut. Stir in the reserved tofu, taking care to coat the tofu thoroughly with the curry sauce. Stir in the tomatoes.

3 Cover and cook over medium heat, stirring occasionally, until the tomatoes are soft, about 5 minutes. If the mixture seems quite dry, stir in ¼ cup water at this point. Add the spinach. (If your pot isn't big enough, you may need to add half, cover, and let it wilt before adding the remainder.) Cover and continue cooking until the spinach is tender, 2 to 3 minutes. Add salt and the cilantro, if you like.

Serves 3

Note: You'll find 10-ounce jars of Patak's curry paste (and a myriad of other pickles and chutneys made by this venerable British company) in any Indian grocery and in many specialty-food shops, or you can order it by mail or substitute your own favorite brand of curry paste.

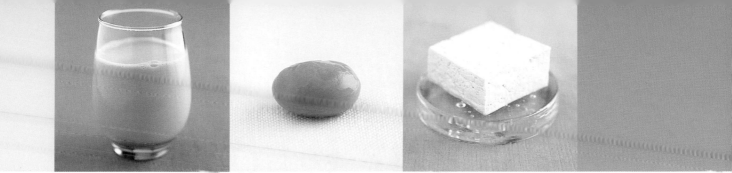

soy on the side

The versatility of soyfoods is perhaps nowhere more in evidence than in this chapter, where it shines in both savory and sweet dishes.

First there's a selection of unusual vegetable side dishes, including Gingered Kabocha Squash with Seasoned Black Soybeans and Garlicky Broccoli Rabe with Tempeh Italiano.

Among the salad recipes, you'll find an Asian Slaw dotted with chewy cubes of Baked Seasoned Tofu and coated with a rich Peanut Miso Dressing. Silken tofu becomes the base for a Creamy Dill Dressing that transforms chopped cauliflower into a crisp, cool slaw. And a Roasted Potato Salad includes bits of seasoned tempeh and marinated artichokes that pop with taste surprises. Serving estimates in these two sections are all for side-dish portions.

I've ended with a few recipes that use soy in unusually delicious ways. There is soymilk in the savory Sage-Scented Cornmeal Scones and in a rich Pineapple-Coconut Rice Pudding laced with rum. Silken tofu is whipped into an elegant Chocolate–Grand Marnier Sauce. A velvet-smooth Pumpkin Tart brings the chapter to a sweet close.

seasoned black soybeans

THE FLAVOR OF HOME-COOKED OR CANNED ORGANIC BLACK SOYBEANS IS ENHANCED BY SIMMERING THEM IN SHOYU AND OTHER SEASONINGS. HERE'S A WAY TO INFUSE THEM DELICATELY WITH FLAVOR SO THAT THEY MAKE MORE OF A STATEMENT WHEN EATEN ON THEIR OWN OR COMBINED WITH OTHER INGREDIENTS, SUCH AS IN THE GINGERED KABOCHA SQUASH ON PAGE 83. IF YOU LIKE THE IDEA OF ADDING A TOUCH OF SWEETNESS, INCLUDE A TABLESPOON OF THE SWEET JAPANESE COOKING WINE CALLED MIRIN.

¾ CUP
soybean cooking liquid (page 9), organic canning liquid, or water

1 TO 1 ½ TABLESPOONS
shoyu (depending upon desired saltiness)

1 ½ CUPS
cooked black soybeans (page 9) or 1 can (15 ounces) organic black soybeans, drained

1 CLOVE
garlic, peeled and minced

3 TABLESPOONS
minced shallot or onion

1 TABLESPOON
mirin (optional)

2 TEASPOONS
finely minced fresh ginger (optional)

2 TABLESPOONS
thinly sliced scallion greens, for garnish

1 In a small, heavy saucepan, heat the liquid over high heat and stir in the shoyu. Add the soybeans, garlic, shallot, mirin, and ginger (if using). Stir gently and remove any loose skins that float to the surface.

2 Reduce heat to medium-low and simmer uncovered, stirring occasionally, until the soybeans become gently infused with flavor and the liquid is some-what reduced, about 25 minutes. Divide the beans and liquid among 3 small bowls and garnish with the scallions.

Serves **2** or **3**
(Makes **1½** cups)

Quick-Seasoned Black Soybeans: If you don't have time to simmer the beans, this technique will enhance the flavor of soybeans. Drain the cooked or canned beans and set them in a 1-quart zipper-top storage bag or lidded container with 1 tablespoon of shoyu per 1½ cups of beans. Marinate the soybeans for 10 minutes or longer (you may refrigerate them overnight), gently shaking from time to time.

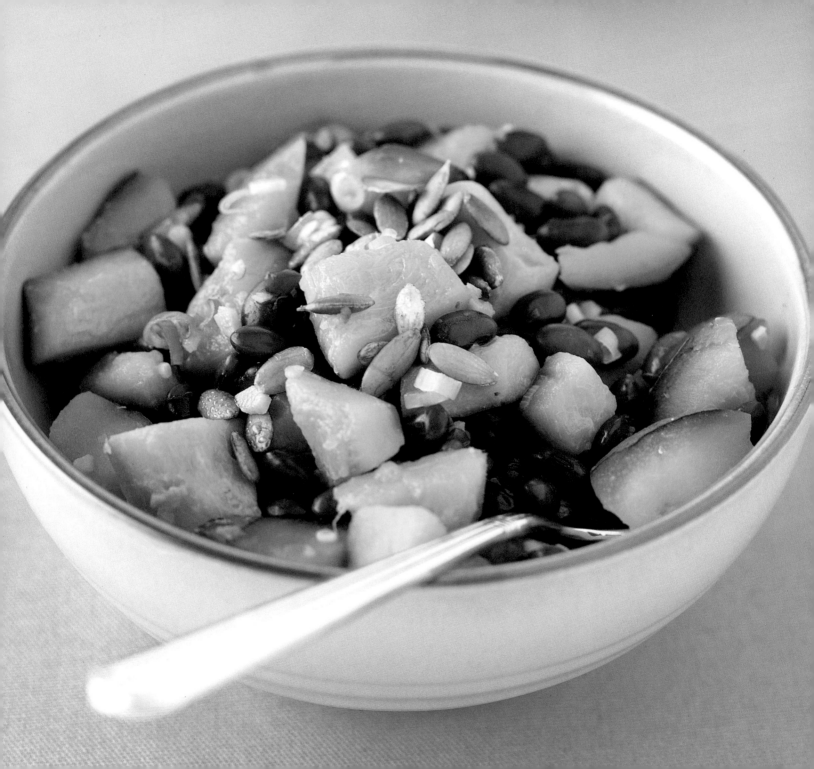

gingered kabocha squash with seasoned black soybeans

WHEN I FIRST TRIED KABOCHA, I THOUGHT IT WAS ONE OF THE BEST THINGS I'D EVER TASTED, AND I STILL DO. WHEN THIS DENSE, INTENSELY FLAVORED SQUASH IS TOSSED WITH SEASONED BLACK SOYBEANS, A TASTY AND STUNNING COMBINATION OF BRIGHT ORANGE AND SLEEK MAHOGANY IS THE HAPPY RESULT.

I STEAM THE SQUASH WITH MINCED GINGER, LIGHTLY COAT THE VEGETABLES WITH THE SOYBEANS' SEASONED COOKING LIQUID, AND ADD FRESHLY TOASTED PUMPKIN SEEDS FOR A GOOD CONTRASTING CRUNCH. IT'S A SIMPLE RECIPE THAT ALLOWS THE KABOCHA'S SUPERB TASTE TO DOMINATE.

1 CUP
water

1 SMALL (ABOUT 1 ½ POUNDS)
kabocha squash, trimmed, seeded, and cut into 1-inch chunks (see note)

2 scallions, thinly sliced (keep white and green parts separate)

1 ½ TABLESPOONS
finely minced fresh ginger

2 TABLESPOONS
shelled pumpkin seeds

1 ½ CUPS
Seasoned Black Soybeans (page 80; prepare without mirin, ginger, and scallion garnish, and reserve seasoned cooking liquid)

1 Pour the water into a large, heavy saucepan. Set as many chunks of kabocha, skin side down, as will fit in the water. Sprinkle half the sliced scallion bulbs and ginger on top. Add the remaining chunks of squash and top with the remaining scallion bulbs and ginger. Bring the water to a boil. Cover and cook over medium heat until the squash is fork-tender but still firm, 8 to 12 minutes. (You can remove pieces as they become tender.) To prevent scorching, be sure to check every few minutes and replenish water if needed.

2 While the squash is cooking, toast the pumpkin seeds in a shallow baking pan in a toaster oven set to 350 degrees until they puff up and begin to pop, 1 to 2 minutes. (Alternatively toast them in a dry skillet over medium heat, stirring constantly, 2 to 3 minutes.) Set aside.

3 When the squash is done, spoon out excess water if there is more than 1 tablespoon or so in the bottom of the pot. Gently stir in the scallion greens and seasoned soybeans plus some (or all) of their seasoned cooking liquid. Cover and cook over medium heat until the beans are good and hot, about 30 seconds. Garnish with pumpkin seeds just before serving.

Serves **4** to **6**

Note: There is really no substitute for kabocha, and fortunately it has become more widely available. I almost always see it in stores that sell organic produce. Don't be fooled: kabocha looks much like a buttercup squash except for its "navel" (opposite the stem end), which has no bump. The attractive rind, with its dark green and bright orange stripes, need not be peeled— just trim off any unsightly rough spots. You'll need your heaviest chef's knife to hack the kabocha into pieces.

diced tempeh italiano

TEMPEH MARINATED WITH OLIVE OIL, VINEGAR, AND ITALIAN SEASONINGS BECOMES INFUSED WITH INTENSE FLAVOR AND MAKES A DELICIOUS ADDITION TO COOKED VEGETABLES AND SALADS. FOR STARTERS, TRY IT WITH BROCCOLI RABE (PAGE 87) AND POTATO SALAD (PAGE 94), AND SEE IF YOU AGREE.

2 TABLESPOONS
olive oil

1 TABLESPOON
balsamic vinegar

1 TABLESPOON
shoyu

1 LARGE CLOVE
garlic, peeled and pushed through a press

2 TEASPOONS
Italian herb blend (see note)

¾ TEASPOON
crushed red pepper flakes

8 OUNCES
tempeh, preferably soy

1 Place the first 6 ingredients in a
1-quart zipper-top storage bag
or lidded container. Seal and
gently shake to blend. If the
tempeh is more than ¾ inch
thick, cut it in half horizontally.
Cut the tempeh crosswise into
"fingers" about ½ inch wide.
Add the tempeh to the marinade,
seal, and shake gently. (The tempeh will quickly absorb most or
all of the marinade.) Set aside
for 1 hour or refrigerate
overnight.

2 Heat a large nonstick skillet over
medium-low heat. Add the tempeh, cover, and cook, turning
the fingers every few minutes,
until both sides are deeply
browned, about 10 minutes.
Transfer to a cutting board.
When cool enough to handle,
cut into ½-inch dice.

Makes about **2¼** cups

Note: You can purchase a
bottled herb blend in any supermarket, but I prefer to make my
own by combining 1 tablespoon
each dried oregano and basil
leaves, 2 teaspoons each dried
thyme and rosemary leaves,
and 2 teaspoons lightly bruised
fennel seeds; you will have a
generous 3 tablespoons. Store
in a well-sealed container in
a cool, dark place for up to
6 months.

garlicky broccoli rabe with tempeh italiano

I LOVE THE BITTER EDGE OF BROCCOLI RABE AND
CAN RARELY RESIST PURCHASING A BUNCH WHEN I SEE ONE IN
THE MARKET. SINCE THIS ASSERTIVE GREEN IS ADORED BY
ITALIANS, IT COMBINES NATURALLY WITH TEMPEH MARINATED
IN ITALIAN SEASONINGS.

LOOK FOR BROCCOLI RABE WITH PERKY LEAVES
AND BRIGHT GREEN FLORETS. ALTHOUGH IT IS A QUICK-
COOKING VEGETABLE, THE STEMS TAKE A FEW MORE MINUTES
THAN THE LEAVES, SO I ADD THEM FIRST.

1 GOOD-SIZED BUNCH (ABOUT 1 POUND)
broccoli rabe

1 TABLESPOON
olive oil

6 LARGE CLOVES
garlic, peeled and thinly sliced

¼ CUP
dry white wine or vermouth

½ TEASPOON
salt, or to taste

Diced Tempeh Italiano (page 85)

1 Holding the broccoli rabe in a bunch, trim off and discard about 1 inch from the bottom of the stems, and cut the remainder of the stems into ½-inch-long slices. Put in a strainer and rinse. Set aside. Still holding the broccoli rabe in a bunch, chop the leaves into 1-inch slices, leaving the small florets whole. Put in a colander, rinse, and set aside separately.

2 In a large skillet or wok, heat the oil over medium-high heat. Sauté the garlic, stirring frequently, until lightly browned, about 1 minute. Add the white wine, broccoli rabe stems, and salt. Cover and cook over medium heat for 2 minutes. Add the leaves and florets and the diced tempeh. If the mixture seems dry at this point, stir in 1 or 2 tablespoons of water. Cover and continue cooking over medium-high heat until the broccoli rabe is tender but still a bit crunchy, 3 to 4 more minutes. Check every minute or so, stir, and add 1 or 2 tablespoons of water if the mixture seems dry.

Serves **3** or **4**

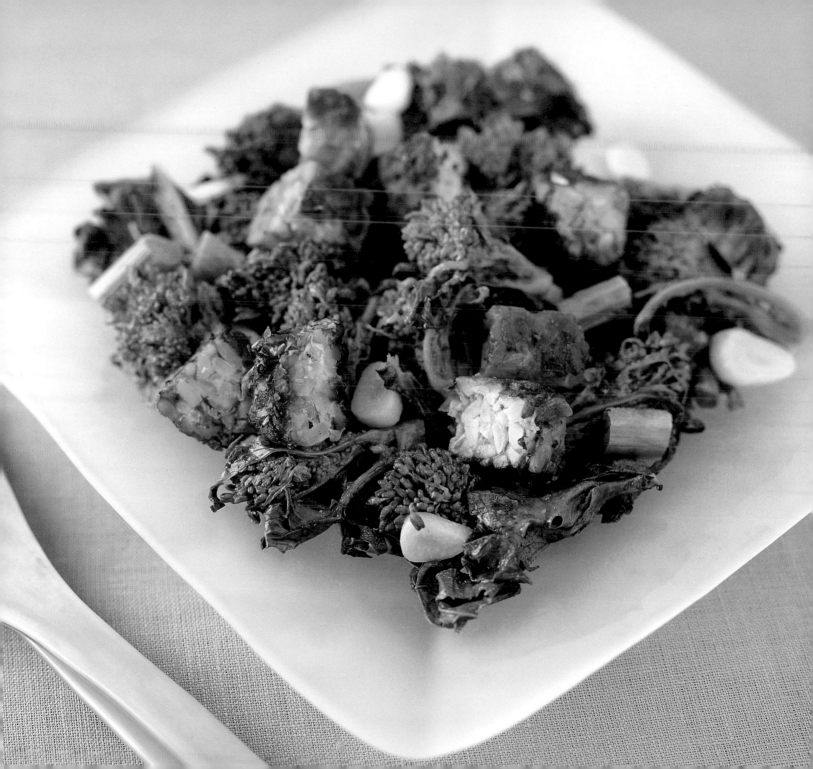

baked seasoned tofu

YOU CAN FIND TASTY, CHEWY SQUARES OF GOLDEN BROWN, PRESSED, SEASONED TOFU IN THE REFRIGERATED SECTION OF MOST CHINESE GROCERIES AND HEALTH-FOOD STORES (SOMETIMES LABELED THAI SPICED OR SICHUAN), BUT IT'S EXPENSIVE AND SOMETIMES A LITTLE TOO SALTY. AFTER MUCH EXPERIMENTATION, I CAME UP WITH THIS TASTY VERSION YOU CAN MAKE AT HOME.

IT'S SIMPLE BUT A BIT TIME CONSUMING TO EXECUTE. TO INSURE GOOD RESULTS, USE ONLY EXTRA-FIRM TOFU. ALSO, MONITOR THE OVEN TEMPERATURE WITH A THERMOMETER TO KEEP IT FROM CREEPING ABOVE 450 DEGREES.

HOMEMADE SEASONED TOFU LASTS AT LEAST A WEEK UNDER REFRIGERATION, AND THE PURCHASED VARIETY LASTS CONSIDERABLY LONGER (CHECK THE EXPIRATION DATE). DICED INTO "CROUTONS," IT ADDS TEXTURE AND PUNCH TO A VARIETY OF DISHES, INCLUDING ASIAN SLAW (PAGE 96) AND DOUBLE-SESAME SKILLET BROWN RICE (PAGE 92).

1 POUND
extra-firm tofu, drained and pressed

1 ¼ CUPS
water

¼ CUP
shoyu

1 TABLESPOON
coarsely chopped fresh ginger

1 TABLESPOON
coarsely chopped garlic

4 star anise, broken into petals (see note; optional)

¼ TEASPOON
crushed red pepper flakes

1 ½ TEASPOONS
toasted Asian sesame oil

2 TEASPOONS
sesame seeds

1 Set the block of tofu on a cutting board with the longer end of the block facing you. Using a serrated knife, cut the tofu crosswise into nine slices, each a scant ½ inch thick. Cut each slice in half to create 2 squares. Set aside.

2 Place a rack in the center of the oven. Preheat the oven to 450 degrees. In a 10- or 12-inch skillet, combine the water, shoyu, ginger, garlic, star anise (if using), and red pepper flakes. Arrange the tofu squares in the marinade in one layer. Over high heat, bring to a boil. Cover, reduce the heat to medium-low, and simmer for 15 minutes.

3 Meanwhile, brush the sesame oil on the bottom of a large, shallow baking dish (about 7 by 11 inches). When the tofu squares are ready, carefully remove them one by one from the simmering marinade, brush off any bits of garlic or ginger, and set in the baking dish. Flip over each piece so that the second side gets a light coating of the oil. Sprinkle with 1 teaspoon of the sesame seeds. Bake uncovered until the top is a deep caramel-brown, 15 to 20 minutes. Flip over, sprinkle with the remaining sesame seeds, and bake until the second side is deeply browned, about 15 minutes more.

4 Remove the baking dish from the oven and set on a rack. (The tofu will become firmer as it cools.) When cool, refrigerate in a tightly sealed container until needed, up to 1 week.

Makes about ¾ pound

Note: Star anise is a characteristic Chinese seasoning for tofu. As the name suggests, it has a flavor akin to licorice. Whole star anise pods are available in Chinese groceries and by mail order. They last a year or so when stored away from heat and light in a well-sealed container.

double-sesame skillet brown rice

I THINK OF MAKING THIS DISH—A HIGHLY PERSONAL RENDITION OF CHINESE FRIED RICE—WHEN MY REFRIGERATOR BOASTS LEFTOVER BROWN RICE AND A SMATTERING OF OTHER COOKED, TASTY MORSELS IN SMALL QUANTITIES, SUCH AS BAKED SEASONED TOFU OR STEAMED VEGETABLES. WHILE IT'S NICE TO TOSS IN SOME DICED COOKED VEGETABLES FOR COLOR, THE DISH TASTES VERY GOOD WITHOUT IT.

THE AMOUNTS ARE ALL APPROXIMATE, SINCE THE IDEA IS TO USE UP WHAT'S ON HAND AND SEASON TO TASTE WITH SHOYU, TOASTED SESAME OIL, AND SESAME SEEDS. IT'S ALSO NICE TO ADD A FEW DROPS OF CHILI OIL, IF YOU CAN TAKE THE HEAT.

COOKED RICE THAT HAS HAD A SOJOURN IN THE REFRIGERATOR IS LIKELY TO BE DRIED OUT AND BRITTLE. TO RESTORE IT TO ITS FRESH-COOKED CHEWINESS, YOUR BEST BET IS TO MICROWAVE IT ON HIGH, LIGHTLY COVERED, UNTIL REHYDRATED, ONE TO TWO MINUTES. IF YOU DON'T OWN A MICROWAVE, SPRINKLE ON TWO TABLESPOONS OF WATER PER CUP OF RICE AND STIR. THEN STEAM THE RICE FOR A MINUTE RIGHT IN THE NONSTICK COVERED SKILLET YOU'LL BE USING TO PREPARE THE RECIPE.

3 CUPS
cooked brown rice

1 TO 2 TABLESPOONS
toasted Asian sesame oil

6 OUNCES
Baked Seasoned Tofu (page 90, or substitute store-bought), cut into ¼-inch dice (1½ cups)

1 CUP
chopped cooked vegetables (optional)

1½ TABLESPOONS
toasted sesame seeds

2 TO 4 TEASPOONS
shoyu

Chili oil or hot pepper sesame oil, to taste (optional)

2 TO 3 TABLESPOONS
chopped scallion greens, for garnish (optional)

1 Put the rice in a large, nonstick skillet and drizzle on 1 table-spoon of the sesame oil while stirring. Turn on the heat to medium, and stir in the tofu and cooked vegetables (if using). Cover and cook, stirring frequently, until the mixture is good and hot, about 3 minutes. (Toasted sesame oil burns more easily than many other oils, so watch closely and reduce the heat if necessary.)

2 Stir in the sesame seeds and enough shoyu, additional toasted sesame oil, and chili oil (if using) to give the mixture a good balance of flavors. Garnish individual portions with chopped scallion, if you wish.

Serves 3 or 4

roasted potato salad with diced tempeh italiano

THERE'S A GOOD DEAL GOING ON IN THIS UNUSUAL POTATO SALAD, WITH EVERY BITE OFFERING SURPRISES. AGAINST THE BACKDROP OF CRISPLY ROASTED POTATOES, THERE ARE HIGHLY SEASONED BITS OF TEMPEH AND MARINATED ARTICHOKE AND THE REFRESHING CRUNCH OF CRISP CELERY AND RED ONION. ALL IN ALL, AN ATTRACTIVE AND MEMORABLE SALAD— GREAT FOR A HOT-WEATHER PICNIC.

1½ POUNDS
thin-skinned potatoes, scrubbed, trimmed, and cut into 1-inch cubes

2 TABLESPOONS
olive oil

2 TABLESPOONS
shoyu

1 CUP
diced celery

Diced Tempeh Italiano (page 85)

GENEROUS ½ CUP
marinated artichoke hearts, coarsely chopped

½ CUP
finely diced red onion

½ CUP
minced parsley

3 TO 5 TABLESPOONS
freshly squeezed lemon juice

Freshly ground black pepper, to taste

1 Place a rack in the center of the oven. Preheat the oven to 425 degrees. Put the potatoes in a large roasting pan. Drizzle on the oil, toss to coat the potatoes well, and arrange the potatoes in one layer. Cover tightly with aluminum foil and roast for 20 minutes.

2 Remove the foil and toss the potatoes, gently prying loose any that are sticking to the pan. Roast uncovered until the potatoes are fork-tender and slightly crusty, about 20 minutes more. Toss every 5 minutes during this time.

3 Remove the pan from the oven and transfer the hot potatoes to a large serving bowl. Drizzle on the shoyu and gently toss.

4 Add the remaining ingredients, using enough lemon juice to give the salad a nice puckery edge. Serve warm or at room temperature. (You'll need to perk up the salad with more lemon juice if it sits for a while.)

Serves **4** to **6**

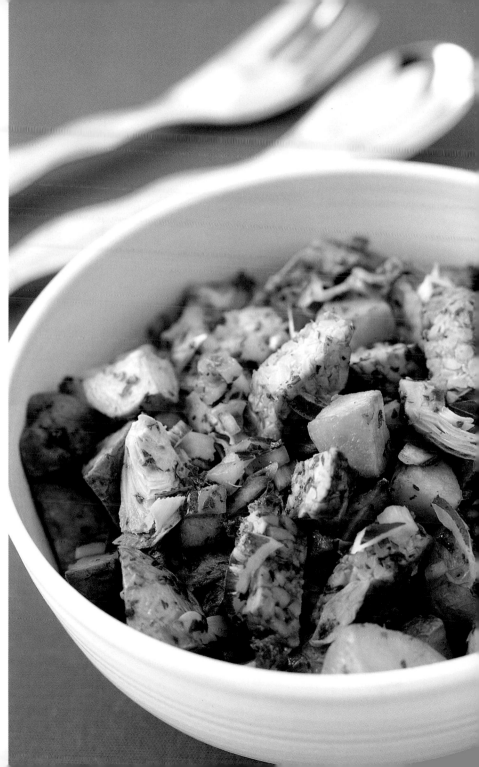

asian slaw with tofu croutons

1 POUND
napa cabbage, shredded
(5 to 6 cups)

1 CUP
finely diced red bell pepper

½ CUP
thinly sliced scallion greens

4 OUNCES
Baked Seasoned Tofu (page 90 or
substitute store-bought), cut into
¼-inch dice (about 1 cup)

⅔ TO ¾ CUP
Peanut Miso Dressing and
Dipping Sauce (page 102)

NAPA CABBAGE IS THE IDEAL CHOICE FOR THIS SIMPLE SLAW, BUT IT'S A BIT DELICATE. FOR OPTIMUM TASTE AND TEXTURE, SPIN THE RINSED LEAVES DRY BEFORE SHREDDING THEM, AND TOSS IN THE DRESSING JUST BEFORE SERVING. A PRACTICAL SOLUTION IS TO DRESS JUST THE AMOUNT YOU'LL BE NEEDING.

FOR A STURDIER SLAW THAT CAN BE REFRIGERATED FOR A FEW DAYS, USE GREEN HEAD CABBAGE, OR A MIXTURE OF GREEN AND RED CABBAGES, INSTEAD OF NAPA.

1 In a large serving bowl or storage container, combine the cabbage, bell pepper, scallions, and diced tofu. Toss in enough dressing to coat the slaw thoroughly.

Serves 4 to 6

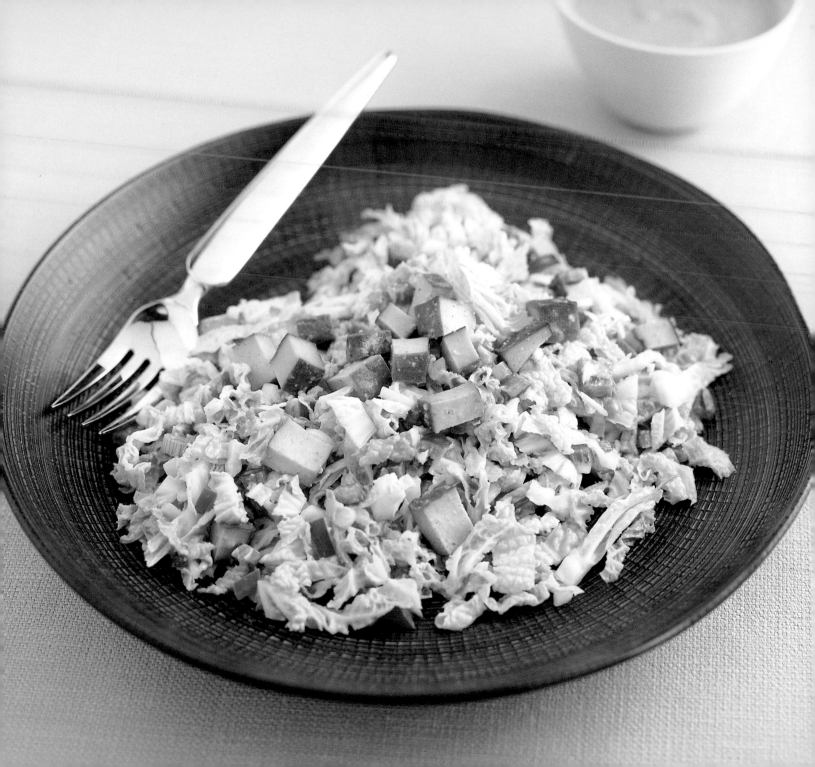

cauliflower slaw with creamy dill dressing

1 MEDIUM HEAD (ABOUT 2 POUNDS) cauliflower

1 LARGE red bell pepper, roasted, peeled, seeded, and finely diced

½ CUP minced red onion

½ TO ⅔ CUP Creamy Dill Dressing (page 100)

Salt and freshly ground black pepper, to taste

Freshly squeezed lemon juice, to taste (optional)

THIS SLAW IS A REFRESHING CHANGE OF PACE. IT'S MADE WITH LIGHTLY STEAMED CAULIFLOWER, WHICH HAS A TEXTURE PLEASANTLY REMINISCENT OF CABBAGE. THE DRESSING WORKS BEAUTIFULLY BECAUSE DILL AND CAULIFLOWER PAIR SO WELL.

THIS SALAD TASTES BEST WHEN FRESHLY MADE. A SPLASH OF LEMON JUICE HELPS REVITALIZE LEFTOVERS.

1 Trim the cauliflower and cut it into small florets. Steam the florets until they lose their raw taste but are still firm and crunchy, 3 to 4 minutes. Run under cold water to stop cooking, then drain thoroughly.

2 Place the florets in the bowl of a food processor and use the pulsing action to chop them coarsely. Transfer to a serving bowl. Toss in the bell pepper, onion, and enough dressing to thoroughly coat the mixture. Adjust the seasonings with salt, pepper, and the lemon juice (if using).

Serves **4**

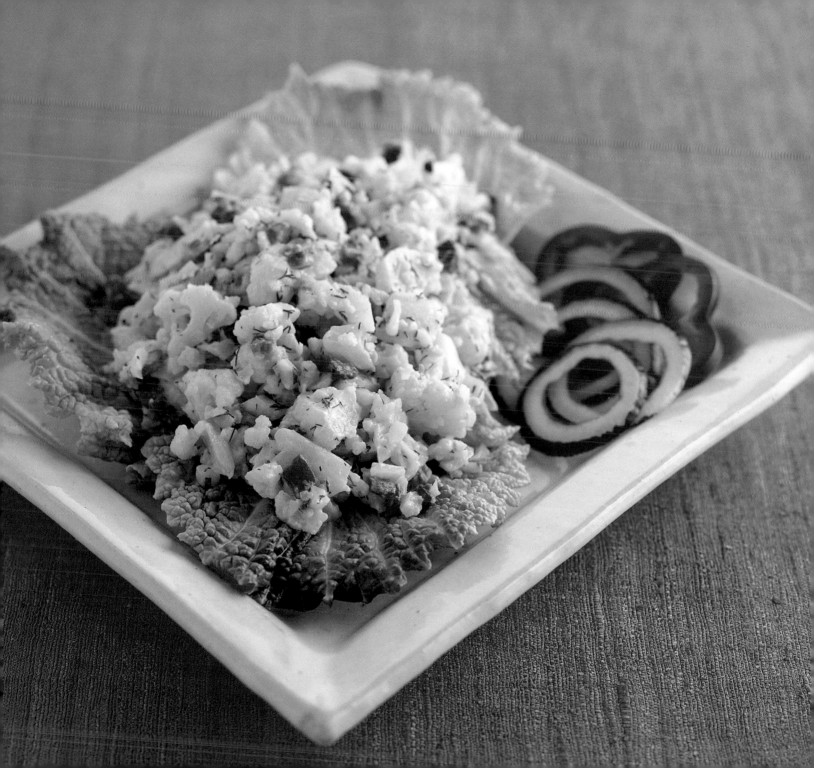

creamy dill dressing

FRESH DILL AND LEMON JUICE COMBINE WITH
SILKEN TOFU TO CREATE A CREAMY HERB DRESSING THAT IS
CHOLESTEROL FREE. WHILE IT'S FINE TO SERVE RIGHT AFTER
YOU MAKE IT, THE FLAVOR ACTUALLY IMPROVES AFTER
OVERNIGHT REFRIGERATION.

    I FIND THIS DRESSING QUITE VERSATILE. YOU'LL
ENJOY IT ON CAULIFLOWER SLAW (PAGE 98), AND IT'S ALSO
TASTY ON STEAMED NEW POTATOES AND SHREDDED CABBAGE.
OR STIR A DOLLOP INTO COLD BEET BORSCHT FOR A BEAUTIFUL
RIBBON OF FLAVOR.

    FOR OPTIMUM TASTE, USE FRESH (REFRIGERATED)
TOFU, NOT ASEPTIC-PACKED. IF YOU'D LIKE TO USE UP THE REST
OF YOUR SILKEN TOFU, TAKE A LOOK AT THE RECIPE ON PAGE 110.

1 CUP (8 OUNCES)
silken soft tofu

1 SMALL CLOVE
garlic, peeled

1 CUP
tightly packed fresh dill
(stems removed)

¼ CUP
freshly squeezed lemon juice

3 TABLESPOONS
olive oil

1 TABLESPOON
Dijon mustard

1 TEASPOON
salt

1 Put the tofu in a fine-mesh
strainer and set aside to drain
for 15 minutes.

2 With the motor of the food
processor running, pop the garlic
through the feed tube. Process
until finely chopped. Remove
the cover, scrape down the sides
of the work bowl, and add the
drained tofu and the remaining
ingredients. Process until
smooth, stopping and scraping
down the work bowl once or
twice as needed. Use immediately or transfer to a tightly
sealed storage container and
refrigerate for up to 5 days.

Makes about **1¼** cups

lime-shoyu vinaigrette

⅓ CUP
freshly squeezed lime juice

¼ CUP
olive oil

2 TABLESPOONS
shoyu

2 TEASPOONS
Dijon mustard

SHOYU ADDS DEPTH OF FLAVOR AS WELL AS SALTINESS TO THIS SIMPLE, VERSATILE DRESSING—A PERSONAL FAVORITE. THE VINAIGRETTE DELIVERS LOTS OF PIZZAZZ TO BLACK SOYBEAN SALSA (PAGE 59) AND TO QUINOA SALAD WITH TEMPEH ADOBO NUGGETS (PAGE 49). IT'S ALSO TERRIFIC ON A MIXED-GREEN SALAD, AS WELL AS ON BEAN AND GRAIN SALADS.

1 Put all the ingredients in a small jar and shake well. Use immediately or refrigerate for up to 5 days. Bring to room temperature and shake well before using.

Makes ¾ cup

peanut miso dressing and dipping sauce

THE COMBINATION OF MISO AND RICH PEANUT BUTTER CREATES AN EXCITING DRESSING AND DIPPING SAUCE THAT CAN BE PREPARED IN A FLASH. I USUALLY USE ONE-THIRD CUP WATER FOR A THICKISH DIPPING SAUCE, AND THIN THE MIXTURE WITH A FEW ADDITIONAL TABLESPOONS OF WATER FOR A DRESSING.

I'M PARTIAL TO THE WAY SWEET WHITE MISO ACCENTUATES THE DELICATE SWEETNESS OF GOOD FRESH PEANUT BUTTER, BUT YOU CAN EXPERIMENT BY SUBSTITUTING THE SALTIER BARLEY MISO AND REDUCING THE SHOYU ACCORDINGLY.

1 LARGE CLOVE
garlic, peeled

2-INCH CHUNK
fresh ginger, trimmed and cut into eighths

⅓ TO ½ CUP
hot water

½ CUP
nonhydrogenated, unsalted peanut butter

2 TABLESPOONS
sweet white miso

ABOUT 1 TABLESPOON
shoyu

3 TABLESPOONS
freshly squeezed lime juice

Chili oil or ground cayenne pepper, to taste (optional)

1 With the motor of the food processor running, pop the garlic and then the ginger through the feed tube and continue to process until they are finely chopped. Remove the lid, scrape down the work bowl, and add ⅓ cup of water, the peanut butter, miso, and shoyu. Blend until smooth.

2 Add the lime juice and a dash of chili oil (if using), and pulse a few times to distribute. Thin with additional water, if you wish. Use immediately or refrigerate for up to 5 days. Shake well before each use and thin with extra lime juice or water if the mixture thickens on standing.

Makes about 1¼ cups

miso pesto

MISO CREATES A REMARKABLY FINE BASE FOR PESTO, LENDING BOTH SALTINESS AND THE KIND OF COMPLEX, AGED FLAVOR TRADITIONALLY PROVIDED BY PARMIGIANO-REGGIANO CHEESE. THE MISO ALSO DOES A GOOD JOB OF PRESERVING THE BASIL'S COLOR AND FLAVOR: UNDER REFRIGERATION, THIS PESTO LASTS BEAUTIFULLY FOR AT LEAST FIVE DAYS. WHENEVER I MAKE PESTO, I LIKE TO ADD A TEASPOON OF FENNEL SEEDS TO ACCENTUATE THE ANISELIKE FLAVOR OF BASIL.

WHAT IS IT ABOUT PESTO THAT BRINGS SUCH ELEGANCE TO EVERYTHING IT GRACES? TRY A DOLLOP IN MINESTRONE OR ON BROILED TOMATOES. OR SEE FOR YOURSELF HOW IT TURNS AN OTHERWISE ORDINARY DISH OF FETTUCCINE AND BROCCOLI (PAGE 74) INTO SOMETHING QUITE SPECIAL.

2 CLOVES
garlic, peeled

2 CUPS
very tightly packed basil leaves, rinsed and spun dry

½ CUP
walnuts, toasted and cooled

2 TABLESPOONS
barley miso

1 TEASPOON
fennel seeds

¼ CUP
olive oil

1 With the motor of the food processor running, pop the garlic cloves through feed tube. Process until finely chopped. Remove the cover, scrape down the sides of the work bowl, and add the basil, walnuts, miso, and fennel seeds. Pulse to create a coarse paste. With the motor running, gradually pour the olive oil through the feed tube and continue processing to create a smooth paste. Stop once or twice to scrape down the sides of the bowl.

2 Set the pesto aside at room temperature if using within the hour. Otherwise refrigerate for up to 5 days and bring to room temperature shortly before needed. Stir well before each use.

Makes about ¾ cup

sage-scented cornmeal scones

THESE CRUMBLY SAVORY SCONES, WITH THEIR CHEERY FLECKS OF CHOPPED SCALLION AND CORN, REQUIRE NO SPECIAL EQUIPMENT TO PREPARE—JUST AN ORDINARY BAKING SHEET. TO MAKE THEM, PAT THE DOUGH INTO A DISK AND THEN CUT INTO WEDGES.

SOYMILK PROVIDES THE LIQUID IN THIS RECIPE. IF YOU WISH, YOU CAN MAKE THE SCONES TOTALLY CHOLESTEROL FREE BY USING A SOY-BASED SHORTENING RATHER THAN BUTTER.

THE SCONES TASTE BEST WHEN FRESHLY MADE AND STILL SLIGHTLY WARM, BUT LEFTOVERS FREEZE QUITE WELL AND MAY BE DEFROSTED AND REWARMED AS NEEDED.

Butter for coating pan (optional)

⅔ CUP
soymilk

1 TABLESPOON
apple cider vinegar or freshly squeezed lemon juice

1 CUP
unbleached white or whole-wheat pastry flour, plus additional for shaping scones

1 CUP
cornmeal

2 TABLESPOONS
sugar or maple sprinkles (see note)

2 TEASPOONS
baking powder

½ TEASPOON
baking soda

¾ TEASPOON
salt

1 ½ TEASPOONS
dried sage leaves, finely crumbled by rubbing between your fingers

⅛ TO ¼ TEASPOON
ground cayenne pepper, to taste

⅓ CUP
Spectrum Spread (see note) or 6 tablespoons chilled butter

½ CUP
frozen corn kernels (defrosting not necessary, but rinse and dry kernels if they are coated with ice crystals)

⅓ CUP
finely chopped scallions

1 Place a rack in the center of the oven. Preheat the oven to 425 degrees. Grease a large baking sheet or line it with parchment paper. Set aside.

2 In a large cup, combine the soymilk and vinegar. Set aside to curdle and thicken slightly.

3 In a large bowl, combine the flour, cornmeal, sugar, baking powder, baking soda, salt, sage, and cayenne. Stir well with a whisk. Using a table knife, cut off tiny bits of shortening and distribute evenly over the flour mixture. With a pastry blender or by rubbing between your fingers, blend in the shortening until the mixture resembles coarse meal. Stir in the corn and scallions.

4 Stir with a fork as you slowly drizzle on ½ cup of the curdled soymilk. Then add just enough additional liquid to make the mixture come together into a mass, forming a soft—but not sticky—dough. (You may use all of the liquid or have a few tablespoons left over, depending upon the condition of the flour and the weather.)

5 Divide the dough in half. Put half on a lightly floured board and, with lightly floured hands, pat into a ¾-inch-thick round. With a floured knife, cut into 6 wedges and transfer to the prepared baking sheet, leaving about 1 inch between the scones. Repeat with the remaining dough.

6 Immediately set the scones in the oven. Bake until the tops have a hint of color and the bottoms are lightly browned, 14 to 15 minutes. Transfer the scones to a wire rack. Cool until just warm, about 3 minutes, and serve.

Makes **12** scones

Notes: Maple sprinkles are made by dehydrating maple syrup. Look for them in natural-food stores.

Spectrum Spread is a gelatinous, nonhydrogenated soy-based shortening stocked in the refrigerator section of most health-food stores. It has a spreadable consistency and a pleasant buttery taste.

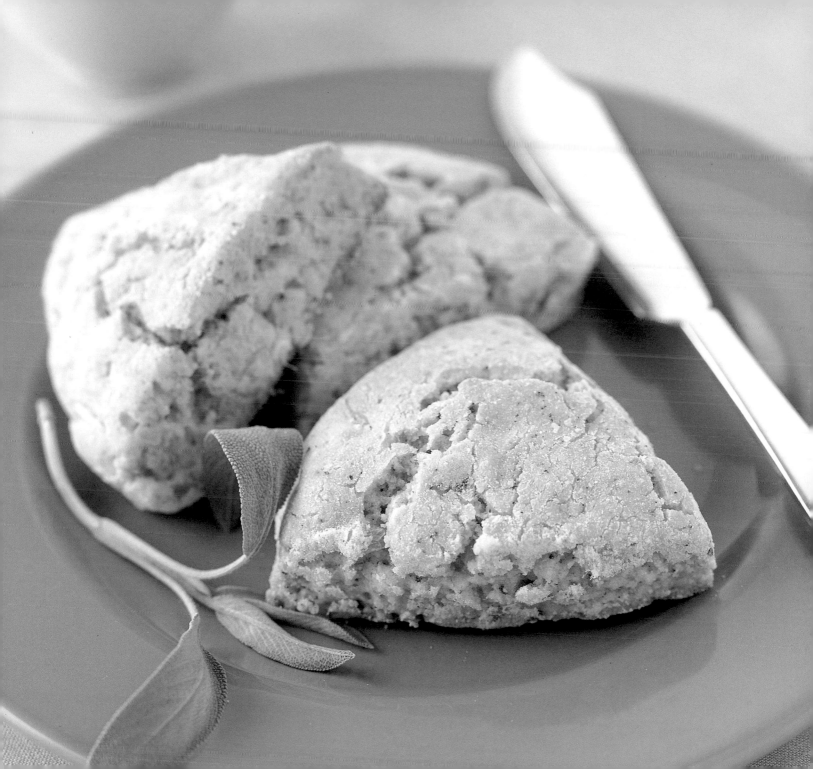

pineapple-coconut rice pudding

I CAN NEVER RESIST EATING A PORTION OF THIS YUMMY RICE PUDDING HOT, JUST AS SOON AS IT'S DONE. THEN I MIGHT HAVE SOME FOR DESSERT. BUT, IN TRUTH, MY FAVORITE TIME TO EAT THIS COMFORTING PUDDING IS FOR BREAKFAST.

THE SOYMILK PLUS A BIT OF GRATED COCONUT CREATE THE RICH, CREAMY TEXTURE COMMONLY ASSOCIATED WITH RICE PUDDING. DRIED PINEAPPLE, MY LATEST GREAT FIND, ADDS A PUNCH OF INTENSE FLAVOR. LEFTOVERS WILL THICKEN WHEN YOU REFRIGERATE THEM; STIR IN A FEW TABLESPOONS OF SOYMILK BEFORE HEATING THEM UP—MOST EFFICIENTLY DONE IN A MICROWAVE.

WHEN SERVING THE RICE PUDDING FOR DESSERT, YOU MIGHT WANT TO SWEETEN IT WITH MAPLE SYRUP OR SUGAR. TO ADD COLOR, GARNISH EACH PORTION WITH A DOLLOP OF YOUR FAVORITE TROPICAL FRUIT ICE OR SOME FRESH BERRIES.

2 CUPS
water

¼ POUND
unsweetened dried pineapple rings (see note)

¼ CUP
rum (optional)

½ TO ⅔ CUP
unsweetened grated dried coconut (use the maximum if you love the coconut flavor)

2 TEASPOONS
ground cinnamon, plus additional for garnish

¼ TEASPOON
salt

1 CUP
white or brown basmati rice

1 LITER
plain or vanilla soymilk

Maple syrup, maple sugar, or brown sugar, to taste (optional)

1 In a large, heavy saucepan, bring the water and dried pineapple to a boil. Cover, turn off the heat, and let sit until the pineapple is soft, about 10 minutes. Remove the pineapple with a slotted spoon and put it on a cutting board. When it is cool enough to handle, chop the pineapple coarsely or snip each ring into seven or eight chunks with a pair of kitchen scissors. Set aside.

2 Return the water to a gentle boil and stir in the rum (if using), coconut, 2 teaspoons cinnamon (make sure it doesn't clump up), salt, rice, and pineapple bits. Add the soymilk and return to a boil. Immediately reduce the heat to low (or the soymilk will froth up and boil over), cover, and simmer until the rice is very tender, 25 to 30 minutes for white rice or 45 to 50 minutes for brown rice.

3 When the rice is tender, turn off the heat. Give the mixture a good stir, and let the pudding sit, uncovered, for a few minutes to cool and thicken slightly. Add maple syrup or another sweetener to taste, if you wish. Top each portion with a light dusting of cinnamon. Serve warm (my preferred way), room temperature, or chilled.

Serves **6**

Note: Dried pineapple rings are sold in natural-food stores. If your pineapple is fairly moist and easy to chop or tear into bits, you can skip the soaking procedure described in the first paragraph; simply add the pineapple bits as directed in the second paragraph.

chocolate–grand marnier sauce

1⅓ CUPS (10 OUNCES)
silken soft tofu

¼ CUP
best-quality unsweetened cocoa
powder

3 TO 4 TABLESPOONS
maple syrup

2 TO 3 TABLESPOONS
Grand Marnier

1 TEASPOON
pure vanilla extract

THIS RICH, VELVETY TOPPING HAS A LOVELY SHEEN AND MAKES AN ELEGANT DESSERT WHEN SPOONED OVER SMALL WHOLE STRAWBERRIES. OR CREATE A POOL OF THE SAUCE ON A DESSERT PLATE AND FAN OUT PERFECTLY RIPE SLICED PEACHES ON TOP. THE SAUCE IS ALSO NICE DRIZZLED DECORATIVELY OVER INDIVIDUAL PORTIONS OF POUND CAKE.

LEFTOVERS? I'VE BEEN KNOWN TO EAT THIS SAUCE STRAIGHT OUT OF THE STORAGE CONTAINER. IT HAS THE SAME IRRESISTIBLE APPEAL AS CHOCOLATE PUDDING, ALTHOUGH IT'S NOT QUITE AS FIRM. INDEED, IT IS LIKELY TO MAKE CHOCOLATE LOVERS VERY HAPPY IF YOU SERVE IT ON ITS OWN AT THE END OF A MEAL.

FOR OPTIMUM TASTE, USE DROSTE COCOA POWDER AND FRESH (REFRIGERATED) SILKEN TOFU (AS OPPOSED TO ASEPTIC-PACKED). IF YOU GET HOOKED AND WANT SOME VARIETY, TRY SUBSTITUTING KAHLUA, COINTREAU, OR AMARETTO FOR THE GRAND MARNIER.

1 Put the tofu in a fine-mesh strainer and set aside to drain for 15 minutes.

2 In a blender or food processor, purée the tofu until creamy, about 30 seconds. Add the cocoa powder, 3 tablespoons of maple syrup, 2 tablespoons of Grand Marnier, and the vanilla extract. Blend thoroughly, stopping once or twice to scrape down the sides of the container. Taste and add more maple syrup and/or Grand Marnier to taste, if you wish. Continue blending until the mixture is extremely smooth.

3 Transfer to a well-sealed storage container or serving glasses and chill at least 1 hour before serving, or refrigerate for up to 3 days.

Makes 1½ cups

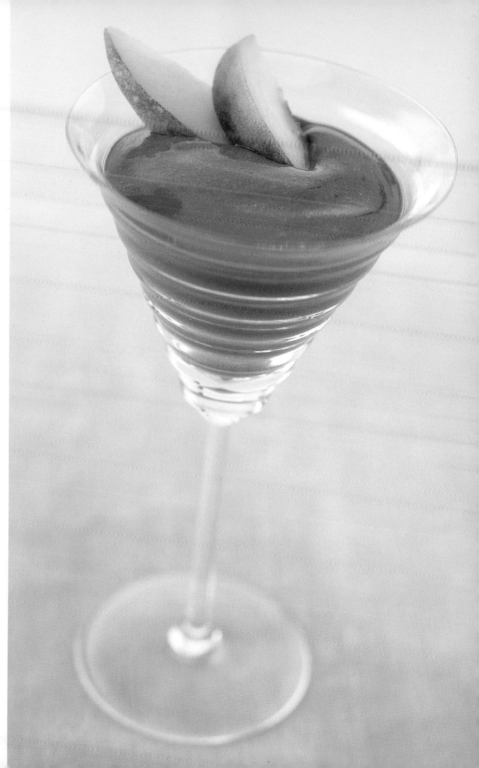

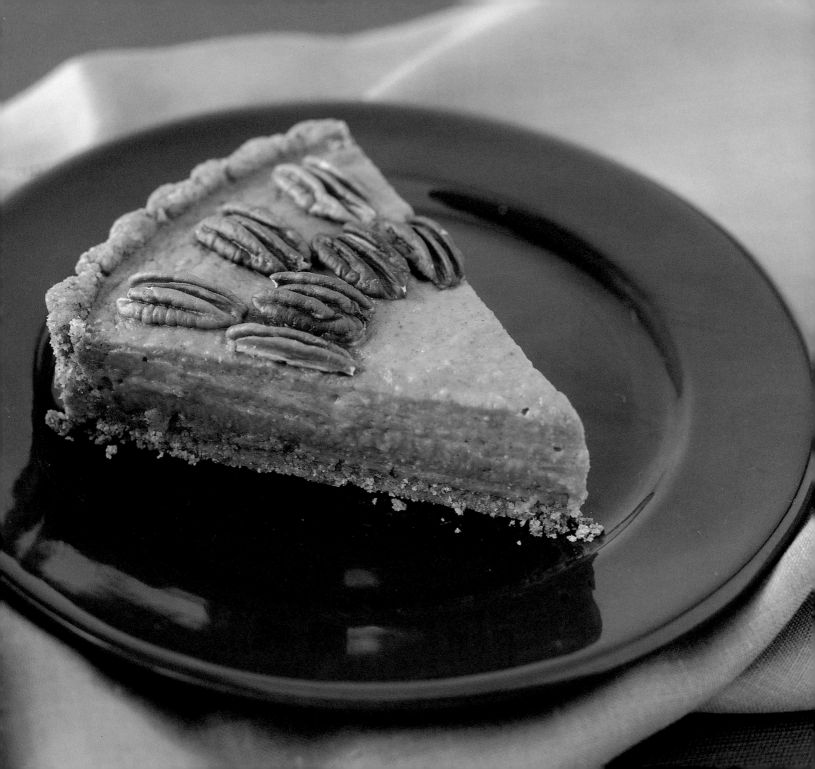

pumpkin tart with pecan crust

PUMPKIN PIE HAS ALWAYS BEEN A PERSONAL FAVORITE, AND THIS LIGHT, SILKY RENDITION IS RIGHT UP THERE WITH THE VERY BEST. IT'S NICE TO HAVE A CHOLESTEROL-FREE ALTERNATIVE FOR THIS ALL-AMERICAN FAVORITE, ONE THAT DOESN'T TASTE FOR A MINUTE LIKE A COMPROMISE. I HAVE MY TALENTED ASSISTANT ROSEMARY SERVISS TO THANK FOR CREATING THIS TERRIFIC RECIPE.

THE TART LOOKS ESPECIALLY PRETTY AND IS EASIER TO SERVE WHEN BAKED IN A TART PAN WITH A REMOVABLE BOTTOM. IF YOU USE A TRADITIONAL PIE PLATE, BE SURE TO GREASE IT THOROUGHLY, SINCE THE CRUST HAS A TENDENCY TO STICK. ALLOW TIME FOR THE PIE TO CHILL THOROUGHLY BEFORE SERVING.

for the crust:

Vegetable oil or butter, for preparing tart pan or pie plate

¾ CUP
rolled oats

¾ CUP
whole-wheat pastry flour or unbleached white flour

½ CUP
pecans, plus 16 pecan halves, lightly toasted, for garnish

½ TEASPOON
ground cinnamon

Pinch of salt

¼ CUP
canola oil

3 TABLESPOONS
maple syrup

for the filling:

1 CUP
soymilk

¼ CUP
arrowroot

1 CAN (16 OUNCES)
solid-pack pumpkin

½ CUP
maple syrup

1 TABLESPOON
grated fresh ginger

1 ½ TEASPOONS
ground cinnamon

½ TEASPOON
salt

¼ TEASPOON
freshly grated nutmeg

⅛ TEASPOON
ground cloves

1 Set a rack in the middle of the oven and preheat the oven to 375 degrees. Lightly oil a 9-inch tart pan with a removeable bottom or thoroughly grease a 9-inch pie plate. Set aside.

2 To prepare the crust, set the oats, flour, ½ cup pecans, cinnamon, and salt in the bowl of a food processor. Pulse until the mixture resembles coarse meal, stopping and scraping down the bowl as needed. Transfer to a medium-sized bowl.

3 In a measuring cup, whisk together the oil and maple syrup. Pour the liquid into the dry ingredients and blend thoroughly with a fork until the mixture forms a soft dough. Press the mixture into the prepared pan or plate. (Crimp the edges if using a pie plate.) Bake for 10 minutes. Set on a rack to cool.

4 To prepare the filling, blend the soymilk and arrowroot in the food processor until the arrowroot is completely dissolved and the mixture is smooth, about 15 seconds. Add all of the remaining ingredients except the pecan halves. Process until thoroughly blended and smooth, stopping

and scraping down the work bowl as needed.

5 Pour the mixture into the crust and smooth the top with a spatula. Bake until the crust is lightly browned and the outside inch of the filling is set, about 35 minutes. (Do not be concerned if the center is still soft; it will firm up as the pie cools.)

6 Remove from the oven and set on the rack. Gently press the toasted pecan halves into the hot filling in 2 concentric circles. Cool to room temperature and then refrigerate until completely chilled, about 3 hours. Serve chilled or at room temperature. Leftovers may be refrigerated for up to 3 days.

Serves **8**

mail-order sources

If you can't locate some of the ingredients used in this book, you can count on finding everything you need through the first three sources listed below. Call and request a catalog, and you will be amazed at the bounty available.

ingredients

Gold Mine Natural Food Co.
3419 Hancock Street
San Diego, CA 92110
800-475-3663
Excellent one-stop shopping for a wide range of unpasteurized misos (Japanese and American) and shoyus, dried and canned organic black soybeans, dried shiitake mushrooms, and toasted Asian sesame oil.

Adriana's Caravan
409 Vanderbilt Street
Brooklyn, NY 11218
800-316-0820
A good source of ethnic condiments and ingredients, such as rice papers, Thai curry paste and fish sauce, Patak's mild curry paste, dried chili peppers, fermented black beans, tahini, dried herbs, and spices.

Penzeys, Ltd.
P.O. Box 1448
Waukesha, WI 53187
414-574-0277
Superior dried herbs and spices with a fascinating catalog full of tips on use and storage.

equipment

Unique Utensils
P.O. Box 3112
Littleton, CO 80161
303-797-6724
Makers of the original Tofu Squeeze, a cleverly designed stainless-steel gizmo for efficiently pressing tofu.

Magefesa Pressure Cookers
North American Promotions, Ltd.
P.O. Box 328
Prospect Heights, IL 60070
888-705-8700
Ask for the Rapid II, rated number one by *Cook's Illustrated* and available only by mail order.

index

table of equivalents

The exact equivalents in the following tables have been rounded for convenience.

liquid and dry measures

U.S.	METRIC
¼ teaspoon	1.25 milliliters
½ teaspoon	2.5 milliliters
1 teaspoon	5 milliliters
1 tablespoon (3 teaspoons)	15 milliliters
1 fluid ounce (2 tablespoons)	30 milliliters
¼ cup	60 milliliters
⅓ cup	80 milliliters
1 cup	240 milliliters
1 pint (2 cups)	480 milliliters
1 quart (4 cups, 32 ounces)	960 milliliters
1 gallon (4 quarts)	3.84 liters
1 ounce (by weight)	28 grams
1 pound	454 grams
2.2 pounds	1 kilogram

length measures

U.S.	METRIC
⅛ inch	3 millimeters
¼ inch	6 millimeters
½ inch	12 millimeters
1 inch	2.5 centimeters

oven temperatures

FAHRENHEIT	CELSIUS	GAS
250	120	½
275	140	1
300	150	2
325	160	3
350	180	4
375	190	5
400	200	6
425	220	7
450	230	8
475	240	9
500	260	10